POCKE

Cultural Assessment

Elaine M. Geissler, PhD, RN, CTN
Tolland, Connecticut

Second Edition

Illustrated

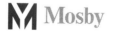

M Mosby

St. Louis Baltimore Boston Carlsbad
Chicago Minneapolis New York Philadelphia Portland
London Milan Sydney Tokyo Toronto

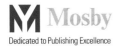

Mosby

Dedicated to Publishing Excellence

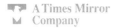

A Times Mirror Company

Publisher: Sally Schrefer
Editor: Michael S. Ledbetter
Associate Developmental Editor: Lisa P. Newton
Project Manager: John Rogers
Associate Production Editor: Mary Turner
Designer: Yael Kats

Special Recognition: Maps reprinted from *The Software Toolworks World Atlas* with permission. The Learning Company, Cambridge, Massachusetts.

Second Edition
Copyright © 1998 by Mosby, Inc.

Printed in the United States of America

Composition by The Clarinda Company
Printing/binding by R.R. Donnelley

Mosby, Inc.
11830 Westline Industrial Drive
St. Louis, Missouri 63146

Library of Congress Cataloging-in-Publication Data
Geissler, Elaine Marie.
    Pocket guide to cultural assessment / Elaine M. Geissler.—2nd ed.
        p.   cm.
    Includes bibliographical references and index.
    ISBN 0-8151-3633-1
    1. Transcultural nursing—Handbooks, manuals, etc.   I. Title.
    [DNLM: 1. Transcultural Nursing handbooks.   WY 49G313p 1998]
    RT86.54.G45   1998
    610.73—dc21
    DNLM/DLC
    for Library of Congress   98-25821
                                                                              CIP

98 99 00 01 02 / 9 8 7 6 5 4 3 2 1

Cultural Assessment

Contributors

Awlasewicz, Anna, RN, BS
Student, University of Connecticut School of Nursing
Storrs, Connecticut
Romania

Ballesteros Plata, Carmen D.U.E.
Diplomada Universitaria en Enfermeria
Almería, Spain
Spain

Bergh, IngaLena, RN, BSc
Head of Planning, Stockholm College of Health and Caring
Sciences
Stockholm, Sweden
Sweden

Birutis, Arunas L.
Nursing Consultant
New York, New York
Lithuania

Brown, Barbara J., RN, EdD, FAAN, FNAP, CNAA
Editor, *Nursing Administration Quarterly;*
Associate Executive Director of Nursing, King Faisal Specialist
Hospital and Research Centre
Riyadh, Saudi Arabia, 1987-1991
Saudi Arabia

Chilicki, Carmen-Rosa, RN, BS
Student, University of Connecticut School of Nursing
Storrs, Connecticut
Poland

Coler, Marga S., RN, CS, CTN, EdD
Professor of Nursing, University of Connecticut
Storrs, Connecticut
Brazil

Dahl, Oyvind, PhD
Associate Professor, Center for Intercultural Communication
Stavanger, Norway
Madagascar, Norway

Dahlen, Tommy
PhD Student, Department of Social Anthropology
Stockholm, Sweden
Sweden

Duncan, Linda, RN, BS
Student, University of Connecticut School of Nursing
Storrs, Connecticut
China

Estrella, Jennifer, MA
Doctoral Candidate, University of Connecticut Department of
Spanish
Storrs, Connecticut
Dominican Republic

Gebrian, Bette Magliore, RN, MPH, PhD
Haitian Health Foundation
Jérémie, Haiti
Haiti

Herrmann, Eleanor Krohn, RN, EdD, FAAN
Professor of Nursing (Retired), University of Connecticut
Storrs, Connecticut
Belize

Karosas, Laima M., APRN, MSN
Doctoral Student, University of Connecticut School of Nursing
Storrs, Connecticut
Lithuania

Kurtz, James R., RN, MPH
Primary Health Care Consultant, Ministry of Health
Lao PDR
Laos

Langer, Carolyn, RN, MS
Student, University of Connecticut
Storrs, Connecticut
South Korea

Platin, Nurgun, RN, DNSc
Professor and Head of Pediatric Nursing Division,
Hacettepe University
Ankara, Turkey
Turkey

Rieke, Hans-Joachim
Berlin, Germany
Participant, Summer Institute for Intercultural Communication,
1991, Portland, Oregon
Germany

Shellenberger, Janet, RN, PhD (Deceased)
Health Education Consultant, Ministry of Education
Lao PDR
Laos

Szwez, Diane, RN, BS
Student, University of Connecticut School of Nursing
Storrs, Connecticut
Russia, Ukraine

Willcoxson, Lesley, PhD
Coordinator, Monash-ANZ Centre for International Briefing
Melbourne, Victoria, Australia
Australia

Foreword

Culture is like a double-edged sword. On the one hand, it allows individuals in social groups to live together in relative harmony through shared values, beliefs, and practices. On the other hand, it creates social disharmony through ethnocentrism or the tendency to judge others based on one's own values, beliefs, and practices that are considered true and just. Compounding its double-edged nature is the fact that the variety of social groups in the world today and diversity of the environmental contexts in which they exist lead to great intergroup variation in the values, beliefs, and practices that arise in an attempt to meet the basic needs of existence, such as kinship and interpersonal relationships, shelter, safety, childbearing and child rearing, food and nutrition, health, and activities of daily living. Likewise, individuals within the same social group have many different life experiences that contribute to intragroup variation in the degree to which they adhere to the norms commonly attributed to their culture. Members of a society often have different perspectives and interpretations of the same situation because of factors such as age, marital status, family structure, gender, income, education level, religious views, and degree of involvement in the situation.

Such intergroup and intragroup variation makes the task that Dr. Geissler has bravely undertaken in this pocket guide a vital necessity and a daunting challenge. It has also presented her with another double-edged sword. On the one hand, health care providers, as well as persons from all walks of life, need quick access to a variety of information to interact effectively with individuals from different cultural groups. However, it is unlikely that anyone, not even an expert in transcultural health care such as Dr. Geissler, can describe all of the permutations of culture and varieties of human experiences that exist in the world. To accommodate both sides of the sword, what Dr. Geissler has wisely done is to compile a resource containing basic cultural, epidemiologic, environmental, and geographic information about cultural groups throughout the world. As with any basic resource, the pocket guide is not intended to be the definitive word on any one cultural group or nation. Its intent is merely to provide us with a snapshot of the cultural diversity that exists and that we must understand to fulfill our dual roles as citizens and providers of culture-competent health care.

Through the pocket guide, Dr. Geissler gives us, the readers, a steppingstone on the path to cultural competence. At the same time, she has placed the onus on the readers to put the other steppingstones in place. As we endeavor to put the next stones in place, we need to heed Dr. Geissler's caution that information in the pocket guide must not be used to stereotype individuals or groups. It is incumbent on us to use the information as a basis for exploring the degree to which people we encounter from the groups and nations represented may or may not adhere to the cultural norms commonly attributed to them.

Another crucial steppingstone is to realize that a group's world view gives rise to culture and therefore their health culture—the values, beliefs, and practices they hold about health promotion and illness prevention; the causation, detection, and treatment of illness; the care of ill and well individuals; whom to go to for assistance; and the social roles, relationships, and expectations that guide the person-provider encounter. As a result, concepts of health, illness, and care cannot readily be separated from general cultural values, beliefs, and practices. This integral relationship is well illustrated when we examine our own behavior as providers of conventional medicine (Western, scientific, biomedicine, or professional medicine). Many of the tenets of conventional medicine and role expectations during the patient-provider encounter are derived from a Northern European world view that espouses individualism, independence, paternalism, reductionism, and belief in the scientific method of finding truth. In the United States, Euro-American health culture promotes individual decision making through informed consent; efficiency based on economy of time, effort, and resources; personal space and privacy; improvement of the human condition through science and technology; the separation of mind, body, and spirit in treatment of illness; and the health care provider as the manager of care. A perusal of the pocket guide reveals that such a health-culture orientation will present problems when we encounter individuals from groups in which the family or community has the decision making responsibilities for its members, emotional and psychologic support are deemed more important than science, technology, and efficiency, and body-mind-spirit cannot be separated or seen as independent from physical and metaphysical forces in the environment.

Another steppingstone is the realization that health behavior is influenced by the situation at hand. As individuals have different experiences with life and health care and are exposed to other health-culture orientations, what they do and believe to be true today about health and illness may be quite different when we next see them. The fluidity of cultural values, beliefs, and practices should again effect caution against stereotyping, analyzing behavior out of context, or interpreting situations from solely our point of view or health-culture orientation.

A fourth crucial steppingstone on the path to cultural competence is to remember what anthropologists learned long ago. The best way to learn about the diverse cultural groups that surround us is through participant-observation. True, we cannot go to each of the places Dr. Geissler takes us in the pocket guide, but we can use a variation of participant-observation to gain a greater depth and breadth of knowledge about the cultural groups in our own region. We can learn about them through the media, including documentaries, novels, newspaper articles, ethnographies, and research studies. We can go to markets and restaurants in ethnic neighborhoods and learn about their foods and the role they play in health and illness. We can experience religious ceremonies at ethnic places of worship and learn the role of rituals and religion in health promotion and treatment of illness. Likewise, we can share the joy of their life celebrations, including marriages, births, and graduations, as well as the sorrow of their losses and misfortunes. We can take time to go back and talk with patients and families about their health concerns and beliefs about care. We can explore ethnic neighborhoods and learn about the cultural symbolism embodied in arts and crafts found there. We can learn ethnic games and gain a beginning understanding about competitiveness and cooperation. In short, we can be like investigative reporters, learning and experiencing the who, what, when, where, and why of the human diversity that surrounds us. When we do that, we will be better able to understand the factors that affect our patients' health behavior and decision making. We will also come to learn more about ourselves and how our behavior affects others.

While the above steppingstones to cultural competence must be put in place independently by each of us, the pocket guide gives us the initial step and makes us aware of the complexity of the task yet before us. However, like most "pockets," it cannot hold everything we need. It is up to the individual reader to use the pocket guide as Dr. Geissler intended, as an introduction to the diversity of values, beliefs, and practices that may affect health care encounters, as a steppingstone to cultural competence in the provision of health care, and to gain a better understanding of ourselves.

Lydia DeSantis, PhD, RN, FAAN, CTN
Professor, University of Miami School of Nursing
Coral Gables, Florida

Preface

The present trend in transcultural theory (and I agree with it) is that individuals within any given culture vary markedly. The earth is populated with a vast mosaic of cultures representing every imaginable variety of learned and environmentally generated beliefs and practices. For each person, his or her own culture is deeply ingrained and comfortable, guiding both the conscious and covert activities and behaviors of daily life, including health and illness. Yet culture is also a dynamic influence, meeting changing needs of groups, as well as individuals within those groups.

In his book *Pandaemonium,* Senator Daniel Patrick Moynihan speculates that in the next 50 years there may be 150 or so new nations on the world map that have been "created for the purpose of giving one or another ethnic group a realm of its own." The most significant change from the first edition of this book reflects Moynihan's prognostication. Twenty-three independent nations have already emerged. The largest number evolved from the dissolution of the Soviet Union. They are as follows:

Armenia
Azerbaijan
Belarus
Bosnia and Herzegovina
Estonia
Georgia
Kazakhstan
Kyrgyzstan
Latvia
Lithuania
Moldova
Tajikistan
Turkmenistan
Ukraine
Uzbekistan

The following nations of the former Yugoslavia and Czechoslovakia:

Croatia

Czech Republic

Macedonia

Serbia and Montenegro (new Yugoslavia)

Slovakia

Slovenia

Two other nations, Eritrea and Palau, have gained independence. Zaire has been renamed "The Democratic Republic of Congo" and must not be confused with its neighbor The Republic of Congo.

Many of these newly independent nations have not yet published professional health literature in the English language that is appropriate to this guide. Other established nations do not have any additional listings since the first edition. This is frustrating for readers who desire equality in the categories and amount of information among countries.

The second edition's immunization schedules from the World Health Organization are much more complete; only a handful of nations have not provided this data. AIDS rates for almost all the countries of the planet are included in this edition; however, they should be considered only as a trend because statistical data change.

The theory about the "melting pot" phenomenon in the United States that expects immigrants to become Americanized linguistically and culturally is passé. Even the theory about the "salad bowl" phenomenon, in which different cultures are expected to live together in peaceful coexistence, is being rejected. At this critical juncture in history the move toward cultural homogeneity is strengthening. Many of the "new" countries previously listed came into existence because of the intense—and for some, deadly—struggle for cultural homogeneity. For many of these nations, little or no information on their health care beliefs and practices exists in the literature to date. This dearth of information will improve over time, and the reader is encouraged to keep abreast of the health care literature for guidance in the delivery of culturally competent health care.

One of the greatest weaknesses of a guide such as this is that of **stereotyping.** The reader is **strongly cautioned against** the false assumption that people from one country or geographic area are clones, holding the same beliefs held by their neighbors. The borders of countries are politically determined and often bear no relationship to cultural values. The differences *within* one culture may be as great as variations between two different cultures. Stewart and Bennett remind us that the tendency to stereotype can be overcome

. . . by approaching every cross-cultural situation as a kind of experiment. They should assume that some kind of cultural difference exists but that the nature of the difference is unclear. Using available generalizations about the other culture, they can formulate a hypothesis and then test it for accuracy. . . The hypothesis should be tested by acting tentatively as if it were accurate and by watching carefully to see what happens. . . (Stewart and Bennett, 1991).

Galanti (1997) makes an effective distinction between stereotyping and generalizing with the story of Rosa, a Mexican woman. "[If] I say to myself, Rosa is Mexican, she must have a large family, I am stereotyping her." Stereotyping closes my mind to potential differences. "But if I think Mexicans often have large families, I wonder if Rosa does, I am asking a generalization," and I remain receptive to further questioning and assessment of Rosa as a unique individual.

I proceeded with this project because of the reality of the work-a-day world. When you have a patient from an unfamiliar culture you can rarely say, "Excuse me. I'll be back in a few hours (or a few days) after I learn about your culture." The information you need to access is scattered throughout a multitude of journals and books, and most are not readily accessible.

This guide places at your fingertips some very basic information about peoples of the countries of our world, *when and where you need it.* I searched the National Library of Medicine's Medline database and the Cumulative Index to Nursing and Allied Health Literature (CINAHL) from their origins. People from various countries and health care professionals who have worked extensively abroad were interviewed and are listed as contributors. The Intercultural Communication Institute's library in Portland, Oregon, provided data not yet "discovered" by health care professionals. Because my search was limited to English language literature and interviews did not always furnish complete data, some categories are missing for many countries. Categories included for the countries often address areas of cultural impact on health care delivery and were gleaned from my transcultural practice and teaching.

Only the dominant culture for a country is included. That limitation was difficult to make. Most countries consist of numerous ethnic and/or racial groups. To include them all would result in a multivolume encyclopedia that is beyond the scope of this guide. Both the United States and Canada are believed to require more comprehensive data for the North American health care professional and, therefore, were not included in this guide.

The purpose of this guide is to help focus your attention on the potential variations a culturally diverse client may, **or may not,** exhibit. It is based on generalizations that must not be mentally converted into stereotypes by the user. Pull out this guide when you are faced with someone from a culture that is unfamiliar to you. Use this guide to start quickly and efficiently increasing your awareness and understanding of *potential* similarities and differences—the generalizations. For unless you are conscious of the cultural patterns of behavior a patient might exhibit, you will not think to address them in your assessment. To be culturally competent with a few cultures that you routinely encounter in your practice is a *must*. To be culturally competent with the many cultures with which you may on occasion be faced is unrealistic. To not use a guide such as this for fear of stereotyping only impedes movement toward delivery of culturally relevant health care. I am willing to risk criticism for stereotyping; but in return, I ask you to thoughtfully build on the information inside these pages with an individualized cultural assessment. Several good assessment guides are available. Examples follow:

Andrews MM, Boyle JS: Andrews/Boyle transcultural nursing assessment guide. In Andrews MM, Boyle JS: *Transcultural concepts in nursing care,* ed 2, Philadelphia, 1995, Lippincott.

Giger and Davidhizar's transcultural assessment model. In Giger JN, Davidhizar RE: *Transcultural nursing: assessment and intervention,* ed 2, St. Louis, 1995, Mosby.

Leininger MM: Leininger's acculturation health care assessment tool for cultural patterns in traditional and non-traditional lifeways, *J Transcultural Nurs* 2(2):40, 1991.

Orque MS, Block B, Monrroy KSA: Block's ethnic-cultural assessment guide. *In Ethnic nursing care: a multicultural approach,* St. Louis, 1983, CV Mosby.

Spector RE: *Guide to heritage assessment and health traditions,* Stamford, Conn, 1996, Appleton & Lange.

Tripp-Reimer T: Cultural assessment. In Bellack JP, Bamford PA: *Nursing assessment: a multidimensional approach,* Monterey, 1984, Wadsworth.

CITED REFERENCES

Galanti GA: *Caring for patients from different cultures,* ed 2, Philadelphia, 1997, University of Pennsylvania Press.

Moynihan DP: *Pandaemonium: ethnicity in international politics,* Oxford, England, 1993, Oxford University Press.

Stewart EC, Bennett MJ: *American cultural patterns: a cross-cultural perspective,* Yarmouth, Me, 1991, Intercultural Press.

Elaine M. Geissler

Special Recognition

The following sources were especially helpful in the preparation of this manuscript and deserve special recognition for their contributions:

Famighetti R, editor: *The world almanac and book of facts,* Wahwah, NJ, 1997, K-III Reference. This source is cited for demographic and geographic data.

Johnson O, editor: *Information please almanac,* Boston, 1997, Houghton Mifflin. This source is cited for demographic and geographic data.

Publications of the STD/AIDS Program of the Pan American Health Organization/World Health Organization

World Health Organization for immunization schedules.

Contents

COUNTRIES

♦ AFGHANISTAN

MAP PAGE (320)

Location: Afghanistan is split east to west by the Hindu Kush mountain range and wedged between the former Soviet Union, China, Pakistan, and Iran. With the exception of the southwest, most of the country is covered by high, snow-capped mountains and deep valleys.

Major Languages	Ethnic Groups		Major Religions	
Pushtu	Pashtun	38%	Sunni Muslim	84%
Dari Persian	Tajik	25%	Shiß	15%
Turkish	Hazara	19%	Other	1%
Baluchi	Uzbek	6%		
Pashai	Other	12%		

Predominant Sick Care Practices: Magico-religious. Charms and amulets are worn to ward off evil spirits. People of this region believe that evil spirits manifest themselves in a number of central nervous system diseases.

Ethnic/Race Specific or Endemic Diseases: ENDEMIC: Chloroquine-resistant malaria, which is limited to a belt in the east and rare in Kabul; gastroenteritis among infants during the summer; and cutaneous leishmaniasis. RISK: Intestinal obstruction caused by ascariasis. AIDS rate per 100,000 is reported by the country as zero.

Health Team Relationships: Women are not allowed to and generally do not wish to be seen and treated by male physicians. Separate buildings for males and females may be required for health and education services. Afghans have no experience with social services, and demanding and giving bribes is part of government business.

Dominance Patterns: Females are subservient to males. Polygamy is practiced. Most women wear the traditional veil. A movement to create a strict Islamic state bars women, including female nurses and doctors, from working, halts education for girls, and forces men to pray in mosques. Family interdependence with strict obedience to elders, particularly the father's authority, is the norm.

Birth Rites: Infant and maternal mortality rates are high. Tetanus neonatorum is one cause of infant death. Most births are assisted by traditional birth attendants (dais); many dais are given some basic training.

Death Rites: Relatives and friends come to the home of the family to express sympathy and, if money is needed, contribute. The body remains in the home with a mullah (priest) or close relatives, who read from the Koran throughout the night. The body is washed by relatives or specialists, wrapped in new white clothing, and placed in a coffin. The body must be buried (not cremated) within 24 hours. Two days after the funeral, a ceremony is held in the mosque or house of the deceased and is followed by a meal.

Food Practices and Intolerances: Because food is not inspected for contaminants, boiled water and milk products are advised. Using the hands to eat is acceptable.

Infant Feeding Practices: Breastfeeding, which is almost universal, continues until the next pregnancy and is sometimes supplemented with bottle feeding (introduced at 6 months). Tea and zoof (fried Linn seeds and cooking oil) provide energy and fat-soluble vitamins. These are given to the majority of infants. Contaminated pacifier nipples contribute to the occurrence of diarrhea and malnutrition. Two thirds of the children show signs of protein-energy malnutrition; one fifth show severe malnutrition.

Child Rearing Practices: Children are an economic asset; they work to supplement the household income. Child labor is common in rural areas and among male children. Girls over 5 are taught by women. Physical punishment for discipline is customary.

National Childhood Immunizations: BCG at birth; OPV at 6, 10, and 14 weeks and 9 months; DPT at 6, 10, and 14 weeks; measles at 9 months.

Other Characteristics: "Afghan" or "Afghanistani" refers to people; "Afghani" is money.

BIBLIOGRAPHY

Carlisle D: Lifting the veil, *Nurs Times* 91(37):22, 1995.
Li GR: Funeral practices, New York, World Relief, n.d.

Lipson JG, Omidian PA: Afghan refugee issues in the U.S. social environment, *West J Nurs Res* 19(1):110, 1997.

Lipson JG, Omidian PA, Paul SM: Afghan health education project, *Public Health Nurs* 12(3):143, 1995.

Singh M: Health status of children in Afghanistan, *J Indian Acad Pediatr* 20(5):317, 1983.

Storti C: *The art of crossing cultures,* Yarmouth, Me, 1990, Intercultural Press.

◆ ALBANIA

MAP PAGE (314)

Location: Situated on the eastern shore of the Adriatic Sea with Greece to the south, Albania is a mountainous (3000 feet [914 m]) country with few roads and a marshy coastal plain.

Major Languages	Ethnic Groups		Major Religions	
Albanian	Albanian	95%	Muslim	70%
Greek	Greek	3%	Albanian Orthodox	20%
	Other	2%	Catholic	10%

Ethnic/Race Specific or Endemic Diseases: AIDS rate per 100,000 is 0.09.

Death Rites: Muslims believe that the human body belongs to God, and organ donations or transplants are forbidden. Muslim physicians may recommend transfusions to save lives. Autopsy is uncommon because the deceased must be buried intact; cremation is not permitted. For Muslim burial the body is wrapped in special pieces of cloth and buried without a coffin in the ground.

National Childhood Immunizations: BCG at birth and 6 years; DPT at 2, 4, 6, and 18 months; DT at 5 years; OPV at 2, 4, 6, and 18 months and 5 years; measles at 9 months.

BIBLIOGRAPHY

Ross HM: Societal/cultural views regarding death and dying, *Top Clin Nurs* 1(1):1, 1981.

Swinburne C: New society, *Nurs Times* 90(29):48, 1994.

USA Today: June 12, 1991.

◆ ALGERIA

MAP PAGE (316)

Location: Located in northern Africa, Algeria is bordered on the west by Morocco and on the east by Tunisia and Libya. Small areas near the Mediterranean coast are low plains. The country is 68% plateau (between 2625 and 5250 feet [800 and 1600 m]).

Major Languages	Ethnic Groups		Major Religions	
Arabic	Arab Berber	99%	Sunni Muslim	99%
French	European and	1%	Other	1%
Berber	Other			

Ethnic/Race Specific or Endemic Diseases: RISK: Schistosomiasis and chloroquine-sensitive malaria, no risk in urban areas, limited risk in the Sahara. AIDS rate per 100,000 is 0.12.

Families' Role in Hospital Care: Family members or close friends, taking a vigilant supervisory role, often accompany the patient and expect to participate in care.

Dominance Patterns: Males dominate; sex roles are clearly and rigidly defined. Women's faces usually are veiled.

Pain Reactions: Those who accept the technology of Western medicine expect and request immediate pain relief. Energy is conserved for recovery; contraindicating therapies often involve exertion. Pain is expressed only in private or with close relatives or friends; pain during labor and delivery is expressive.

Birth Rites: Fathers are not present during delivery. Babies are wrapped tightly in swaddling clothes to protect them physically and psychologically.

Death Rites: Muslim belief forbids organ donations or transplants. Muslim physicians may recommend transfusions to save lives. Autopsy is uncommon because the deceased must be buried intact; cremation is not permitted. For Muslim burial the body is wrapped in special pieces of cloth and buried without a coffin in the ground.

Food Practices and Intolerances: Lamb and chicken are eaten frequently. Pork, carrion, and blood are forbidden. Food is usually spicy. Ramadan fasting is practiced, with exemptions for the sick and children.

Infant Feeding Practices: Breastfeeding is common. Mothers may wean the infant abruptly.

National Childhood Immunizations: BCG at birth; DPT at 3, 4, 5, and 18 months and 6 years; OPV at 3, 4, and 5 months; measles at 9 months.

Other Characteristics: Hope, optimism, and the positive advantages of treatment should be stressed when discussing outcomes.

BIBLIOGRAPHY

Green J: Death with dignity—Islam, *Nurs Times* 85(5):56, 1989.

Reizian A, Meleis AI: Arab-Americans' perceptions of and responses to pain, *Crit Care Nurse* 6(6):30, 1986.

Ross HM: Societal/cultural views regarding death and dying, *Top Clin Nurs* 1(1):1, 1981.

Taylor VL, editor: *Culturgrams: the nations around us,* Provo, Utah, 1987, Brigham Young University, David M Kennedy Center for International Studies.

Zémor O: Midwives in Algeria, *World Health,* Dec 1988, p 15.

◆ ANDORRA

MAP PAGE (314)

Location: Andorra is a coprincipality situated high in the Pyrenees Mountains on the French/Spanish border.

Major Languages	Ethnic Groups		Major Religions	
Catalan	Spanish	61%	Catholic	99%
French	Andorran	30%	Other	1%
Castilian Spanish	French	6%		
	Other	3%		

Ethnic/Race Specific or Endemic Diseases: No AIDS data in WHO statistics.

BIBLIOGRAPHY

No data located.

◆ ANGOLA

MAP PAGE (317)

Location: Angola extends for more than 1000 miles (1609 km) along the South Atlantic in southwestern Africa. A plateau averaging 6000 feet (1829 m) in height rises abruptly from the coastal lowlands. Most of the land is desert or savanna.

Major Languages	Ethnic Groups		Major Religions	
Portuguese	Ovimbundu	37%	Catholic	38%
Bantu Languages	Kimbundu	25%	Protestant	15%
	Bakongo	13%	Other	47%
	Mestizo	2%		
	European and Other	24%		

Ethnic/Race Specific or Endemic Diseases: ACTIVE: Cholera and yellow fever. **ENDEMIC:** Chloroquine-resistant malaria. **RISK:** Schistosomiasis. AIDS rate per 100,000 is 2.90.

Birth Rites: Nurses and midwives perform most maternity care.

National Childhood Immunizations: BCG at birth; DPT at 2, 3, and 4 months; OPV at 2, 3, and 4 months; measles at 9 months.

BIBLIOGRAPHY

Farrell M: The price of war, *Nurs Health Care* 13(8):414, 1992.
Raisler J: Anatomy of a training seminar: teaching and learning in Angola, *J Nurse Midwife* 34(1):36, 1989.

◆ ANTIGUA AND BARBUDA

MAP PAGE (313)

Location: Antigua, the larger of these two eastern Caribbean islands, is low lying, deforested, and subject to droughts. Barbuda is a wooded, coral island.

Major Languages	Ethnic Groups		Major Religions	
English	African	96%	Anglican	98%
Local Languages	Other	4%	Other	2%

Ethnic/Race Specific or Endemic Diseases: AIDS rate per 100,000 is 7.58.

National Childhood Immunizations: DPT at 3, 4, 5, and 18 months; OPV at 3, 4, 5, and 18 months; MMR at 15 months.

Other Characteristics: Several people may engage in simultaneous conversations with frequent interruptions, loud verbal battles, repetition, cursing, and boasting. Such discourse is valued as a normal part of interpersonal relationships.

BIBLIOGRAPHY

Menyuk P, Menyuk D: Communicative competence: a historical and cultural perspective. In Wurzel JS: *Toward multiculturalism,* Yarmouth, Me, 1988, Intercultural Press.

◆ ARGENTINA

MAP PAGE (314)

Location: Argentina, a land of plains from the Atlantic to the Chilean border, also has the high peaks of the Andes. The north is swampy, and the central populated area has fertile land used for agriculture or grazing. The south boasts Patagonia, with its cool, arid steppes. Many Argentineans are of Italian descent. Life expectancy is one of the highest in South America; the standard of living is generally high.

Major Languages	Ethnic Groups		Major Religions	
Spanish	White	85%	Catholic	90%
English	Native American	15%	Protestant	2%
Italian	and Mestizo		Jewish	2%
German			Other	6%
French				

Ethnic/Race Specific or Endemic Diseases: ENDEMIC: Chloroquine-sensitive malaria is present; however, it is not found in urban areas. RISK: Argentine hemorrhagic fever in four provinces. The AIDS rate per 100,000 is 4.72.

Health Team Relationships: It may be more ethical to protect the patient from knowing diagnosis, prognosis, and treatment reality than to be truthful.

Dominance Patterns: Society is generally patriarchal, with deference given to the father; however, he considers the opinions of the rest of the family.

Eye Contact Practices: Eye contact is maintained.

Touch Practices: Males may touch while in conversation.

Perceptions of Time: A relaxed attitude toward punctuality exists.

Food Practices and Intolerances: The staple food for many is beef; it is eaten 3 times a day.

National Childhood Immunizations: BCG at birth, between 6 and 7 years, and at 16 years; DPT at 2, 4, 6, and 18 months; Td at 7 and 16 years; OPV at 2, 4, 6, and 18 months and between 6 and 7 years; measles at 12 months.

BIBLIOGRAPHY

Johnson GA: Palliative care in Argentina: a gringo's perspective, *Am J Hospice Palliat Care* 10(4):11, 1993.

Latin America: intercultural experiential learning aid, Provo, Utah, 1976, Language Research Center, Brigham Young University.

Taylor VL, editor: *Culturgrams: the nations around us,* Provo, Utah, 1987, Brigham Young University, David M Kennedy Center for International Studies.

U.S. Agency of International Development: Agency program fights Argentine virus, *Front Lines* 31(10):4, 1991.

◆ ARMENIA

MAP PAGE (315)

Location: The smallest of the former Soviet republics, Armenia achieved independence in 1991. It is a landlocked country located in the southern Caucasus. The terrain is rugged mountains and excellent pastures. It has a recent history of a devastating earthquake that destroyed its infrastructure and left approximately 500,000 people handicapped, orphaned, and/or homeless.

Major Languages	Ethnic Groups		Major Religions	
Armenian	Armenian	93%	Armenian	94%
	Azeri	3%	Orthodox	
	Other	4%	Other	6%

Health Care Beliefs: A former recognition of the importance of health promotion and disease prevention has become stagnant due in part to the lack of infrastructure needed to provide public health services. Alcohol consumption is viewed as part of the social and cultural behavior of males.

Ethnic/Race Specific or Endemic Diseases: The AIDS rate per 100,000 reported by the country is zero.

Health Team Relationships: The health care system is centralized, bureaucratic, medically oriented, and male dominated despite a good number of female physicians, who occupy positions with less power. Communication among health care personnel is generally unidirectional, from physicians to therapists and nurses, and takes the form of instructions and orders. Some physicians and nurses take bribes from patients for services that might include basics, for example, bathing, turning, and feeding. Because hospitals are paid by the government based on the amount of time a bed is occupied, length of stay may be somewhat extended.

Dominance Patterns: Males are dominant.

Birth Rites: Abortion is the primary birth control method, with an average of 15 abortions for a 35-year-old woman. Vasectomy is not generally a culturally acceptable option for the Armenian male. As many as one in three women are infertile from the results of sexually transmitted diseases and unsafe abortions.

Infant Feeding Practices: Breastfeeding practices declined after the 1988 earthquake.

National Childhood Immunizations: BCG at birth and 7 and 12 years; DPT at 3, 4½, 6, and 18 months; DT/Td at 6, 16, 26, 36, and 46 years; OPV at 3, 4½, 6, 18, and 20 months and 6 years; measles at 12 months; mumps at 15 months.

BIBLIOGRAPHY

Bernal H et al.: Community health nursing in a former Soviet Union republic: a case study of change in Armenia, *Nurs Outlook* 43(2):78, 1995.

Hertzberg DL: The interdisciplinary team: the experience in the Armenia pediatric rehabilitation program . . . Project HOPE Pediatric Rehabilitation Education Program, *Holistic Nurs Practice* 7(4):42, 1993.

Kalayjian AS: Mental health outreach program following the earthquake in Armenia, *Issues Ment Health Nurs* 15(6):533, 1994.

◆ AUSTRALIA

MAP PAGE (311)

Location: Australia is the only country that occupies a complete continent. Its western half is a desert plateau that includes the Great Victoria Desert to the south and the Great Sandy Desert to the north. The Great Barrier Reef, 1245 miles (2000 km) long, lies along the northeast coast. Aborigines were the only inhabitants when the Dutch discovered parts of the continent in 1623.

Major Languages	Ethnic Groups		Major Religions	
English	White	95%	Anglican	26%
Aborigine	Asian	4%	Catholic	26%
	Aborigine	1%	Other	24%
	and Other		Christian	
			Other	24%

With large numbers of aboriginals and immigrants, many Australians come from a non–English-speaking background.

Predominant Sick Care Practices: Biomedical and other public institutions tend to follow Anglo-Saxon/Celtic beliefs and values. Health promotion is not a significant component of health care counseling.

Health Care Beliefs: Active involvement is the norm; health promotion is important.

Ethnic/Race Specific or Endemic Diseases: The AIDS rate per 100,000 is 3.81.

Health Team Relationships: National socialized medicine is in force, with health care available to all; it is funded by a levy on salaries. The government functions as provider, financier, and regulator and constitutes the major influence on health care services. Respect for authority figures (physicians, in particular) is not strong. Patients may question diagnoses. Physicians encourage patients to express their feelings. Nurses may lack assertiveness skills essential for effective communication.

Families' Role in Hospital Care: To maintain the family atmosphere, families are encouraged to feed, bathe, and care for their children in some hospitals.

Dominance Patterns: The male has a strong role, especially in making decisions for the family. The female is the primary child care giver, even though she may be working. The term *mate* is used to indicate camaraderie among males.

Eye Contact Practices: A combination of direct eye contact and looking away shows interest.

Touch Practices: Demonstrations of familiarity, for example, hugging, are generally avoided, especially among males. Today females touch frequently when greeting or at departure.

Perceptions of Time: Being punctual for appointments is important; being punctual for social functions is viewed more leniently. Orientation lies in the present, with less worrying about the future. Long-term health promotion activities such as smoking cessation or reducing high cholesterol levels are not associated with future benefits.

Pain Reactions: Pain is expressed verbally within limits.

Birth Rites: A physician usually delivers, but home birth, alternative birthing centers, and use of midwives are increasing. Lamaze method and Alexander's technique are common. The father is usually present at the birth.

Death Rites: Cremation and burial are both practiced. The family usually does not see the body; no wake is held. Grieving is reserved: crying with no wailing. Health care practitioners are expected to help the family through the stages of grief; to provide privacy; and to be sensitive to the family's desires regarding arrangements for an autopsy, for the mortuary, for viewing the body (if desired), and for the funeral.

Food Practices and Intolerances: Large amounts of beef and dairy products are consumed, with a current tendency toward ingesting less in dairy fats and more in polyunsaturated fats. The consumption of beer is one of the highest per capita.

Infant Feeding Practices: Breastfeeding is widely recommended until 4 to 6 months and practiced by more than 80% of mothers on discharge from the hospital. This figure drops to 50% at 3 months and 40% at 6 months.

Child Rearing Practices: Emphasis is placed on discipline. Children are encouraged to develop independence within clearly defined limits and controls.

National Childhood Immunizations: BCG at birth and 6 years; DPT at 2, 4, 6, and 18 months; OPV at 2, 4, and 6 months; measles at 12 months; hep B at birth and only the risk groups at 6 weeks and 6 months.

Other Characteristics: Large teeth, with as many as four extra molars, are present. Incidence of skin cancer is one of the highest in the world. Open expression (bordering on the confrontational) or critical questioning during interactions is commonplace. Disagreement is often a valued basis for conversations, eliciting real interest and respect in the participants. Positioning the thumbs upward is a rude gesture; curling the index finger inward is used only to call animals.

BIBLIOGRAPHY

Ashby MA et al.: An inquiry into death and dying at the Adelaide Children's Hospital: a useful model? *Med J Aust* 154(3):165, 1991.

Davis AJ, Slater PV: U.S. and Australian nurses' attitudes and beliefs about the good death, *IMAGE: J Nurs Sch* 21(1):34, 1989.

Gorman D: Multiculturalism and transcultural nursing in Australia, *J Transcultural Nurs* 6(2):27, 1995.

Indrus L: Transcultural nursing in Australia: response to a changing population base, *Recent Adv Nurs* 20:81, 1988.

Kanitsaki O: Transcultural nursing: challenge to change, *Aust J Adv Nurs* 5(3):4, 1988.

Lawson K, Tulloch MI: Breastfeeding duration: prenatal intentions and postnatal practices, *J Adv Nurs* 22:841, 1995.

McCallum LW et al.: The Ankall project: a model for the use of volunteers to provide emotional support in terminal illness, *Med J Aust* 151(1):33, 1989.

McKenna B: *Aboriginal culture in the Kimberley region: a guide for health practitioners,* Perth, Australia, 1987, Health Department of Western Australia.

Oldenburg B, Owen N: Preventive care in general practice in Australia: a public health perspective, *Patient Educ Counseling* 25(3):305, 1995.

Overfield T: *Biologic variation in health and illness,* Menlo Park, Calif, 1985, Addison-Wesley.

Page L: Impressions of midwifery in New Zealand & Australia, *Midwives* 109(1299):88, 1996.

People to have a voice in health care, Health Victoria Supplement, 1985.

People To People International Citizen Ambassador Program, J People Transcultur Nurs Deleg Australia & New Zealand, Spokane, 1987.

Poroch D, Mcintosh W: Barriers to assertive skills in nurses, *Aust NZ J Ment Health Nurs* 4(3):113, 1995.

Redman S et al.: Evaluation of an Australian intervention to encourage breast feeding in primiparous women, *Health Promot Int* 10(2):101, 1995.

Renwick GW: *Australians and North Americans,* Yarmouth, Me, 1980, Intercultural Press.

Singh B, Raphael B: Postdisaster morbidity of the bereaved: a possible role for preventive psychiatry, *J Nerv Ment Dis* 169(4):203, 1981.

Sleed J: Manners abroad need study, Portland, Ore, Newhouse News Service, n.d.

Storti C: *The art of crossing cultures,* Yarmouth, Me, 1990, Intercultural Press.

Taylor VL, editor: *Culturgrams: the nations around us,* Provo, Utah, 1987, Brigham Young University, David M Kennedy Center for International Studies.

Westbrook MT, Nordholm LA, McGee JE: Cultural differences in reactions to patient behaviour: a comparison of Swedish and Australian health professionals, *Soc Sci Med* 19(9):939, 1984.

Willcoxson L: Contributor.

Wilson JM, Retsas AP: Personal constructs of nursing practice: a comparative analysis of three groups of Australian nurses, *Int J Nurs Stud* 34(1):63, 1997.

◆ AUSTRIA

MAP PAGE (314)

Location: This landlocked nation in central Europe includes much of the mountainous territory of the eastern Alps, with many snowfields, glaciers, and snowcapped peaks.

Major Language	Ethnic Groups		Major Religions	
German	German	99%	Catholic	85%
	Croatian and	1%	Protestant	6%
	Slavic		Other	9%

Health Care Beliefs: Active involvement.

Ethnic/Race Specific or Endemic Diseases: RISK: Rett syndrome in girls. The AIDS rate per 100,000 is 2.40.

Health Team Relationships: Patients may consider titles more important than names and use the term *doctor* or *nurse* in reference to a health professional. Dependence on the physician is typical, initiative is not rewarded, and nurses are expected to follow orders for everything except basic nursing care. Patients receive sufficient oral drugs for 24 hours and are responsible for taking them. Psychologists enjoy a strong role as health care administrators and teachers.

Dominance Patterns: Because the society is patriarchal, women are influenced by husbands or fathers in areas such as politics.

Touch Practices: Privacy curtains between hospital beds are rare because of the communal living styles.

Perceptions of Time: The past is valued. Traditional approaches to healing are more readily accepted than new procedures or medications. The people also value punctuality.

Birth Rites: Natural childbirth and the father's presence in the delivery room are becoming more popular.

Food Practices and Intolerances: The main meal is at midday, and a light meal is eaten in early evening, with another at the end of the day.

National Childhood Immunizations: DPT at 3, 4, and 5 months and between 16 and 18 months; DT/Td at 7 years and between 14 and 15 years; OPV at 4 months, between 5 and 6 months, at 7 months, 7 years, and between 14 and 15 years; MMR at between 2 and 7 years; measles for girls at 13 years.

BIBLIOGRAPHY

Boerckel K: Childbirth education in Austria, *Int J Childbirth Educ* 6(1):39, 1991.

Clift JM: Nursing and health services in Austria, *Nurs Adm Q* 16(2):60, 1992.

Clift JM: Nursing education in Austria, Germany, and Switzerland, *IMAGE: J Nurs Sch* 29(1):89, 1997.

Cochrane L: Vienna—psychiatry in a "cultured" city, *Psychiatr Nurs* 26(1):1985.

Galanti GA: *Caring for patients from different cultures,* ed 2, Philadelphia, 1997, University of Pennsylvania Press.

Language Research Center: *German-speaking people of Europe,* Provo, Utah, 1976, Brigham Young University.

Morris J: Rett's syndrome: a case study, *J Neurosci Nurs* 22(5):285, 1990.

Reeser DS: An international experience: studying health care systems in Austria and Yugoslavia, *Imprint* 32(1):46, 1985.

Taylor VL, editor: *Culturgrams: the nations around us,* Provo, Utah, 1987, Brigham Young University, David M Kennedy Center for International Studies.

◆ AZERBAIJAN

MAP PAGE (315)

Location: This mountainous country is located on the western shore of the Caspian Sea; only about 7% of its land is arable. Independence was achieved with the dissolution of the former Soviet Union.

Major Languages	Ethnic Groups		Major Religions	
Azeri	Azeri	90%	Muslim	93%
Russian	Russian	3%	Other	7%
Armenian	Armenian	2%		
	Other	5%		

Ethnic/Race Specific or Endemic Diseases: The AIDS rate per 100,000 is 0.01.

National Childhood Immunizations: BCG at 7 days and 8, 13, 24, and 31 years; DPT at 3 and 4½ months, between 6 and 7 months, and at 3 years; OPV at 3 and 4½ months, between 6 and 7 months, and at 2, 3, 8, and 14 years; measles at 12 months and 7 years; mumps at 18 months.

Other Characteristics: Azerbaijan is noted for the longevity of its people, with approximately 48:100,000 over 100 years of age.

BIBLIOGRAPHY

No data located.

◆ BAHAMAS

MAP PAGE (313)

Location: The Bahamas include about 700 relatively flat islands (22 are inhabited) off the east coast of Florida, with no freshwater streams.

Major Languages	Ethnic Groups		Major Religions	
English	Black	85%	Baptist	32%
Creole	White	15%	Anglican	20%
			Catholic	19%
			Other	29%

Ethnic/Race Specific or Endemic Diseases: The AIDS rate per 100,000 is 141.82.

National Childhood Immunizations: DPT at 3, 5, 7, and 18 months; Td at 6 years; OPV at 3, 5, and 7 months and between 4 and 5 years; measles at 12 months.

BIBLIOGRAPHY

Adler MW, editor: Statistics from the World Health Organization and the Centers for Disease Control, *AIDS* 6(10):1229, 1992.

◆ BAHRAIN

MAP PAGE (318)

Location: An archipelago in the Persian Gulf off the eastern coast of Saudi Arabia, the islands are level expanses of sand and rock.

Major Languages	Ethnic Groups		Major Religions	
Arabic	Bahraini	63%	Shi'a Muslim	70%
English	Asian	13%	Sunni Muslim	30%
Farsi	Other Arab	10%		
Urdu	Iranian	8%		
	Other	6%		

Ethnic/Race Specific or Endemic Diseases: The AIDS rate per 100,000 is 1.41.

Families' Role in Hospital Care: Family members or close friends participate in the patient's care or take a vigilant and supervisory role.

Pain Reactions: Patients expect immediate pain relief and may request it persistently. Therapies requiring exertion are in conflict with the belief in energy conservation for recovery. Pain is expressed only privately or in the company of close relatives and friends. During labor and delivery, pain is expressed.

Death Rites: Muslim belief forbids organ donations and transplants. Muslim physicians may recommend transfusions to save lives. Autopsy is uncommon because the deceased must be buried intact. Cremation is not permitted. For Muslim burial the body is wrapped in special pieces of cloth and buried without a coffin in the ground.

Food Practices and Intolerances: Pork, carrion, and blood are forbidden. Food tends to be spicy. Ramadan fasting is carried out between sunrise and sunset. The sick and children are exempt.

National Childhood Immunizations: BCG at birth and between 4 and 6 years; DPT at 2, 4, 6, and 18 months and between 4 and 6 years; OPV at 2, 4, 5, and 18 months and between 4 and 6 years; measles at 9 and 15 months; hep B at birth and 2 and 6 months.

Other Characteristics: Hope, optimism, and the positive advantages of treatment should be stressed when discussing outcomes.

BIBLIOGRAPHY

al Gasseer NH: Experience of menstrual symptoms among Bahraini women, doctoral dissertation, Chicago, 1990, University of Illinois.

Green J: Death with dignity—Islam, *Nurs Times* 85(5):56, 1989.

Morris S, executive producer: *Bahrain: land of life-giving water,* June 12, 1997, Discovery Channel.

Reizian A, Meleis AI: Arab-Americans' perceptions of and responses to pain, *Crit Care Nurse* 6(6):30, 1986.

Ross HM: Societal/cultural views regarding death and dying, *Top Clin Nurs* 1(1):1, 1981.

◆ BANGLADESH

MAP PAGE (320)

Location: Formerly East Pakistan, Bangladesh is on the northern coast of the Bay of Bengal and is surrounded primarily by India. The country is low lying (less than 600 feet [183 m]) and subject to tropical monsoons, frequent floods, and famine. It is one of the most heavily populated and poorest countries in the world.

Major Languages	Ethnic Groups		Major Religions	
Bangla (Bengali)	Bengali	98%	Muslim	83%
English	Bihari and Other	2%	Hindu	16%
			Other	1%

Predominant Sick Care Practices: Biomedical; magicoreligious. Evil spirits and God's will are suspected causes of illness. Injections are perceived as a cure for illness. Faith healers, called fakirs, are used to exorcise the evil air. Fakirs may be preferred because they spend time with patients and do not always charge a fee. They encourage modern treatment as needed.

Health Care Beliefs: Acute sick care.

Ethnic/Race Specific or Endemic Diseases: ENDEMIC: Chloroquine-resistant malaria. RISK: Japanese encephalitis; iodine deficiency disease is severe, resulting in goiter and mental and physical retardation. Acute respiratory tract infections, low birth weight, and dehydration from diarrhea cause many deaths in those under age 5. Vitamin A deficiency is the most common cause of childhood blindness. The AIDS rate per 100,000 is reported by the country as zero.

Dominance Patterns: In this patriarchal society women's activities may be severely restricted; physical seclusion often results.

Birth Rites: Contraceptive practices have increased in recent years. Rural, traditional custom requires the mother to reach a water source unaided and to wash herself and her clothing immediately after delivery. The umbilical cord may be cut with the clean inner strip of a bamboo stalk. After delivery, rituals are performed. The mother chants prayers and stays indoors. Traditionally this rest period of 7, 21, or even 40 days for the mother after birth is practiced depending on the economic means and the degree of traditional values of the family. Only the husband may visit. Plum branches are placed on the door of the home to protect against evil spirits, and the Muslim holy Iman chants the birth announcement.

Death Rites: Muslim belief forbids organ donations or transplants. Muslim physicians may recommend transfusions to save lives. A holy Iman does not have to be present at death; however, a Muslim may recite the Declaration of the Faith: "There is no God but God and Muhammad is his Messenger." Family members wash the body according to Islamic tradition. Autopsy is uncommon because the deceased must be buried intact. Cremation is not permitted. For Muslim burial the body is wrapped in special pieces of cloth and buried without a coffin in the ground.

Food Practices and Intolerances: Rice gruel is commonly used during illness. Deficiency of iodine in the water and lack of iodized salt cause many children to show signs of iodine deficiency. People in Bangladesh are among the most malnourished in the world.

Infant Feeding Practices: Breastfeeding is almost universal and usually continues until the child is 1 year of age. For the first 3 days the infant is spoon-fed sugar water. Economically deprived families breastfeed male and female infants the same until supplementary foods are introduced; then male children may receive higher quality supplementary nutrition.

Child Rearing Practices: Economic and cultural influences prompt the allocation of sparse family nutritional and health care resources to boys, resulting in an increased mortality rate in 1- to 4-year-old female children.

National Childhood Immunizations: BCG at birth; DPT at 6, 10, and 14 weeks; OPV at birth, 6, 10, and 14 weeks and 9 months; measles at 9 months.

BIBLIOGRAPHY

Ahmed S: A birth in Bangladesh, *Midwives Chron Nurs Notes* 101(1203):98, 1988.

Ahmet L: A model for midwives: support for ethnic breast-feeding mothers, *Midwives Chron Nurs Notes* 103(1224):5, 1990.

Chowdhury AM et al.: Oral rehydration therapy: a community trial comparing the acceptability of homemade sucrose and cereal-based solutions, *Bull World Health Organ* 69(2):229, 1991.

Koenig MA, D'Souza S: Sex differences in childhood mortality in rural Bangladesh, *Soc Sci Med* 22(1):15, 1986.

Lally MM: Last rites and funeral customs of minority groups, *Midwife Health Visit Comm Nurse* 14(7):224, 1978.

Long N: Mission of the month: Bangladesh, *Front Lines* 32(1):8, 1992.

Nafisa M: Exorcising the evil air, *Nurs Times* 84(27):50, 1988.

Ross HM: Societal/cultural views regarding death and dying, *Top Clin Nurs* 1(1):1, 1981.

Rowell M: Eradication of Vitamin A deficiency, *J Ophthalmic Nurs Tech* 12(5):217, 1993.

State of the natural world: children of the monsoon, May 29, 1992, Discovery Channel.

◆ BARBADOS

MAP PAGE (313)

Location: An Atlantic island, Barbados lies 300 miles (483 km) north of Venezuela. The island is 21 miles (34 km) long and 14 miles (23 km) at its widest point. The country is one of the better developed English-speaking Caribbean nations, with a high population density and demographic characteristics consistent with developed countries.

Major Language	Ethnic Groups		Major Religions	
English	African	80%	Anglican	70%
	Mixed	16%	Methodist	9%
	European	4%	Catholic	4%
			Other	17%

Health Care Beliefs: Active involvement.

Ethnic/Race Specific or Endemic Diseases: The AIDS rate per 100,000 is 35.98.

Dominance Patterns: Some women and their children may be subject to high levels of physical, emotional, and sexual abuse. The assumption that strong extended family support systems exist here may not be true. The elderly are cared for in institutions or small one- or two-person households.

Child Rearing Practices: The majority of adults generally approve of corporal punishment, unless it is excessive or self-serving.

National Childhood Immunizations: BCG at 4½ and 10 years; DPT at 3, 4½, and 6 weeks, 18 months, and 4½ years; OPV at 3, 4½, and 6 weeks, 18 months, and 4½ years; measles at 12 months.

BIBLIOGRAPHY

Adler MW, editor: Statistics from the World Health Organization and the Centers for Disease Control, *AIDS* 6(10):1229, 1992.

Brathwaite FS: The elderly in Barbados: problems and policies, *Bull Pan Am Health Organ* 24(3):314, 1990.

Handwerker WP: Gender power differences between parents and high-risk sexual behavior by their children: AIDS/STD risk factors extend to a prior generation, *J Women's Health* 2(3):301, 1993.

Lyte V: Island of innovation: nurse training in Barbados, *Nurs Times* 86(49):44, 1990.

Payne MA: Use and abuse of corporal punishment: a Caribbean view, *Child Abuse Negl* 13(3):1389, 1989.

Rosenkoetter MM et al.: The Barbados project: an experience in collaboration and mutuality, *Nurs Health Care* 14(10):528, 1993.

◆ BELARUS

MAP PAGE (315)

Location: Located in eastern Europe with Poland on the west and Russia on the east, Belarus is one of the co-founders of the Commonwealth of Independent States. It contains hilly lowlands with forests, swamps, peat marshes, rivers, and lakes.

Major Languages	Ethnic Groups		Major Religion
Belarussian	Belarussian	78%	Eastern Orthodox
Russian	Russian	13%	
	Polish	4%	
	Ukrainian	3%	
	Other	2%	

Ethnic/Race Specific or Endemic Diseases: Since the nuclear power station disaster in Chernobyl in 1986 there has been an increase in the incidence of thyroid cancer, common oral health diseases, gastroduodenal pathology, hematologic diseases, and disturbances of the immune system. The AIDS rate per 100,000 is 0.03.

National Childhood Immunizations: BCG at between 3 and 5 days, at 7 days, between 11 and 12 years, and between 16 and 17 years; DPT at 3, 4½, and 6 months and 3 years; OPV at 3, 4½, and 6 months and 2, 3, 8, and 14 years; measles at 12 months.

BIBLIOGRAPHY

Leous PA: Chernobyl "fall-out" on oral health, *World Health* 47(1):24, 1994.

◆ BELGIUM

MAP PAGE (314)

Location: Belgium, a neighbor of France, Germany, the Netherlands, and Luxembourg, has an opening onto the North Sea. The land is generally flat with a system of dikes and sea walls along the coast that prevent tidal flooding. Regionalism based on language (Flemish [Dutch] in the north and French in the south) remains the most powerful issue in contemporary Belgium.

Major Languages	Ethnic Groups		Major Religions	
Flemish	Fleming	55%	Catholic	75%
French	Walloon	33%	Protestant	25%
German	Other	12%		

Belgians are divided into French-speaking Walloons and Flemish-speaking Flemings.

Health Care Beliefs: The majority of people contribute to health insurance plans.

Ethnic/Race Specific or Endemic Diseases: The AIDS rate per 100,000 is 2.14.

Health Team Relationships: Patients may choose their own health care providers, and they may see several providers simultaneously for the same health problem.

Touch Practices: A handshake or three kisses on the cheek for greeting and leave-taking is common.

Perceptions of Time: Punctuality is practiced.

Birth Rites: Deliveries are usually assisted by physicians, with midwives responsible for postnatal care.

Food Practices and Intolerances: The main meal is the evening meal. Staples include cheese, bread, fruit, and vegetables, with wine a common beverage.

National Childhood Immunizations: DPT at 3, 4, 5, and 13 months; DT/Td at 6 years; OPV at 3, 5, and 13 months and 6 years; MMR at 15 months.

Other Characteristics: Carrying on a conversation while hands are in the pockets or pointing with a finger is not acceptable.

BIBLIOGRAPHY

Axtell RE, editor: *Do's and taboos around the world,* ed 2, New York, 1990, A Benjamin Book, John Wiley & Sons.

Glen S: A family affair: the health of children and their families: paediatric nurses in Denmark, France, Belgium, and Holland, *Nurs Mirror* 155(24):24, 1982.

Nonneman W, van Doorslaer E: The role of the sickness funds in the Belgian health care market, *Soc Sci Med* 39(10):1483, 1994.

Smoyak S: Psychosocial nursing in Belgium, *J Psychosoc Nurs Ment Health Serv* 22(5):35, 1984.

Szpalski M et al.: Health care utilization for low back pain in Belgium: influence of sociocultural factors and health beliefs, *Spine* 20(4):431, 1995.

Taylor VL, editor: *Culturgrams: the nations around us,* Provo, Utah, 1987, Brigham Young University, David M Kennedy Center for International Studies.

Wilson H: Community nursing in Belgium, *Nurs Times* 86(29):56, 1990.

◆ BELIZE

MAP PAGE (312)

Location: This Central American nation (formerly British Honduras) faces the Caribbean Sea to the east and is bounded by the Republics of Mexico and Guatemala. The coastline, just a few feet above sea level, is flat, swampy, and fringed by islets (called "cayes") and a barrier reef—the longest in the Western Hemisphere. In the west and south the terrain rises gradually to its highest peak at 3559 feet (1085 m). In this subtropical climate the rivers are numerous. Although it is surrounded by Spanish-speaking Central American countries, Belize's links to English-speaking eastern Caribbean islands and to Britain remain strong.

Major Languages	Ethnic Groups		Major Religions	
English	Mestizo	44%	Catholic	62%
Spanish	Creole	30%	Protestant	30%
Garifuna	Maya	11%	Other	8%
Maya	Garifuna	7%		
Ketchi	Other	8%		
Creole				

Predominant Sick Care Practices: Biomedical; magico-religious. Women of obeah belief read cards. Dream books may be consulted to interpret the significance of dreams. The evil eye, mal ojo, is a commonly held belief. Among women the expression "cut your eye at someone" means casting the evil eye. Family herb recipes are often tried before or with biomedical treatment. Nurses and physicians are sought for advice and care.

Health Care Beliefs: Passive role; acute sick care. Regular physical examinations are usually not practiced.

Ethnic/Race Specific or Endemic Diseases: ENDEMIC: Chloroquine-sensitive malaria is found (no risk in urban areas). RISK: Schistosomiasis, keloids, sickle cell anemia, and hypertension are reported. The AIDS rate per 100,000 is 12.84.

Health Team Relationships: The physician usually is not questioned by patients. Physician/nurse relationships are superior/subordinate (respectively) relationships. Female chaperons are often present when female patients have physical examinations by male physicians. Male nurses usually do not give intimate physical care to females.

Families' Role in Hospital Care: Families are encouraged to assist with the patient's care and act as advocates. Some families bring food to the patient daily. Chronically ill elderly are often cared for at home; however, they are hospitalized in acute illness. The mentally ill are hospitalized because families are hesitant to care for them at home.

Dominance Patterns: This society is a matriarchal one.

Eye Contact Practices: Many persons do not maintain direct eye contact, especially with authority figures.

Touch Practices: Greetings are usually formal.

Perceptions of Time: The people adhere to schedules.

Pain Reactions: Expressive reactions predominate. Cancer is usually suspected if a reason for the pain cannot be found. It is believed that if pain is denied, it will go away. Before medical aid is sought, home remedies or over-the-counter medications are used. Some people believe that dark rum relieves headaches and hot Coca-Cola or pure lime juice relieves diarrhea. Hot food, cold drink, and heavy food are avoided at night to ward off colic and nightmares. Bones of spoiled fish are used to make a soup believed to cure sickness caused by having ingested spoiled fish.

Birth Rites: Half of children are born out of wedlock and are called "outside children." Until the early 1960s newborn babies were christened before relatives or friends were allowed to visit because it was believed that babies not yet christened could be "overlooked" or given the bad eye. In addition to nurse midwives, Belize has a 4-month program for traditional birth attendants (nannies), who are recognized as primary health care workers by the Ministry of Health.

Death Rites: People are demonstrative in their expressions of grief. A spectacular funeral procession includes many cars and people.

Food Practices and Intolerances: Rice, red beans, and fish are food staples that are highly seasoned with pepper. The diet is high in carbohydrates.

Infant Feeding Practices: Although breastfeeding is encouraged, bottle feeding for 3 years is preferred.

Child Rearing Practices: Children are raised with strict discipline until the boys are 13 years old and the girls are 16 years old. Grandmothers are frequently involved in child care. Disposable diapers are used; however, in rural areas cloth diapers or bare bottoms are the custom. Toilet training begins as soon as the child can sit up. In school, sex education is presented co-educationally to 10- to 12-year-old boys and girls.

National Childhood Immunizations: BCG at birth; DPT at 3 weeks, between 4 and 4½ weeks, between 5 and 5½ weeks, and between 4 and 5 years; OPV at 3 weeks, between 4 and 4½ weeks, between 5 and 5½ weeks, and between 4 and 5 years; measles at 9 and 15 months. The belief persists that immunizations make children ill.

Other Characteristics: In 1990 the population estimate was 184,000 people; 44% were 14 years old or younger, and 5.6% were 65 years old or older. The country has neither medical schools nor national health insurance. Skin color and/or physical features may influence status and opportunity.

BIBLIOGRAPHY

Belize Information Service and Central Statistics Office: *Belize in figures,* Belize, 1991, Government Printery.

Buhler RO: Belizean folk remedies, *Natl Studies* 3(2):17, 1975.

Cody E: Belize: a different beat, The Washington Post, Sept 30, 1991, p. A14.

Dobson N: *History of Belize,* Port of Spain, 1973, Longman Caribbean.

Fact Sheet: Belize, Belize, 1989, Government Information Service.

Herrmann EK: Contributor.

Herrmann EK: *Origins of tomorrow: a history of Belizean nursing education,* Belize, 1985, Ministry of Health.

Holland J: Promoting primary health in Belize, *Health Visit* 56(11):400, 1983.

Johnson JD et al.: Communication factors related to closer international ties: an extension of a model in Belize, *Int J Intercult Relations* 13(1):1, 1989.

Johnson L, Belizean medical student at the University of the West Indies: Personal communication to Herrmann EK, 1989.

Johnson S, principal nursing officer, Belize: Personal communication to Herrmann EK, Feb 1990, July 1991.

Robbins W: Health care Belize style: have clinic, will travel, *Front Nurs Serv Q Bull* 63(2):12, 1987.

Wolfson E: Nursing in Indian Church, Belize, *Minn Nurs Accent* 67(1):4, 1995.

◆ BENIN

MAP PAGE (316)

Location: Benin (formerly Dahomey), located in West Africa on the Gulf of Guinea, is one of the smallest and most densely populated countries in Africa. A narrow coastal strip of land rises to a swampy, forested plateau, with highlands to the north.

Major Languages	Ethnic Groups		Major Religions	
French	African	99%	Indigenous	70%
Fon	European	1%	Beliefs	
Yoruba			Muslim	15%
Other			Christian	15%

Predominant Sick Care Practices: Magico-religious. The practice of folk healers (medicine people) is often specialized.

Ethnic/Race Specific or Endemic Diseases: ENDEMIC: Yellow fever; chloroquine-resistant malaria. The AIDS rate per 100,000 is 3.96.

Birth Rites: Indigenous and government-trained nurse midwives provide care during deliveries; however, some indigenous midwives exclude duties that involve washing the baby or cutting the umbilical cord. During birth the kneeling position is used; most deliveries take place at home. Female circumcision may be performed; infanticide may occur in rural areas if an infant displays signs of witchcraft.

Infant Feeding Practices: Infant diarrhea may be the result of teething and is perceived as normal or related to bewitchment or other physical or medical causes; medical causes are the only ones for which oral rehydration therapy is seen as appropriate. For diarrhea caused by bewitchment a traditional healer is consulted.

Child Rearing Practices: Female circumcision and excision is widespread in some groups.

National Childhood Immunizations: BCG at birth; DPT at 6, 10, and 14 weeks and 1 year; OPV at birth and 6, 10, and 14 weeks; measles at 9 months.

BIBLIOGRAPHY

Hounsa AM et al.: An application of Ajzen's theory of planned behaviour to predict mothers' intention to use oral rehydration therapy in a rural area of Benin, *Soc Sci Med* 37(2):253, 1993.

Murphy JE: Bush nursing in Benin, *JCN* 10(4):15, 1993.

Sargent C: The implications of role expectations for birth assistance among Bariba women, *Soc Sci Med* 16:1483, 1982.

Wright J: Female genital mutilation: an overview, *J Adv Nurs* 24:251, 1996.

◆ BHUTAN

MAP PAGE (320)

Location: Bhutan is a mountainous country on the southeast slope of The Himalayas, bordering Tibet and India. A succession of lofty and rugged mountains reaches 24,000 feet (7315 m), separated by deep and sometimes high valleys. A subtropical zone of humid plains exhibits thick tropical forests.

Most people live in the intermediate areas between the plains and the high mountains.

Major Languages	Ethnic Groups		Major Religions	
Dzongkha	Bhote	50%	Buddhist	75%
Nepalese	Nepalese	35%	Hindu	25%
Tibetan Dialects	Other	15%		

Predominant Sick Care Practices: Traditional. People believe that sickness comes to those who have engaged in evil actions. Indian ayurvedic medicine and Tibetan herbal medicine are practiced. People have faith in the local healers.

Health Care Beliefs: Passive role; acute sick care. Events are determined by the Fates or the deities and cannot be changed.

Ethnic/Race Specific or Endemic Diseases: ENDEMIC: Chloroquine-resistant malaria in rural areas; respiratory diseases, including tuberculosis; iodine deficiency goiter; leprosy; and vitamin A deficiency in certain areas. RISK: Gastrointestinal diseases are found in young children; parasites are common. Hand washing and sanitary waste disposal are not practiced in some areas, contaminating drinking water. Young women self-inflict burns in response to family quarrels. The AIDS rate per 100,000 is reported by the country as zero.

Food Practices and Intolerances: Rice is a staple.

National Childhood Immunizations: BCG at birth and 1 year; DPT at 6, 10, and 14 weeks and 18 months; OPV at 6, 10, and 14 weeks and 9 and 18 months; measles between 9 and 12 months; and hep B at 6, 10, and 14 weeks. Because good health results from past virtue, immunizations are not perceived as being able to affect future health.

BIBLIOGRAPHY

Bibbings J: VSO nursing in Bhutan, *Nurs J Clin Pract Educ Manage* 3(47):9, 1989.

Bibbings J: Wound care in a developing country, *Nurs J Clin Pract Educ Manage* 4(41):29, 1991.

Clinchy RA: Emergency medicine comes to the Himalayas, *Emergency* Oct 1984, p 42.

◆ BOLIVIA

MAP PAGE (314)

Location: Bolivia is landlocked in the heart of South America, with high, cold, dry mountains (altiplanos) in the west, medium-elevation valleys in the middle, and low, wet, hot, forested plains in the east.

Major Languages	Ethnic Groups		Major Religions	
Spanish	Quechua	30%	Catholic	95%
Quechua	Mestizo	30%	Indigenous and	5%
Aymara	Aymara	25%	Protestant	
	European	15%		

Ethnic/Race Specific or Endemic Diseases: ENDEMIC: Congenitally transmitted Chagas' disease. RISK: Yellow fever; chloroquine-resistant malaria is present, with no risk in urban areas. Infant mortality can reach 100/1000. The AIDS rate per 100,000 is 0.15.

Health Team Relationships: Physicians expect nurses to assume a traditional, passive role.

Eye Contact Practices: Avoiding eye contact during conversations is considered insulting. Eyes and facial expressions often are used to communicate.

Touch Practices: Females who are friends may walk arm-in-arm or hold hands.

Perceptions of Time: Punctuality is flexible.

Death Rites: The Aymara's (a cultural [Indian] group living in mountainous areas) life is built around an acceptance of death.

National Childhood Immunizations: BCG at birth; DPT at 2, 4, and 6 months and 1½ years; OPV at birth and 2, 4, and 6 months; measles at 9 months.

Other Characteristics: Bolivians believe that their country's system of social welfare is one of the best in the world because their benefits are clearly spelled out in the constitution; however, they are not unduly concerned if people do not receive the benefits the constitution promises.

BIBLIOGRAPHY

Azogue E: Women and congenital Chagas' disease in Santa Cruz, Bolivia, *Soc Sci Med* 37(4):503, 1993.

Bahr J, Wehrhahn R: Life expectancy and infant mortality in Latin America, *Soc Sci Med* 36(10):1373, 1993.

Bastien JW: The making of a community health worker, *World Health Forum* 11(4):368, 1990.

Fryer ML: Health education through interactive radio: a child-to-child project in Bolivia, *Health Educ Q* 18(1):65, 1991.

Perry HB: Simon Saavedra: pioneering Bolivian midlevel health professional, *J Am Acad Physician Assist* 6(1):48, 1993.

Ross HM: Societal/cultural views regarding death and dying, *Top Clin Nurs* 1(1):1, 1981.

Savino MM: The professional nursing role in Cochabamba, Bolivia: clinical nurses' and physicians' perceptions about ideal and actual functioning; identified role problems; and leadership recommendations, doctoral dissertation, Ithaca, NY, 1988, Cornell University.

Stewart EC, Bennett MJ: *American cultural patterns: a cross-cultural perspective,* rev ed, Yarmouth, Me, 1991, Intercultural Press.

Taylor VL, editor: *Culturgrams: the nations around us,* Provo, Utah, 1987, Brigham Young University, David M Kennedy Center for International Studies.

◆ BOSNIA AND HERZEGOVINA

MAP PAGE (314)

Location: Formerly part of Yugoslavia, Bosnia and Herzegovina is located on the Balkan Peninsula in southeastern Europe. The country is hilly with some mountains. The Bosnian region is heavily forested, whereas the Herzegovina region in the south has rugged, flat farmland.

Major Languages	Ethnic Groups		Major Religions	
Serbo-Croatian	Serbian	40%	Muslim	40%
	Muslim	38%	Orthodox	31%
	Croatian	22%	Catholic	15%
			Other	14%

Reports of ethnic cleansing and religious differences do not reflect the fact that the mixed populations work, go to school, and have coffee side by side.

Ethnic/Race Specific or Endemic Diseases: Posttraumatic stress syndrome as the aftermath of war. The AIDS rate per 100,000 is 0.17.

National Childhood Immunizations: BCG at birth, 7 years, and between 13 and 14 years; DPT at 3, 4, 6, and 18 months; OPV at 3, 4, 6, and 18 months; MMR at 1 year.

BIBLIOGRAPHY

Etherington C: Working in international war zones: a personal account, *Tenn Nurse* 58(5):14, 1995.
Walker G: In the line of fire . . . Post-traumatic stress disorder, *Nurs Times* 91(11):44, 1995.
Weaver K: A Serb in Sarajevo . . . Conditions in the hospital are appalling, *Nurs Standard* 8(22):18, 1994.
Weaver K: Nursing the peace, *Nurs Standard* 10(25):26, 1996.

◆ BOTSWANA

MAP PAGE (317)

Location: This south-central African country is a sparsely populated near-desert region, with salt lakes in the north and the Kalahari Desert in a basin in the plateau region. The climate is subtropical. Rural people live in large villages. Most people live in the eastern part of the nation, where greater rainfall produces better grazing land.

Major Languages	Ethnic Groups		Major Religions	
English	Botswana	95%	Indigenous	50%
se Tswana	Bushmen	4%	Beliefs	
	European	1%	Christian	50%

Predominant Sick Care Practices: Biomedical; traditional. Herbalists and diviners are common folk healers; however, herbs are not used for common illnesses. People seek spiritual healers at African Christian churches. The people believe in the practice of sorcery and take daily precautions to protect themselves against jealousy. Folk healers have special areas of expertise, and treatments from two or more systems are not used simultaneously because they can cancel out each other.

Health Care Beliefs: Acute sick care; health promotion important. Nurses promote preventive, diagnostic, and curative skills.

Ethnic/Race Specific or Endemic Diseases: ENDEMIC: Chloroquine-resistant malaria; schistosomiasis. RISK: Children: malnutrition, acute respiratory infections, gastrointestinal diseases, and other infectious diseases. Adults: tuberculosis, heart disease, parasitic infections, injuries, burns, and digestive diseases. The AIDS rate per 100,000 is 35.93.

Health Team Relationships: Nurses have an important role because of the shortage of physicians. The government bears primary responsibility for health care delivery in remote areas and to the poor.

Birth Rites: Eating eggs is avoided during pregnancy. Massage is an assessment procedure used in the perinatal period. Approximately one third of the births occur at home and are often assisted by female family members or traditional, untrained midwives. Animal fat is used to oil the newborn, and the baby's head is shaved after the umbilical cord falls off.

National Childhood Immunizations: BCG at birth; DPT at 2, 3, and 4 months; DT at 6 years; measles at 9 months; OPV at 2, 3, and 4 months; hep B at birth and 2 and 9 months.

Other Characteristics: One of the highest life expectancy rates in Africa at 59 for men and 65 for women. The infant mortality rate is one of the lowest in Africa at 43/1000.

BIBLIOGRAPHY

Acheson E: Notes on nursing from Botswana, Africa, *Oklahoma Nurse* 37(6):14, 1992.

Acheson E: Notes on nursing from Botswana, Africa, Part II, *Oklahoma Nurse* 38(1):6, 1993.

Anderson S: Traditional maternity care within a bio-social framework, *Int Nurs Rev* 33(4):102, 1986.

Barbee EL: Tensions in the brokerage role: nurses in Botswana, *West J Nurs Res* 9(2):244, 1987.

Beardslee C et al.: Nursing care of children in developing countries: issues in Thailand, Botswana, and Jordan, *Recent Adv Nurs* 16:31, 1987.

Kupe SS: A history of the evolution of nursing education in Botswana, 1922-1980, doctoral dissertation, New York, 1987, Columbia University Teachers College.

Manyeneng WG: Leadership issues for nurses in primary health care in Botswana, *Nurs Health Care* 16(4):214, 1995.

Mmtli K, Mossieman DS: A model of distance education for nurses: the Botswana experience, *Nurs Health Care* 16(4):221, 1995.

Ngcongco VN, Stark R: Family nurse practitioners in Botswana: challenges and implications, *Int Nurs Rev* 37(2):239, 1990.

◆ BRAZIL

MAP PAGE (314)

Location: Covering nearly half of South America, Brazil is the fifth largest and the sixth most populous country in the world. Forests cover 60% of the country. The Amazon River (3912 miles [6296 km]) and the world's largest tropical rain forest are in Brazil. It reflects African, Indian, and Dutch cultures in the north and northeast and German and Italian influences in the south. São Paulo has one of the largest Japanese communities in the world. A developed country, Brazil has two distinct classes—rich and poor—as well as a small middle class.

Major Languages	Ethnic Groups		Major Religions	
Portuguese	White	55%	Catholic	70%
Spanish	Mulatto	38%	Other	30%
English	African	6%		
French	Other	1%		
German				

Predominant Sick Care Practices: Biomedical; holistic; magico-religious (extensive in interior Brazil). Pharmacies run by doctors of homeopathy are common. The government, following the DRG classification system, pays about 80% of hospital costs. Self-dosage with over-the-counter medications, including antibiotics, is practiced.

Health Care Beliefs: The recently inaugurated Unified Health System (SUS) places emphasis on primary health care. Active involvement is practiced by the small middle-class element, with a more passive role among the poor.

Ethnic/Race Specific or Endemic Diseases: ACTIVE: Cholera. ENDEMIC: Chloroquine-resistant malaria. RISK: Dengue fever; cholera; yellow fever; schistosomiasis; leprosy; diarrhea; parasites; malnutrition. Many people attribute health problems to a malfunctioning liver. Vitamin A deficiency is the most common cause of childhood blindness. The AIDS rate per 100,000 is 5.99.

Health Team Relationships: The term *doctor (dotor)* is used indiscriminately to express respect and affection. Nurses are addressed by a title followed by their first name. Within the patriarchal and capitalist health care system, nurses tend to internalize an oppressed role. Concepts of class and social status are strong. Some women may prefer a female caregiver.

Families' Role in Hospital Care: The family assumes some responsibility for direct care; family members may bring food or take turns staying with the patient 24 hours a day.

Dominance Patterns: The extended family includes godparents and godchildren. When speaking in the third person, people refer to parents as "senhor" or "senhora." When more than one last name is used, the mother's name comes first.

Eye Contact Practices: Direct eye contact predominates, especially from a lower social class.

Touch Practices: Women greet by kissing on both cheeks, and men shake hands and embrace; however, greeting a professional is limited to a handshake.

Perceptions of Time: Brazilians are casual about punctuality and oriented to the present. The future is measured in decades or generations, and definitions of early and late are flexible. Arriving late may indicate a successful social standing. Current rewards for activity are preferred over delayed gratification.

Pain Reactions: Pain is expressed vocally. Persons from the interior part of the country tend to somatize problems.

Birth Rites: Fathers are not usually present during labor and delivery. Circumcision is not routinely done at birth. Girls may have their ears pierced soon after birth. A rest period of 40 days after birth is acceptable for the mother.

Food Practices and Intolerances: Yams, bread, and couscous are common for breakfast. The main meal, which is eaten at noon, consists of rice, beans, mashed potatoes, and meat or fish. A light meal is taken around 8 pm. Sandwiches are categorized as a snack, not a meal. In both children and adults, weight gain is considered healthy.

Infant Feeding Practices: Breastfeeding is short term; São Paulo women breastfeed for a longer term. The attitude of the father may be the most significant factor in breastfeeding.

Child Rearing Practices: Children are treated affectionately; kissing a child is preceded by inhaling (smelling). Pacifiers are tied to the diaper or kept on a cord around the infant's neck. Grandmothers play an active role in caregiving, especially for working mothers. Students attend public high schools for half a day (morning, afternoon, or evening). Children in the lowest socioeconomic bracket often work rather than going to school; homeless children are a major concern in large cities.

National Childhood Immunizations: BCG at birth; DPT at 2, 4, and 6 months; OPV at 2, 4, and 6 months; measles at 9 months.

Other Characteristics: The finger sign for OK in the United States is a crude sexual invitation in Brazil. The thumbs-up sign indicates fine, OK, or great.

BIBLIOGRAPHY

Angels with wet wings won't fly: maternal sentiment in Brazil and the image of neglect, *Cult Med Psychiatry* 12:141, 1988.

Angerami ELS, Puntel de Almeida MC: Nursing administration trends in Brazil, *Nurs Adm Q* 16(2):47, 1992.

Beasley A: Breastfeeding studies: culture, biomedicine, and methodology, *J Hum Lact* 7(1):7, 1991.

Beckmann CA: Maternal-child health in Brazil, JOGNN 16(4):238, 1987.

Coler MS: Contributor.

Coler MS, Hafner LP: An intercultural assessment of the type, intensity, and number of crisis precipitating factors in three cultures: United States, Brazil and Taiwan, *Int J Nurs Stud* 28(3):223, 1991.

Coler MS et al.: Justification for mental health services at the department of nursing, Universidade Federal da Paraiba-Brasil through the utilization of nursing diagnoses and diagnostic categories, Classif Nurs Diagn Proc Eighth Conf, 165, 1989.

Coler MS et al.: A Brazilian study of two diagnoses in the NANDA human response pattern: moving, a transcultural comparison, Classif Nurs Diagn Proc Ninth Conf, 255, 1991.

Condon JC, Yousef F: *An introduction to intercultural communication,* New York, 1975, Macmillan.

Galanti GA: *Caring for patients from different cultures,* ed 2, Philadelphia, 1997, University of Pennsylvania Press.

Giugliani ERJ et al.: Effect of breastfeeding support from different sources on mothers' decisions to breastfeed, *J Human Lact* 10(3):157, 1994.

Gorayeb R: Child rearing patterns in Brazil, *Acta Psychiatr Scand Suppl* 344:147, 1988.

Green HB: Temporal attitudes in four Negro subcultures, *Studium Generale* 23(6):571, 1970.

Hartz J: *Children in exile,* March 8, 1992, NBC-TV.

Hoy R: Health care in Brazil, *Nurs Lond* 3(47):12, 1989.

Kurian GT, editor: *Encyclopedia of the third world,* ed 4, vol 1, New York, 1992, Facts of Life.

Language Research Center: *Brazil: intercultural experiential learning aid,* Provo, Utah, 1976, Brigham Young University.

Language Research Center: *Latin America: intercultural experiential learning aid,* Provo, Utah, 1976, Brigham Young University.

McGreevey WP: The high costs of health care in Brazil, *Int Nurs Rev* 36(1):13, 1989.

Meleis AI et al.: Veiled, voluminous, and devalued: narrative stories about low-income women from Brazil, Egypt, and Colombia, *Adv Nurs Sci* 17(2):1, 1994.

Messias DKH: Brazilians. In Lipson JG, Dibble SL, Minarik PA: *Culture & nursing care: a pocket guide,* San Francisco, 1996, UCSF Nursing Press.

Monteiro CA et al.: The recent revival of breast-feeding in the city of São Paulo, Brazil, *Am J Public Health* 77(8):964, 1987.

Pannuti CS, Grinbaum RS: Global aspects of infection control: Part 1. An overview of nosocomial infection control in Brazil, *Infect Control Hosp Epidemiol* 16(3):170, 1995.

Reis HT: Perceptions of time and punctuality in the United States and Brazil, *J Pers Soc Psychol* 38(4):541, 1980.

Rowell M: Eradication of vitamin A deficiency, *J Ophthalmic Nurs Tech* 12(5):217, 1993.

Schreuders T: Treating leprosy in Amazonas, *Nurs Times* 86(35):60, 1990.

Stewart EC, Bennett MJ: *American cultural patterns: a cross-cultural perspective,* rev ed, Yarmouth, Me, 1991, Intercultural Press.

Trevizan MA, Mendes IAC: Administration of patient care: theoretical aspects, *Int Nurs Rev* 40(1):25, 1993.

Waldow VR: The conscientization of oppression in Brazilian nursing through feminist pedagogy: a case study, doctoral dissertation, New York, 1992, Columbia University Teachers College.

◆ BRUNEI

MAP PAGE (321)

Location: A thinly populated independent sultanate on the northwest coast of the island of Borneo, Brunei is covered with tropical rain forest.

Major Languages	Ethnic Groups		Major Religions	
Malay	Malay	64%	Muslim	67%
English	Chinese	20%	Buddhist	13%
Brunei-Chinese	Other	16%	Christian	10%
			Other	10%

Ethnic/Race Specific or Endemic Diseases: The AIDS rate per 100,000 is reported by the country as zero.

Death Rites: Muslim belief forbids organ donations or transplants. Muslim physicians may recommend transfusions to save lives. Autopsy is uncommon because the deceased must be buried intact. Cremation is not permitted. For Muslim burial the body is wrapped in special pieces of cloth and buried without a coffin in the ground.

National Childhood Immunizations: BCG at birth and 6 years; DPT at 6, 12, and 18 weeks; DT at 5 years; OPV at 6, 12, and 18 weeks and 5 years; measles at 12 months; hep B at birth and 1 and 5 months.

BIBLIOGRAPHY

Burnard P, Zakiah HRB: Interpersonal skills training in Brunei, *Br J Nurs* 1(8):416, 1992.

Ross HM: Societal/cultural views regarding death and dying, *Top Clin Nurs* 1(1):1, 1981.

◆ BULGARIA

MAP PAGE (314)

Location: Bulgaria is situated on the Black Sea in the eastern part of the Balkan Peninsula. Plains cover two thirds of Bulgaria, and mountains cover one third.

Major Language	Ethnic Groups		Major Religions	
Bulgarian	Bulgarian	85%	Bulgarian	85%
	Turkish	8%	Orthodox	
	Gypsy	3%	Muslim	13%
	Macedonian	3%	Other	2%
	Armenian and	1%		
	Other			

Ethnic/Race Specific or Endemic Diseases: The AIDS rate per 100,000 is 0.01.

Food Practices and Intolerances: Large meals are taken at midday and in the evening. Cheese, yogurt, lamb, and mutton are popular foods.

National Childhood Immunizations: BCG at birth, 7 months, between 6 and 7 years, between 11 and 12 years, and at 17 years; DPT at 2, 3, 4, and 24 months; OPV at birth, 2, 3, 4, and 24 months and 7 and 12 years; MMR at 14 months; measles at 12 years; hep B at birth and 1 and 6 months.

Other Characteristics: The head motions for yes and no are the opposite of those used in the United States.

BIBLIOGRAPHY

Axtell RE, editor: *Do's and taboos around the world,* ed 2, New York, 1990, John Wiley & Sons.

East meets west: Georgi Georgev talks with Shirley Smoyak: exchanges about the state-of-the-art in mental health, *J Psychosoc Nurs Ment Health Serv* 21(11):35, 1983.

Taylor VL, editor: *Culturgrams: the nations around us,* Provo, Utah, 1987, Brigham Young University, David M Kennedy Center for International Studies.

◆ BURKINA FASO

MAP PAGE (316)

Location: Burkina Faso (formerly Upper Volta) is land-locked in West Africa and consists of plains, low hills, and high savannas, with desert in the north.

Major Languages	Ethnic Groups		Major Religions	
French	Mossi	36%	Muslim	50%
Sudanic	Other	64%	Indigenous Beliefs	40%
Languages			Christian	10%

Ethnic/Race Specific or Endemic Diseases: ENDEMIC: Chloroquine-resistant malaria. The AIDS rate per 100,000 is 16.30.

National Childhood Immunizations: BCG at birth; DPT at 2, 3, and 4 months; yellow fever and measles at 9 months; OPV at birth and 2, 3, and 4 months; measles at 9 months.

BIBLIOGRAPHY

Riesman P: On the irrelevance of child rearing practices for the formation of personality: an analysis of childhood, personality, and values in two African communities, *Cult Med Psychiatry* 7(2):103, 1983.

◆ BURUNDI

MAP PAGE (317)

Location: Burundi is a high plateau divided by several deep valleys in east central Africa; it is close to the equator. Bantu tribes densely populate the area, and ethnic strife and violence exist between the Tutsi and Hutu groups. Burundi is an agricultural nation that experiences famine at times.

Major Languages	Ethnic Groups		Major Religions	
Kirundi	Hutu	85%	Catholic	62%
French	Tutsi	14%	Indigenous	32%
Swahili	Twa and	1%	Beliefs	
	Other		Protestant	5%
			Muslim	1%

Ethnic/Race Specific or Endemic Diseases: ENDEMIC: Yellow fever. RISK: Cholera; chloroquine-resistant malaria. The AIDS rate per 100,000 is 7.73.

National Childhood Immunizations: BCG at birth; DPT at 6, 10, and 14 weeks and 18 months; OPV at birth and 6, 10, and 14 weeks; measles at 9 months.

Other Characteristics: When a person is accused, skillful deception is highly valued.

BIBLIOGRAPHY

Condon JC, Yousef F: *An introduction to intercultural communication,* New York, 1975, Macmillan.

◆ CAMBODIA (KAMPUCHEA)

MAP PAGE (321)

Location: A large alluvial plain on the Indochinese peninsula, Cambodia is ringed by mountains.

Major Languages	Ethnic Groups		Major Religions	
Khmer	Khmer	90%	Theravada	95%
French	(Cambodian)		Buddhist	
	Vietnamese	5%	Other	5%
	Chinese	1%		
	Other	4%		

Predominant Sick Care Practices: Biomedical; holistic; magico-religious; traditional. Biomedical medicine is practiced; however, it does not replace traditional beliefs. Herbal medicine is important in regard to tradition. Most herbal medicines are classified as "cool," whereas most Western medicines are considered "hot." An imbalance in the hot/cold theory is believed to be one cause of disease. Traditionally, illness is dealt with through self-care and self-medication. Folk remedies include variations of acupuncture, massage, herbal remedies, and dermabrasive practices such as cupping, pinching, rubbing, and burning.

Health Care Beliefs: Active involvement; acute sick care. Health promotion is important. Energizing hot forces and calming cool forces restore equilibrium in the body and are the treatment goals. The belief in the balance between work and leisure supports laughter as healthy. Unhealthy air currents (bad winds) are thought to get caught inside the body and cause illness. Pinching, scratching, or rubbing the area with a coin releases the bad winds, leaving marks or red lines on the skin. These actions are thought to restore health.

Accidents are believed to be caused by fate as punishment for past sins; therefore emergency intervention may be considered inappropriate. Traditionally, mental illness is met with denial. According to common belief, thinking too much (koucharang), particularly in periods of stress, creates mental imbalance. Self-treatment strategies include suppressing sad thoughts, forgetting about it, being sheltered and protected by family, being encouraged to laugh, and not being left alone. Sleeping pills, alcohol, and suicide ideology are sometimes involved, as well. Somatization of koucharang is common.

Ethnic/Race Specific or Endemic Diseases: ENDEMIC: Chloroquine-resistant malaria. **RISK:** Japanese encephalitis; schistosomiasis; posttraumatic stress syndrome. The AIDS rate per 100,000 is 0.89.

Health Team Relationships: Because physicians are considered experts and authority figures, patients are given little information. Health care professionals are respected, and patients do not question or oppose them openly; however, patients may not comply with recommended medical regimens. Patients may hide their true feelings to avoid disagreement and to appear compliant. This behavior is thought to protect the patients' self-esteem and the health professionals' status. Noncompetitive and nonconfrontational approaches by health professionals are indicated. An open show of impatience or anger is culturally inappropriate. Female patients' questions may be answered by their husbands. Traditionally, the oldest male in the family makes decisions about health care. A female patient may refuse care from a male health care giver.

Families' Role in Hospital Care: The family is highly valued, and membership within the family is flexible. An understanding of this tradition is helpful for health care professionals. Status is based on membership within the family, age, and gender.

Dominance Patterns: Decision making is influenced by the astrologic/lunar calendar. Women defer to men; however, women often control the men, the home, the acute care decisions, and the economic power of the community. The traditional extended family is more important than the individual. The husband is responsible for matters concerning the outside world, and the wife, with all household affairs. Men practice polygamy if the first wife agrees in writing. Some men may believe that if they are sufficiently strong, powerful, and healthy, STDs and HIV will be unable to infect them.

Eye Contact Practices: Continuous direct eye contact is disrespectful.

Touch Practices: The head is considered the center of life. It is revered, and invasive procedures frighten the patient. Touching the head is offensive to many. Only parents may be permitted to touch the heads of their children. Touch is a demonstration of love from the family; affection may be expressed through various means such as massage or rubbing coins against the skin. Handshaking has gained wide acceptance among men; however, it is not customary among women.

Perceptions of Time: Time is flexible. Planning for the future and keeping appointments are not valued. Taking scheduled medication is not understood; pills are taken only if the patient feels ill.

Pain Reactions: Pain may be severe before relief is requested.

Birth Rites: Prenatal care is not the norm. Pregnancy may not be announced to avoid tempting spirits. Prenatal care may not be sought until 5 or 6 months into the pregnancy. The desire is for a small fetus to ease delivery; therefore prenatal vitamins may be rejected. Relatives' children, abandoned children, or children given to an infertile couple who are part of the household may be inadvertently added to the obstetrical history. Because childbirth is thought to be a cold condition, warmth is needed to replace lost heat and energy. The mother's head is often covered with blankets or towels. After delivery the woman may refuse to bathe, drink ice water, or hold her baby and may experience "toa": the period of collapse treated by the restoration of humoral balance and mind/body equilibrium. The family is expected to care for the baby and mother immediately after the birth. The woman may have a lying-in period of 1 week to 3 months. Newborns are not given compliments so that they will not be captured by evil spirits. Buddhist belief in past and future lives places the blame for birth defects on mistakes made in past lives.

Death Rites: The people prefer quality in life rather than quantity because Buddhists believe in reincarnation. They expect less suffering in the next life. Patients prefer to die at home rather than in the hospital. Jewels or portions of rice (depending on the family's financial standing) are placed in the deceased's mouth to help the soul encounter gods or devils and to ensure that the deceased will be wealthy in the next life. Cremation in the temple is preferred, and the deceased's ashes are kept in a pagoda or at home. Immediately following death, monks are called to pray. Neighbors join in the celebrations and may bring small money gifts. The longer and more elaborate a funeral, the more respect is paid to the deceased. White clothes are worn during the 3-month mourning period. Afterward a black armband or black clothing is worn. Some mourners may shave their heads.

Food Practices and Intolerances: Families demonstrate love through food.

Infant Feeding Practices: The female breast is accepted dispassionately as the means of infant feeding; however, colostrum is considered dirty. Breastfeeding may continue up to 3 years, with solids introduced early on. In traditional families male children may breastfeed as many years as they like to enhance their power and energy, whereas females may be weaned around 2 years to avoid developing these male characteristics. Weaning usually means the end of milk intake because of the high incidence of lactose intolerance. Many believe that fluids should be withheld with diarrhea because it is a cold disease.

Child Rearing Practices: The character of an infant's personality is thought to be partially determined by the year and time of day at birth. Methods for calculating the age of an infant may vary by as much as 2 years. Babies are frequently fondled, cared for, and carried about by the mother or another woman in the family. Parents are relaxed and enjoy children under 6 years old. After that, strict upbringing begins, independence is discouraged, and parents demand obedience. The oldest child, boy or girl, is responsible for younger siblings if the parents die, are old, or are ill. Large families are valued.

Between puberty and marriage the traditional girl spends 1 month in seclusion. She observes many rites, eats a vegetarian diet, remains in her room in the dark, and is visited only by her mother. A child's name may be changed to confuse potential evil spirits.

National Childhood Immunizations: BCG at birth; DPT at 6, 10, and 14 weeks; OPV at birth and 6, 10, and 14 weeks; measles at 9 months.

Other Characteristics: It is believed that a heated coin or one smeared with oil and rubbed vigorously over the body, causing red welts, will draw out illness. The red marks are thought to be evidence that illness is being brought to the surface of the body, proving that those who sustain the marks are indeed ill. Injections also are used and are considered more beneficial to recovery than pills. Wrist strings are worn to prevent soul loss—a state that resolves itself into illness. Infants may wear the strings around the neck, ankles, or waist. Emotional disturbances may manifest themselves somatically because shame is connected to mental illness in this culture. Speaking loudly, yelling, snapping fingers under the nose, pointing, beckoning with finger, or holding hand outstretched with palm up offends others. The woman officially uses her husband's last name, and names are written in the following order: family name, middle name, and given name. The woman's lower torso is extremely private; the area between waist and knees is kept covered.

BIBLIOGRAPHY

Crow GK: Toward a theory of therapeutic syncretism: the Southeast Asian experience: a study of the Cambodians' use of traditional and cosmopolitan health systems, doctoral dissertation, Salt Lake City, 1988, University of Utah.

D'Avanzo CE: Bridging the cultural gap with Southeast Asians, *MCN Am J Matern Child Nurs* 17:204, 1992.

Dunn JD: Educating sex workers in Cambodia, *Community Nurse* 1(3):29, 1995.

Frye BA: The process of health care decision making among Cambodian immigrant women, *Appl Res Eval* 10(2):113, 1989-1990.

Frye BA: The Cambodian refugee patient: providing culturally sensitive rehabilitation nursing care, *Rehab Nurs* 15(3):156, 1990.

Frye BA: Cultural themes in health-care decision-making among Cambodian refugee women, *J Community Health Nurs* 8(1):33, 1991.

Frye BA, D'Avanzo C: Cultural themes in family stress and violence among Cambodian refugee women in the inner city, *Adv Nurs Sci* 16(3):64, 1994.

Frye BA, D'Avanzo C: Themes in managing culturally defined illness in the Cambodian refugee family, *J Community Health Nurs* 11(2):89, 1994.

Galanti GA: *Caring for patients from different cultures,* ed 2, Philadelphia, 1997, University of Pennsylvania Press.

Kelly BR: Cultural considerations in Cambodian childrearing, *J Ped Health Care* 10(1):2, 1996.

Kulig JC: Contraception and birth control use: Cambodian refugee women's beliefs and practices, *J Community Health Nurs* 5(4):235, 1988.

Lawson LV: Culturally sensitive support for grieving parents, *MCN Am J Matern Child Nurs* 15:76, 1990.

Lenart JC, St. Clair PA, Bell MA: Childrearing knowledge, beliefs, and practices of Cambodian refugees, *J Pediatr Health Care* 5(6):299, 1991.

Li GR: Funeral practices, New York, World Relief, n.d.

Miles G: Community spirit, *Internat Perspect* 91(40):44, 1995.

Miller JA: Caring for Cambodian refugees in the emergency department, *J Emerg Nurs* 21(6):498, 1995.

Muecke MA: Caring for Southeast Asian refugee patients in the USA, *Am J Public Health* 73(4):431, 1983.

Nguyen A, Bounthinh T, Mum S: *Folk medicine, folk nutrition, superstitions,* Washington, DC, 1980, Team Associates.

Rasbridge LA, Kulig JC: Infant feeding among Cambodian refugees, *MCN Am J Matern Child Nurs* 20(1):213, 1995.

Rosenberg J: Cambodian children integrating treatment plans, *Pediatr Nurse* 12:118, 1986.

Schreiner D: S.E. Asian folk healing practices—child abuse? Eugene, Ore, 1981, Indochinese Health Care Conference.

Stewart EC, Bennett MJ: *American cultural patterns: a cross-cultural perspective,* rev ed, Yarmouth, Me, 1991, Intercultural Press.

Uland E, Smith S: Southeast Asian mental health issues, unpublished manuscript, 1984.

U.S. Department of Health, Education, and Welfare, Social Security Administration Office of Family Assistance, SSA 77-21013: A guide to two cultures: Indochinese, Washington, DC, n.d.

Vandeusen J et al.: South East Asian social and cultural customs: similarities and differences, *J Refugee Resettlement* 1:20, 1980.

◆ CAMEROON

MAP PAGE (316)

Location: Cameroon is a West African nation with a high plateau in the interior and swamps and plains along the coast of the Gulf of Guinea. English and French are the official languages, with over 200 vernacular languages spoken.

Major Languages	Ethnic Groups		Major Religions	
English	Cameroon	31%	Indigenous	51%
French	Highlander		Beliefs	
African	Equatorial	19%	Christian	33%
Languages	Bantu		Muslim	16%
	Kirdi	11%		
	Fulani	10%		
	N.W. Bantu	29%		
	and Other			

Predominant Sick Care Practices: Biomedical; magico-religious.

Health Care Beliefs: Passive role; acute sick care. A primary health care policy was enacted in 1982; however, the people and the majority of health care practitioners still operate on a curative model.

Ethnic/Race Specific or Endemic Diseases: ENDEMIC: Yellow fever; chloroquine-resistant malaria. RISK: Cholera; schistosomiasis; intestinal parasites; diarrhea. The AIDS rate per 100,000 is 20.90.

Families' Role in Hospital Care: Relatives provide routine bedside care for hospitalized patients.

Child Rearing Practices: Female circumcision and excision are widespread in some groups.

National Childhood Immunizations: BCG at birth; DPT at 6, 10, and 14 weeks; OPV at birth and 6, 10, and 14 weeks; measles at 9 months.

BIBLIOGRAPHY

Awasum HM: Health and nursing services in Cameroon: challenges and demands for nurses in leadership positions, *Nurs Adm Q* 16(2):8, 1992.

Jato MN: Teaching future nursing teachers primary health care, *Int Nurs Rev* 29(6):189, 1982.

Jato MN et al.: Community participation in rural health care, *Int Nurs Rev* 31(6):180, 1984.

Wright J: Female genital mutilation: an overview, *J Adv Nurs* 24:251, 1996.

◆ CAPE VERDE

MAP PAGE (316)

Location: These mountainous Atlantic islands are 385 miles (620 km) off the coast of Senegal in Africa.

Major Languages	Ethnic Groups		Major Religions	
Portuguese	Creole	71%	Catholic	65%
Crioulo	African	28%	Indigenous	35%
	European	1%	Beliefs	

Regardless of the color of their skin, people often categorize themselves as white.

Predominant Sick Care Practices: Biomedical; traditional. Mixing traditional beliefs and modern concepts, Cape Verdeans believe that illness may be caused by neglecting social norms; therefore healthy people may seek medical care because they think they may be causing a family member's disease. The "patient" may never mention these family-related problems. A black bead with an odd number of white dots provides protection against the evil eye.

Ethnic/Race Specific or Endemic Diseases: ENDEMIC: Chloroquine-sensitive malaria; yellow fever. The AIDS rate per 100,000 is 5.37.

Death Rites: Some believe that the spirits of the dead wander about from midnight to 1 AM.

Infant Feeding Practices: A belief exists that after delivery, sexual contact between the mother and a man other than the newborn's father results in a mixing of the adults' blood, poisoning the mother's milk. The poison's effect on the infant may be delayed.

National Childhood Immunizations: BCG at birth; DPT at 6, 10, and 14 weeks; OPV at birth and 6, 10, and 14 weeks; measles at 9 months.

BIBLIOGRAPHY

Campinha-Bacote J: Transcultural psychiatric nursing: diagnostic and treatment issues, *J Psychosoc Nurs Ment Health Serv* 32(8):41, 1994.

Reitmaier P: The death of Amilcar: a case study from Santo Antao/Cabo Verde, *Ann Soc Belg Med Trop* 67(suppl 1):111, 1987.

◆ CENTRAL AFRICAN REPUBLIC

MAP PAGE (316)

Location: A landlocked republic 500 miles (805 km) north of the African equator, the country is covered with tropical forest in the south and semidesert land in the east. It is one of the 25 poorest countries in the world.

Major Languages	Ethnic Groups		Major Religions	
French	Baya	34%	Muslim	26%
Sangho	Banda	27%	Protestant	25%
Arabic	Mandjia	21%	Catholic	25%
Hunsa	Sara	10%	Indigenous	24%
Swahili	Mboum and Other	8%	Beliefs	

Ethnic/Race Specific or Endemic Diseases: ENDEMIC: Chloroquine-resistant malaria; yellow fever. RISK: Schistosomiasis. AIDS rate per 100,000 is 19.56.

Child Rearing Practices: Female circumcision and excision are widespread in some groups.

National Childhood Immunizations: BCG at birth; DPT at 6, 10, and 14 weeks; OPV at birth and 6, 10, and 14 weeks; measles at 9 months.

BIBLIOGRAPHY

Adler MW, editor: Statistics from the World Health Organization and the Centers for Disease Control, *AIDS* 6(10):1229, 1992.

Wright J: Female genital mutilation: an overview, *J Adv Nurs* 24:251, 1996.

◆ CHAD

MAP PAGE (316)

Location: Chad is a landlocked country in north central Africa, with a northern desert that runs into the Sahara. Chad is one of the poorest countries in the world; most of its population live in poverty and are without easy access to safe water and basic sanitation facilities. Most of its 186 miles (300 km) of paved roads are impassable during and after the rainy season (June through September).

Major Languages	Ethnic Groups		Major Religions	
French	Muslim Groups	44%	Muslim	50%
Arabic	Non-Muslim	25%	Christian	25%
Sara	Groups		Indigenous	25%
Sango	Other	31%	Beliefs	
Other				

Ethnic/Race Specific or Endemic Diseases: ENDEMIC: Yellow fever; schistosomiasis; chloroquine-resistant malaria. **RISK:** Cholera. The AIDS rate per 100,000 is 9.31.

Death Rites: For Muslim burial the body is wrapped in special pieces of cloth and buried without a coffin in the ground. Cremation is not permitted.

Child Rearing Practices: Female circumcision and excision are widespread in some groups.

National Childhood Immunizations: BCG at birth; DPT at 6, 10, and 14 weeks; OPV at birth and 6, 10, and 14 weeks; measles at 9 months.

BIBLIOGRAPHY

Ross HM: Societal/cultural views regarding death and dying, *Top Clin Nurs* 1(1):1, 1981.
Stiegler KS: All-out effort thwarts Chad cholera crisis, *Front Lines* 31(11):10, 1991.
Wright J: Female genital mutilation: an overview, *J Adv Nurs* 24:251, 1996.

◆ CHILE

MAP PAGE (314)

Location: The country fills a narrow 1800 mile (2897 km) strip between the Andes mountains and the Pacific Ocean. One third of Chile is covered by towering mountain ranges, and the southernmost city in the world is located at its tip. A 700 mile (1127 km) valley in the center is thickly populated, and in the north is the Atacama Desert.

Major Language	Ethnic Groups		Major Religions	
Spanish	European and	95%	Catholic	89%
	Mestizo		Protestant and	11%
	Native	3%	Other	
	American			
	Other	2%		

Health Care Beliefs: Acute sick care only.

Ethnic/Race Specific or Endemic Diseases: RISK: Malnutrition in poor areas; digestive problems in summer. The AIDS rate per 100,000 is 1.87.

Birth Rites: Use of contraceptives is limited. Rhythm is a popular birth control practice. Many believe that a woman should have as many children as God gives her. Abortion is illegal.

Child Rearing Practices: Up to three fourths of older individuals are involved in providing care and education and entertaining children.

National Childhood Immunizations: BCG at birth and 6 years; DPT at 2, 4, 6, and 18 months and 4 years; OPV at 2, 4, 6, and 18 months and 4 years; MMR at 12 months and 6 years.

BIBLIOGRAPHY

Anderson F: Chilean midwifery: under the jackboot, *Nurs Times* 85(31):74, 1989.

Burkhalter BR, Marin PS: A demonstration of increased exclusive breastfeeding in Chile, *Int J Gynaecol Obstet* 34(4):353, 1991.

Kaiser MA: The productive roles of older people in developing countries, *Generations,* Winter 1993, p 65.

Perez A, Valdes V: Santiago breastfeeding promotion program: preliminary results of an intervention study, *Am J Obstet Gynecol* 165 Part 2:2039, 1991.

Ringeling I, Herrera G: Chile's rural nurses, *World Health* Sept-Oct 1992, p 8.

Scarpaci JL: Help-seeking behavior, use, and satisfaction among frequent primary care users in Santiago de Chile, *J Health Soc Behav* 29(3):199, 1988.

Valenzuela MS et al.: Survey of reproductive health in young adults, Greater Santiago, *Bull Pan Am Health Organ* 25(4):293, 1991.

◆ CHINA

MAP PAGE (319)

Location: The world's third largest country, China, occupies the eastern part of Asia. Western China is mountainous, arid, and isolated, whereas the eastern third has fertile agricultural land and river deltas. Tibet and Taiwan are part of the People's Republic of China; however, Taiwan is currently not subject to mainland China. Occupied Hong Kong was returned to China in 1997.

Major Languages	Ethnic Groups		Major Religions	
Mandarin	Han Chinese	92%	Atheist and	97%
Yue	Other	8%	Eclectic	
Wu			Other	3%
Hakka				
Xiang and Other				

Predominant Sick Care Practices: Holistic; traditional. Medical pluralism is common. Chinese medicine is one of the oldest types of medicine that are practiced in the world; it has a theoretical base and diagnostic and treatment modalities that are still in use today. Traditional health care includes moxibustion (cupping), acupuncture, and herbal medicine. Formerly free, the health care system is in transition, with an option for fee-for-service choices.

Health Care Beliefs: Health promotion is important. The Chinese are the first to attribute an upset in body energy to the cause of disease. Health is believed to be a state of spiritual and physical harmony with nature; health and illness are not separate but part of a lifelong continuum. Some resist surgery because of a religious belief that they do not own their physical bodies and that the soul or spirit will escape from the body and be lost forever if surgery should be performed. Drawing blood may be resisted because of the belief that blood does not regenerate; blood is perceived as the source of life. Taking medications while feeling well is an alien concept to some Chinese. Stigma is attached to mental illness; therefore severe personality disorganization is the only criterion for entering the health care system, and emotional problems are somatized.

Ethnic/Race Specific or Endemic Diseases: ENDEMIC: Chloroquine-sensitive; resistant malaria. RISK: Japanese encephalitis; schistosomiasis; adult lactase deficiency; alpha-thalassemia; Chinese-type G6PD deficiency; viral hepatitis. Neurasthenia (nervous exhaustion) is a common modern Chinese psychiatric disorder; psychologic symptoms include anxiety states, depression, and hypochondria. Hypertension, diabetes, and cancer are the leading causes of death. The AIDS rate per 100,000 is reported by the country as zero.

Health Team Relationships: Most nurses are female. Male nurses usually work in urology or psychiatric services. Nurses serve in roles that are supplementary to physicians, and social assertiveness is not emphasized. Nurses and physicians are authority figures or experts, and patients are not given much information about their illnesses, medicines, or diagnostic procedures. Patients do not express their concerns about prescribed interventions or treatments. Thoughts are expressed politely and with restraint through language that is indirect. The listener is expected to understand. The expectation that when people are ill, others are obliged to care for them minimizes people's problem solving and active involvement in their own health restoration. Physicians rely heavily on inspection and palpation in making diagnoses.

Families' Role in Hospital Care: A family member may be given leave from work to care for an aged relative. The family members traditionally remain with the patient during hospitalization; they supply food and clean clothing and assist with feeding, bathing, and keeping the patient comfortable.

Street clothes are worn, and personal belongings are stored under the bed.

Dominance Patterns: The family unit is more important than the individual. Marked role differentiation is based on age, birth order, gender, generation, and social status. The aged are not segregated and have high status. Older Chinese parents take pride in being supported and cared for by their children. However, the migration of children for better work opportunities, the one-child policy, and a decline in multigenerational families' living together may influence this responsibility. In this patrilineal culture father/son relationships are strong and upon marrying, the daughter becomes part of her husband's family. Devotion to parents includes caring for them physically and psychologically. In decision making, the young defer to the old; both parents make decisions concerning the child.

Eye Contact Practices: Gazing around and looking to one side when listening to another are polite. With the elderly, however, direct eye contact is used.

Touch Practices: Chinese do not like to be touched by strangers. Introductions elicit a nod or a slight bow. Personal space and confidentiality during caregiving, however, do not appear important in clinics.

Perceptions of Time: An inexact, patient, and broad orientation is taken toward time. The past is valued, and traditional approaches to healing are preferred over new procedures or medications. Recently China seems to be shifting to a more futuristic orientation. There is no difference between the past and present verb tenses.

Pain Reactions: Strong negative feelings such as anger and pain are often suppressed. A display of emotion is considered a weakness of character. Because it is considered impolite to accept something the first time it is offered, pain relief interventions must be offered more than once. A residual of the long-ago opium war still finds the government limiting the manufacture of morphine, thus limiting its availability to patients in pain.

Birth Rites: Amniocentesis may be used to determine the sex of a fetus. The government limitation of one child per family causes some to consider abortion if the fetus is female. Premature birth weight is suggested at 2300 g. Fathers are not seen in labor rooms, delivery rooms, or postpartum areas. Women labor fully clothed and deliver in the low lithotomy position. Acupuncture is used during labor induction, stimulation, and caesarean section. After childbirth the mother is separated from her baby for 12 to 24 hours and does not bathe for 7 to 30 days; she is permitted to eat only certain foods. Keeping warm is important. Mothers with one child use IUDs. National regulations forbid removal of the birth control device. The newborn is considered 1 year old at birth.

Death Rites: The Chinese have an aversion to death and anything concerning death. Autopsy and disposal of the body are individual preferences; they are not prescribed by religion. Euthanasia is permitted, and donation of body parts is encouraged. The eldest son is responsible for all arrangements for the deceased. The deceased is initially buried in a coffin. After 7 years the body is exhumed and cremated and the urn is reburied in a tomb. White or yellow and black clothing are worn as a sign of mourning. Very traditional people may hire professional criers for funerals.

Food Practices and Intolerances: The diet is low in fat and concentrated sugars. Excessive amounts of soy sauce and dried and preserved foods contribute to high sodium intake. Herbs are used to treat symptoms, wounds, and diseases. The ginseng root is widely used. Raw vegetables and meats are usually not eaten. Hot and warm beverages are preferred. A common meal is rice, which is a "neutral" food, as are fish and noodles.

Infant Feeding Practices: Breastfeeding is encouraged and may be continued for 4 to 5 years. Cow milk and goat milk are not acceptable alternatives for breast milk.

Child Rearing Practices: Parents rear young children in a permissive environment but constantly care for them. When children are old enough, repressive authority is encountered; the children are expected to develop self-control. Until school age, children are placed in a day care facility or with family elders. Children are taught to show respect and deference to parents and authority figures. To discipline them, the parents shame the children or make them feel guilty; these tactics may be followed by reasoning. Children learn to control their emotions; aggressive behavior is undesired and suppressed. Child abuse is rare. Children are taught to be unselfish and to function competitively in a group. Fathers are less involved in child rearing than are mothers. Mother/son relationships are close and long-lived. In education, students are not free to choose their professions but are placed where the government believes they can best serve the nation.

National Childhood Immunizations: BCG at birth and 7 and 12 years; DPT at 3, 4, and 5 months and between 1½ and 2 years; OPV at 3, 4, and 5 months and 4 years; measles at 8 months.

Other Characteristics: The belief that illness needs to be drawn out of the body is practiced through coin rubbing. A heated coin or one smeared with oil is vigorously rubbed over the body, producing red welts. It is believed that the red welts will only appear if people are ill.

BIBLIOGRAPHY

Andrews MM, Boyle JS: *Transcultural concepts in nursing care,* ed 2, Philadelphia, 1995, Lippincott.

Bowling SK: International psychiatric nursing delegates: a visit to China, *Kansas Nurse* 66(4):14, 1991.

Breiner SJ: Early child development in China, *Child Psychiatry Hum Dev* 11(2):87, 1980.

Brower HT: Culture and nursing in China, *Nurs Health Care* 5(1):27, 1984.

Brown BS: Growing up healthy, the Chinese experience, *Pediatr Nurs* 9(4):255, 1983.

Chae M: Older Asians, *J Gerontol Nurs* 13(11):11, 1987.

Chan JYK: Dietary beliefs of Chinese patients, *Nurs Standard* 9(27):2, 1995.

Chinese revolutions—health care overseas, *Nurs Times* 85(29):48, 1989.

Condon JC, Yousef F: An introduction to intercultural communication, New York, 1975, Macmillan.

DeSantis L: Bridging the gap: cultural diversity in nursing. Paper presented to the Florida Nurses Association, 1990.

Dirschel KM: International nursing exchange: the United States and China. In *Perspectives in nursing—1985-1987,* New York, 1985, National League for Nursing.

Dollar B: The child care in China. In Wurzel JS, editor: *Toward multiculturalism: a reader in multicultural education,* Yarmouth, Me, 1988, Intercultural Press.

Douglas J: Impressions of nursing in China, *J Transcultural Nurs* 6(1):26, 1994.

Duncan L: Contributor.

Eisenbruch M: Cross-cultural aspects of bereavement, Part 2, Ethnic and cultural variations in the development of bereavement practices, *Cult Med Psychol* 8(4):315, 1984.

Ekblad S: Social determinants of aggression in a sample of Chinese primary school children, *Acta Psychiatr Scand* 73(5):515, 1986.

Ekblad S: Influence of child-rearing on aggressive behavior in a transcultural perspective, *Acta Psychiatr Scand Suppl* 344:133, 1988.

Elder SP, Hsia L: Women's health care and the workplace and the People's Republic of China, *J Nurse Midwifery* 31(4):182, 1986.

Farb P: Man at the mercy of language. In Wurzel JS, editor: *Toward multiculturalism: a reader in multicultural education,* Yarmouth, Me, 1988, Intercultural Press.

Fisher P: Chinese population crises. Paper submitted for Sociology 107W, Storrs, 1989, University of Connecticut.

Galanti GA: *Caring for patients from different cultures,* ed 2, Philadelphia, 1997, University of Pennsylvania Press.

Greenhalgh S, Bongaarts J: Fertility policy in China: future options, *Science* 235:1167, 1987.

Hoeman SP, Ku YL, Ohl DR: Health beliefs and early detection among Chinese women, *West J Nurs Res* 18(5):518, 1996.

Holroyd EA, Mackenzie AE: A review of the historical and social processes contributing to care and caregiving in Chinese families, *J Adv Nurs* 22:473, 1995.

Holtzen VL: A comparative study of nursing in China and the United States, *Nurs Forum* 22(3):86, 1985.

Horn BM: Cultural concepts and postpartal care, *Nurs Health Care* 2(9):516, 1981.

Hsiao WC: Transformation of health care in China, *N Engl J Med* 310(14):932, 1984.

Human rights in China, *Beijing Review* 34(44):8, 1991.

Iorio J, Nelson MA: China: caring's the same, *Nurs Outlook* 31(2):100, 1983.

Jang Y: Chinese culture and occupational therapy, *Br J Occup Ther* 58(3):103, 1995.

Jung M: Structural family therapy: its application to Chinese families, *Fam Process* 23(3):365, 1984.

Kong DS et al.: Child-rearing practices of Chinese parents and their relationship to behavioural problems in toddlers, *Acta Psychiatr Scand Suppl* 344:127, 1988.

Kuo C, Kavanagh KH: Chinese perspectives on culture and mental health, *Issues Ment Health Nurs* 15:551, 1994.

Liu YC: China: health care in transition, *Nurs Outlook* 31(2):94, 1983.

Lockhart JD: The children of China, *Hosp Pract* 14(2):118, 1979.

Mackenzie AE, Holroyd EF: An exploration of the carers' perceptions of caregiving and caring responsibilities in Chinese families, *Int J Nurs Stud* 33(1):1, 1996.

Martinelli AM: Pain and ethnicity: how people of different cultures experience pain, *AORN J* 46(2):273, 1987.

McKay S: Maternity care in China: report of a tour of Chinese medical facilities, *Birth* 9(2):105, 1982.

Morrisey S: Attitudes on aging in China, *J Gerontol Nurs* 9(11):589, 1983.

Muecke MA: Caring for Southeast Asian refugee patients in the USA, *Am J Public Health* 73(4):431, 1983.

Novajosky M, Schulze M: The birth of homecare in China, *Int Perspect* 11(10):72, 1992.

Overfield T: *Biologic variation in health and illness,* Menlo Park, Calif, 1985, Addison-Wesley.

Paice JA: Teaching cancer pain relief in China, *Am Nurse* 24(10):8, 1992.

A planet for the taking, March 15, 1989, Discovery Channel.

Prosser MH: *The cultural dialogue,* Washington, DC, 1985, SIETAR.

Randolph G: The yin and yang of clinical practice, *Top Clin Nurs* 1(1):31, 1979.

Rosenthal TH: East meets west: health care delegation visits China, *Hosp News CT* 14(3):5, 1997.

Sawyer F: *ABC News,* June 2, 1991.

Spector RE: *Cultural diversity in health & illness,* ed 4, Stamford, Conn, 1996, Appleton & Lange.

Stewart EC, Bennett MJ: American cultural patterns: a cross-cultural perspective, rev ed, Yarmouth, Me, 1991, Intercultural Press.

Teeng WS et al.: Family planning and child mental health in China: the Nanjing survey, *Am J Psychiatry* 145(11):1396, 1988.

Tien-Hyatt JL: Keying in on the unique care needs of Asian clients, *Nurs Health Care* 8(5):269, 1987.

Tseng V, Hsu J: The Chinese attitude toward parental authority as expressed in Chinese children's stories, *Arch Gen Psychiatry* 26(1):28, 1972.

Xiangdong M, Blum RW: School health services in the People's Republic of China, *J Sch Health* 60(10):483, 1990.

Yeh M, Gift AG, Soeken KL: Coping in spouses of patients with acute myocardial infarction in Taiwan, *Heart Lung* 23(2):106, 1994.

Zhan L: guest lecture, NURS 285, Storrs, 1991, University of Connecticut.

◆ COLOMBIA

MAP PAGE (314)

Location: Colombia is the only country in South America that borders the Atlantic and Pacific Oceans. It is composed of low coastal plains along the oceans and three parallel mountain ranges running north to south, which are part of the

Andes. The climate is dependent on altitude. At the end of the 1980s about one fifth of the population lived in poverty.

Major Languages	Ethnic Groups		Major Religions	
Spanish	Mestizo	58%	Catholic	95%
Indian Dialects	White	20%	Other	5%
	Mulatto	14%		
	African	4%		
	Native American and Other	4%		

Predominant Sick Care Practices: Biomedical; magico-religious. Illness may be caused by punishment from God for transgressions. The mestizo believe that people are controlled by environment, nature can be dangerous, and nature is animated by the presence of spirits. A common folk healer is called a "curandero"/"curandera" and may be used concurrently with biomedical medicine. Most medications can be purchased in pharmacies over the counter.

Ethnic/Race Specific or Endemic Diseases: ENDEMIC: Chloroquine-resistant malaria. RISK: Yellow fever; dengue fever; cholera; mild protein deficiency malnutrition; iron deficiency anemia. The AIDS rate per 100,000 is 2.55.

Health Team Relationships: Clients may be very modest with care providers of the opposite sex. Hospitalized patients expect to be passive, and family members provide for most self-care activities at home.

Families' Role in Hospital Care: Female family members may wish to provide so much care that it can become problematic for encouraging basic self-care activities. Many visitors may be anticipated.

Dominance Patterns: The father or oldest sibling is spokesperson, with adult family members' being part of decision making. The extended family is important.

Eye Contact Practices: Direct eye contact may not be used with authority figures or elders or in awkward situations.

Touch Practices: Touch is important and used when giving bad news. Hugs are used in greeting others. Handshaking is common, although among women some may grasp wrists instead of hands. With close friends and relatives a narrow space is maintained between people.

Perceptions of Time: Relaxed. Short-term planning is more common than long-term planning. People may be a little late for appointments, or appointments may be canceled without warning.

Birth Rites: During labor, pain relief is welcome but not expected by women of lower socioeconomic groups. The father or family members are not usually present during delivery. Traditional Catholics believe that abortion is a sin. If the father is consulted, his decision about continuing or terminating the pregnancy is usually followed. Significant numbers of women use contraceptives; however, sterilization is preferred. Male circumcision is a personal not a religious choice and is usually done at the time of birth.

Death Rites: Family members may wish to view the body before it is removed to the morgue, and burial often takes place within 24 to 36 hours. Cremation is not common.

Food Practices and Intolerances: The main meal is in late evening, but for some, lunch with the staples of rice, potatoes, and/or soup may be bigger than dinner. Sandwiches are not a substitute for meals. Fruit juice may be diluted with water and is only taken with meals. Catholics may prefer fish on Fridays during the season of Lent. A drink of unprocessed sugar and water is believed helpful when ill with respiratory or flu symptoms. Diarrhea is defined as loose stools in any form.

Child Rearing Practices: A dependent role is common, and children may live with parents until they marry. Punishment and threats, including the threat of being given an injection in a health care environment, are used to influence behavior. Children are expected to be obedient, respectful, and quiet with adults.

National Childhood Immunizations: BCG at birth; DPT at 2, 4, and 6 weeks; OPV at 2, 4, and 6 weeks; measles at 9 months.

Other Characteristics: Injections of oil are used to treat infections and cause hard lumps under the skin. To indicate a person's height by extending the arm with the palm down is an insulting gesture. The city of Bogotá created international interest in its system of Kangaroo Care for treatment of premature (low birth weight) infants.

BIBLIOGRAPHY

Anderson GC, Marks E, Wahlberg V: Kangaroo care for premature infants, *Am J Nurs* 86(7):807, 1986.

Browner C: The role of faculty development in multicultural education, Los Angeles, Prism Publishing of Mount St. Mary's College, n.d.

de Lima L, Bruera E: Palliative care in Colombia: program in "La Viga," *J Palliat Care* 10(1):42, 1994.

de Orjuella ML: Evolution of nursing: its influence and commitment in the social development of Colombia, *J Prof Nurs* 5(6):330, 1989.

de Pheils PB: Colombians. In Lipson JG, Dibble SL, Minarik PA: *Culture & nursing care: a pocket guide,* San Francisco, 1996, UCSF Nursing Press.

de Prjuela ML: Evolution of nursing: its influence and commitment in the social development of Colombia, *J Prof Nurs* 5(6):330, 1989.

Geissler EM: Personal journal, 1967.

Hollerbach P: The impact of national policies on the acceptance of sterilization in Colombia and Costa Rica, *Stud Fam Plann* 20(6):308, 1989.

Irujo S: An introduction to intercultural differences and similarities in non-verbal communication. In Wurzel JS, editor: *Toward multiculturalism,* Yarmouth, Me, 1988, Intercultural Press.

Stewart EC, Bennett MJ: American cultural patterns: a cross-cultural perspective, rev ed, Yarmouth, Me, 1991, Intercultural Press.

Virgin C, Jacobsen U: More female warmth and less high technology. Paper presented at the Fifth International Council on Women's Health Issues, Copenhagen, 1992.

World Monitor TV, April 11, 1991.

◆ COMOROS

MAP PAGE (317)

Location: The three volcanic islands of Comoros (Grande Comoro, Anjouan, and Mohéli) are located in the Mozambique Channel of the Indian Ocean between Madagascar and Africa.

Major Languages	Ethnic Groups		Major Religions	
Arabic	Arab	40%	Sunni Muslim	86%
Malagasy	African	38%	Catholic	14%
French	East Indian	22%		
Comorian	and Other			

Ethnic/Race Specific or Endemic Diseases: ENDEMIC: Chloroquine-resistant malaria. The AIDS rate per 100,000 is 0.31.

Death Rites: The Muslim belief forbids organ donations or transplants. Muslim physicians may recommend transfusions to save lives. Autopsy is uncommon because the deceased must be buried intact. Cremation is not permitted. For Muslim burial the body is wrapped in special pieces of cloth and buried without a coffin in the ground.

National Childhood Immunizations: BCG at birth; DPT at 6, 10, and 14 weeks; OPV at 6, 10, and 14 weeks; measles at 9 months.

BIBLIOGRAPHY

Ross HM: Societal/cultural views regarding death and dying, *Top Clin Nurs* 1(1):1, 1981.

◆ CONGO, THE REPUBLIC OF

MAP PAGE (317)

Location: Not to be confused with its neighbor Zaire, which recently changed its name to "The Democratic Republic of Congo," this west central African nation (formerly the French Congo) lies astride the equator. It is covered by thick tropical rain forests.

Major Languages	Ethnic Groups		Major Religions	
French	Kongo	48%	Christian	50%
Lingala	Sangha	20%	Animist	42%
Kikongo	Teke	17%	Muslim	2%
Other	M'Bochi	12%	Other	6%
	Other	3%		

Ethnic/Race Specific or Endemic Diseases: ENDEMIC: Yellow fever; chloroquine-resistant malaria. RISK: Schistosomiasis; Crimean-Congo hemorrhagic fever. The AIDS rate per 100,000 is 94.56.

National Childhood Immunizations: BCG at birth; DPT at 2, 3, 4, and 16 months; OPV at birth and 2, 3, and 4 months; measles at 9 months.

BIBLIOGRAPHY

Adler MW, editor: Statistics from the World Health Organization and the Centers for Disease Control, *AIDS* 6(10):1229, 1992.

Paverd N: Crimean-Congo haemorrhagic fever: a nursing care plan, *Nurs Rsa Verpleging* 3(4):33, 1988.

Paverd N: Crimean-Congo haemorrhagic fever: a protocol for control and containment in a health care facility, *Nurs Rsa Verpleging* 3(7):33, 1988.

Pittsburgh Post-Gazette, May 23, 1997.

◆ COSTA RICA

MAP PAGE (312)

Location: Costa Rica spans the width of a narrow section of Central America in the tropical zone. Most people live at the higher, temperate altitudes. This country has one of the lowest death rates in the world and has achieved a relatively high standard of living and social services. Costa Ricans call themselves "Ticos."

Major Languages	Ethnic Groups		Major Religions	
Spanish	European	96%	Catholic	95%
Creole	Black	3%	Other	5%
	Native American	1%		

Most indigenous Indian people have become assimilated into the dominant culture.

Predominant Sick Care Practices: Biomedical; magico-religious; traditional. The people frequently use traditional medicinal plants (bush medicines) along with over-the-counter Western medicines. Some believe that one type of medicine cannot cure many different diseases.

Health Care Beliefs: Health promotion is important and includes strong programs addressing environmental preservation of land, rain forests, and other ecosystems. State-of-health population indicators are similar to those of developed nations. Infant mortality has dropped 75% with the introduction of primary and secondary health care. Morbidity and mortality rates have been lowered. Applying the hot/cold theory and keeping the body in balance promote preventive health care. By 1984 Costa Rica had exceeded most of the objectives of the World Health Organization.

Ethnic/Race Specific or Endemic Diseases: RISK: Chloroquine-sensitive malaria; parasite infestation; malnutrition. The AIDS rate per 100,000 is 5.77.

Dominance Patterns: A patriarchal society with belief in machismo influencing behavior. Women are generally viewed as morally and spiritually superior.

Touch Practices: Costa Ricans touch frequently.

Food Practices and Intolerances: Plantains are plentiful. Black bean soup and tortillas are staples. The main meal of the day is lunch, and a late dinner is eaten. Children overall appear well nourished.

Child Rearing Practices: In 1982 contraception by sterilization was rendered illegal. Education is valued, and the country has a very high literacy rate.

National Childhood Immunizations: BCG at birth; DPT at 2, 4, 6, and 18 months and 4 years; OPV at 2, 4, 6, and 18 months and 4 years; MMR at 18 months and 7 years.

BIBLIOGRAPHY

Bähr J, Wehrhahn R: Life expectancy and infant mortality in Latin America, *Soc Sci Med* 36(1):1373, 1993.

Diamond DLM: Latin American food: more than beans and rice, *Top Clin Nurs* 11(4):57, 1996.

Finn J: A transcultural nurse's adventures in Costa Rica: using Leininger's sunrise model for transcultural nursing discoveries, *J Transcultural Nurs* 4(2):1993.

Giger JN, Davidhizar RE: *Transcultural nursing: assessment and intervention,* ed 2, St. Louis, 1995, Mosby.

Hill CE: Local health knowledge and universal primary health care: a behavioral case from Costa Rica, *Med Anthropol* 9(1):11, 1985.

Hollerbach P: The impact of national policies on the acceptance of sterilization in Colombia and Costa Rica, *Stud Fam Plann* 20(6):308, 1989.

Mohs E: General theory of paradigms in health, *Scand J Soc Med Suppl* 46:14, 1991.

Pezza PE: Health education and primary health care in Costa Rica: the role of the health assistant, *Health Promot Int* 10(2):143, 1995.

◆ CROATIA

MAP PAGE (314)

Location: Croatia is a parliamentary democracy that declared independence from Yugoslavia in 1991. It is located on the Balkan Peninsula in southeastern Europe. The country includes fertile agricultural areas, and a third is forested. The land stretches from the Alps down to the Mediterranean, with numerous islands along the coastline.

Major Language	Ethnic Groups		Major Religions	
Croatian	Croat	78%	Catholic	77%
	Serb	12%	Orthodox	11%
	Other	10%	Other	12%

Ethnic/Race Specific or Endemic Diseases: RISK: Posttraumatic stress syndrome from the aftermath of war. The AIDS rate per 100,000 is 0.33.

Health Team Relationships: Physicians earn just slightly more than nurses.

Food Practices and Intolerances: Bread is a dietary staple.

National Childhood Immunizations: BCG at birth and 2, 8, and 13 years; DPT at 3, 4, 5, and 12 months and 4 years; OPV at 3, 4, 5, and 12 months and 4, 6, and 14 years; MMR at 2 years; measles at 6 years and girls again at 14 years.

BIBLIOGRAPHY

McGorry ME: Sarajevo: an RN volunteer's reflection, *Tex Nurs* 69(4):8, 1995.

Simunec D: Letter from Croatia, *Nurs Times* 91(34):149, 1995.

Welsh J: Volunteering in Croatia, *Can Nurse* 90(5):51, 1994.

◆ CUBA

MAP PAGE (313)

Location: Cuba, the largest and westernmost island of the West Indies, is located 90 miles (145 km) south of the southern tip of Florida.

Major Language	Ethnic Groups		Major Religions	
Spanish	Mulatto	51%	Catholic	85%
	White	37%	Other	15%
	Black	11%		
	Chinese	1%		

Predominant Sick Care Practices: Biomedical; magico-religious. Santeria is a blend of African and Catholic religions and health care beliefs. The use of some alternative therapies increased with shortages of medicines.

Health Care Beliefs: Active involvement; health promotion important. Supernatural forces such as those involved in the "evil eye" are thought to cause some illnesses that must be cured by ethnic treatments or magic spells. Amulets on a bracelet or necklace or pinned to clothing provide some protection against the evil eye. Illness prevention and health promotion programs and facilities are in place nationwide. Cuba has already achieved "health for all" as defined by the World Health Organization. Mortality and morbidity rates rival and sometimes exceed those of Western nations.

Ethnic/Race Specific or Endemic Diseases: Polio, malaria, and diphtheria have been eradicated. The risks in Cuba, like most developed nations, are for chronic rather than infectious diseases. The AIDS rate per 100,000 is 0.97.

Health Team Relationships: Physicians and nurses visit the homes of the ill. Such programs strengthen relationships between the health care professionals and the community.

Families' Role in Hospital Care: Patients assume a passive role and expect care that is provided by family to include bathing, toileting, and feeding if possible. Parents can stay overnight and give personal care to hospitalized children.

Dominance Patterns: Traditionally a male-dominated culture with strong interdependent family networks for love, emotional support, material assistance, and overall well-being.

Eye Contact Practices: Direct eye contact. Looking away may be interpreted as disrespect or dishonesty.

Touch Practices: Close contact and touching are acceptable. Among men the handshake is common.

Pain Reactions: Verbal expression is acceptable.

Birth Rites: Close to 100% of births occur in health institutions. During pregnancy loud noises and looking at people with deformities are avoided. The woman's mother is present whenever possible during labor and delivery, whereas the traditional male is not. Male circumcision is common. Following delivery, traditional mothers and infants are not allowed out of the house for 41 days, and female family members will care for them during that time.

Death Rites: Agreeing to DNR (do not resuscitate) indicates giving up hope and possibly abandonment. Fear of death is common. Family and friends remain with the deceased through the night. Burial takes place within 24 hours. After the burial, family and friends stay up for 9 consecutive days; less traditional people replace this with a holy hour each evening.

Food Practices and Intolerances: The adult diet tends to be high in fat, cholesterol, sugar, and fried foods and low in vegetables and fiber. Economic blockades have resulted in food shortages. Meat and milk may be available only to pregnant women, the elderly, and the sick and not to children over 5 years old unless these items can be purchased with dollars. Fried rice and beans are common, and meat is preferred with all meals. Intake of sweets is high. Taboos include drinking water with fish or beer with bananas.

Infant Feeding Practices: Breastfeeding may be stopped as early as 3 months, at which time solid foods are introduced. If affordable, vitamin and mineral preparations supplement the diet. Traditionally, plump babies and young children are idealized.

Child Rearing Practices: Crying is an undesirable behavior because a happy, contented child is perceived as a quiet one. The mother explains and reasons as she rears her child. Physical punishment is common. These methods anticipate and prepare the child for developmental tasks. Toilet training begins as early as when the child can sit up, with bladder control expected by 1 to 2 years and bowel control by 2 years. Mothers or parents should be included in health education programs. The school system provides health teaching and assumes much of the child-rearing responsibilities. Child dependency may go considerably beyond the legal age of independence.

National Childhood Immunizations: BCG at birth; DPT at 3, 4, 5, and 17 months; DT at 6 years; OPV at 2, 3, 6, and 18 months and 4 years; MMR at 12 months.

BIBLIOGRAPHY

DeSantis L, Thomas JT: Parental attitudes toward adolescent sexuality: transcultural perspectives, *Nurse Pract* 12(8):43, 1987.

DeSantis L, Thomas JT: Childhood independence: views of Cuban and Haitian immigrant mothers, *J Pediatr Nurs* 9(4):258, 1994.

Guttmacher S: The prevention of health risks in Cuba, *Int J Health Serv* 17(1):179, 1987.

Guttmacher S: Minimizing health risks in Cuba, *Med Anthropol* 11:167, 1989.

Li GR: Funeral practices, New York, World Relief, n.d.

Martinson IM et al.: The block nurse program, *J Community Health Nurs* 2(1):21, 1985.

Pasquali E: Santeria: a religion and health care system for Long Island Cuban-Americans, *Cult Connections* 7(3):1, 1987.

Ruiz P: Cultural barriers to effective medical care among Hispanic-American patients, *Annu Rev Med* 36:63, 1985.

Swanson JM: Nursing in Cuba: population-focused practice, *Public Health Nurs* 4(3):183, 1987.

Swanson JM: Health-care delivery in Cuba: nursing's role in achievement of the goal of "health for all," *Int J Nurs Stud* 25(1):11, 1988.

Swanson KA et al.: Primary care in Cuba: a public health approach, *Health Care Women Int* 16(4):299, 1995.

Thomas JT, DeSantis L: Feeding and weaning practices of Cuban and Haitian immigrant mothers, *J Transcultural Nurs* 6(2):34, 1995.

Varela L: Cubans. In Lipson JG, Dibble SL, Minarik PA: *Culture & nursing care: a pocket guide,* San Francisco, 1996, UCSF Nursing Press.

◆ CYPRUS

MAP PAGE (318)

Location: Cyprus is a Mediterranean island off the southern coast of Turkey; it has a broad central plain between mountain ranges.

Major Languages	Ethnic Groups		Major Religions	
Greek	Greek	78%	Greek	78%
Turkish	Turkish	18%	Orthodox	
English	Armenian	4%	Muslim	18%
	and Other		Other	4%

Ethnic/Race Specific or Endemic Diseases: The AIDS rate per 100,000 is 0.40.

National Childhood Immunizations: DPT at 2, 4, and 6 months, between 18 and 24 months, and between 5 and 6 years; Td at between 14 and 15 years; OPV at 2, 4, and 6 months, between 18 and 24 months, and between 5 and 6 years; measles at 15 months; hep B at birth, 1 and 5 months, and between 5 and 6 years.

BIBLIOGRAPHY

Angel JL: Genetic and social factors in a Cypriote village, *Hum Biol* 44(1):53, 1972.

Volkan VD: Mourning and adaptation after a war, *Am J Psychother* 31(4):561, 1977.

◆ CZECH REPUBLIC

MAP PAGE (314)

Location: This landlocked, mountainous country is located in central Europe. Formerly part of Czechoslovakia, it separated from Slovakia in 1993.

Major Languages	Ethnic Groups		Major Religions	
Czech	Czech	94%	Atheist	40%
Slovak	Slovak	3%	Catholic	40%
	Other	3%	Protestant	5%
			Other	15%

Ethnic/Race Specific or Endemic Diseases: The AIDS rate per 100,000 is 0.13.

Health Team Relationships: Insurance from employers is compulsory, with the government responsible for children, students, pensioners, the unemployed, and the disabled.

Child Rearing Practices: Dependency, security, obligation, and reciprocity within the extended family are valued.

National Childhood Immunizations: BCG at birth and 14 years; DPT at between 2 and 3 months, between 4 and 5 months, between 10 and 11 months, at 3 years, and between 6 and 7 years; OPV at between 2 and 14 months, between 15 and 26 months, and at 13 years; measles at 15 months, between 21 and 25 months, and at 15 years.

BIBLIOGRAPHY

Gallagher G: A bright future, *Nurs Times* 88(22):42, 1992.
Misconiova B: Healing a sick society, *World Health* 1:4, 1992.
Murer CG: Sweeping up the rubble, *Rehab Manage Int* 4(1):40, 1994.
Stein F: The Slovak-American swaddling ethos: homeostate for family dynamics and cultural continuity, *Fam Process* 17(1):31, 1978.
Utley G: *NBC-TV Nightly News,* July 19, 1992.

◆ DENMARK

MAP PAGE (314)

Location: Denmark is situated on the Jutland Peninsula and on neighboring islands that separate the North and Baltic Seas in northern Europe. It is the smallest and flattest of the Scandinavian countries. Its highest point is 570 feet (174 m) above sea level.

Major Languages	Ethnic Groups		Major Religions	
Danish	Danish	99%	Lutheran	91%
Faroese	Other	1%	Other Christian	9%

Predominant Sick Care Practices: Biomedical; magico-religious; traditional.

Health Care Beliefs: Active involvement; passive role; health promotion important.

Ethnic/Race Specific or Endemic Diseases: RISK: Krabbe's disease; phenylketonuria. The AIDS rate per 100,000 is 4.13.

Health Team Relationships: Collegial relationships may exist among nurses and physicians, or physicians may expect nurses to fulfill service roles.

Families' Role in Hospital Care: Nurses provide all patient care; however, families may help with children.

Dominance Patterns: Some males have a slight dominant edge.

Eye Contact Practices: Direct eye contact is expected and is held.

Touch Practices: Touching is infrequent and is used with friends and associates only.

Perceptions of Time: Promptness is valued.

Pain Reactions: Patients are willing to inform the health care professional that they are in pain.

Food Practices and Intolerances: Breakfast may consist of combinations of yogurt products, white bread, coffee, corn flakes, cheese, and orange juice. The largest meal is taken between 6 and 8 PM. Spaghetti is currently a popular food among young people.

Infant Feeding Practices: Breastfeeding is most common.

National Childhood Immunizations: Pertussis at 5 and 9 weeks and 10 months; DT at 5, 6, and 15 months; IPV at 5, 6, and 15 months; MMR at 15 months and 12 years; OPV at 2, 3, and 4 years.

Other Characteristics: During conversation, periods of silence are valued.

BIBLIOGRAPHY

Andrews MM, Boyle JS: *Transcultural concepts in nursing care,* ed 2, Philadelphia, 1995, Lippincott.

Geissler EM: Personal observations and communications, Aug 22-29, 1992.

Larsen AS: Helping patients avoid readmission to hospital: a health behaviour study, *Recent Adv Nurs* 22:62, 1988.

Lindquist GJ: Primary health care in four countries, *J Prof Nurs* 2(4):203, 1986.

Menyuk P, Menyuk D: Communicative competence: a historical and cultural perspective. In Wurzel JS: *Toward multiculturalism,* Yarmouth, Me, 1988, Intercultural Press.

Merrick J: Physical punishment of children in Denmark: an historical perspective, *Child Abuse Negl* 10(2):263, 1986.

Wagner L: A proposed model for care of the elderly, *Int Nurs Rev* 36(2):50, 1989.

◆ DJIBOUTI

MAP PAGE (316)

Location: Formerly French Somaliland (and from 1967 to 1977 the Territory of the Afars and Issas), this sparsely populated, small country lies in northeast Africa at the southern entrance to the Red Sea. The area is arid, sandy, and desolate.

Major Languages	Ethnic Groups		Major Religions	
French	Somali Issa	60%	Muslim	94%
Arabic	Afar	35%	Christian	6%
Issa	Other	5%		
Afar				

Ethnic/Race Specific or Endemic Diseases: ENDEMIC: Yellow fever; chloroquine-sensitive malaria. The AIDS rate per 100,000 is 40.17.

Death Rites: Muslim belief forbids organ donations or transplants. Muslim physicians may recommend transfusions to save lives. Autopsy is uncommon because the deceased must be buried intact. Cremation is not permitted. For Muslim burial the body is wrapped in special pieces of cloth and buried without a coffin in the ground.

Child Rearing Practices: Circumcision is done on almost all females.

National Childhood Immunizations: BCG at birth; DPT at 6, 10, and 14 weeks; OPV at birth and 6, 10, and 14 weeks; measles at 9 months.

BIBLIOGRAPHY

Adler MW, editor: Statistics from the World Health Organization and the Centers for Disease Control, *AIDS* 6(10):1229, 1992.

Ross HM: Societal/cultural views regarding death and dying, *Top Clin Nurs* 1(1):1, 1981.

Wright J: Female genital mutilation: an overview, *J Adv Nurs* 24:251, 1996.

◆ DOMINICA

MAP PAGE (313)

Location: An eastern Caribbean island discovered by Columbus in 1493.

Major Languages	Ethnic Groups		Major Religions	
English	Black	98%	Catholic	80%
French Patois	Other	2%	Protestant	20%

Ethnic/Race Specific or Endemic Diseases: The AIDS rate per 100,000 is 7.04.

National Childhood Immunizations: BCG at 3 months; DPT at 3, 4½, and 6 months; DT at 3 years; Td at 11 years; OPV at 3, 4½, and 6 months; MMR at 12 months.

BIBLIOGRAPHY

No data located.

◆ DOMINICAN REPUBLIC

MAP PAGE (313)

Location: This country occupies the eastern two thirds of the Caribbean island of Hispaniola, sharing it with Haiti.

Major Language	Ethnic Groups		Major Religions	
Spanish	Mixed	73%	Catholic	95%
	White	16%	Other	5%
	Black	11%		

Predominant Sick Care Practices: Magico-religious; traditional.

Health Care Beliefs: The hot/cold balance theory is a factor in the cause of disease.

Ethnic/Race Specific or Endemic Diseases: ENDEMIC: Chloroquine-sensitive malaria below 400 m. RISK: Dengue fever; schistosomiasis. An estimated 60% of the population have parasites. Diarrhea and dehydration are the leading causes of death among children, accidents are second, and mal ojo (the evil eye) is third. High rates of poverty and malnutrition contribute to health risks and death rates. The AIDS rate per 100,000 is 4.92.

Health Team Relationships: Patients, in part deferring to the physicians' knowledge and learning, may ask few or even no questions of physicians. Patients tend to feel more comfortable with nurses and communicate more openly with them. They may appear to agree with suggested treatment but not be able to follow it for economic or family reasons and use home remedies or seek help from a folk healer (curandero).

Families' Role in Hospital Care: Families often provide food, linen, and clothing and purchase medicines for the sick family member.

Dominance Patterns: The traditional pattern is a matriarchal society within the home because men are not always present. Everyday decisions fall to the oldest women in the family. Men usually decide how the household income is spent, though this is changing as more women enter the workforce.

Eye Contact Practices: Eye contact is dependent on the situation, social standing, and gender of the individuals involved. Men are more apt to sustain direct eye contact than women.

Touch Practices: Direct touch is acceptable among members of the same sex. Men embrace and pat each other on the shoulder as a greeting and often touch each other's arms to get attention. Women are very openly affectionate among themselves, holding hands in public, touching each other's hair, embracing, and kissing. When greeting males, however, women only kiss on the cheek.

Perceptions of Time: A now-oriented view of the world is common, with putting things off until tomorrow practiced.

Pain Reactions: Loud, expressive reactions are seen, along with praying and complaining. Pain is perceived as an inevitable part of illness or injury by many and as a punishment from God by others. Pain medicines may not be available or may be in limited amounts in some health care facilities.

Birth Rites: Surgical sterilization is the most common birth control method, but often it is not categorized as a contraceptive method. It is believed that cravings during pregnancy should be satisfied. Newborns may be kept indoors for a month. The traditional mother may not wish to bathe, wash her hair, or have intercourse for 40 days after giving birth. Protection of the child from the evil eye may take the form of wearing red clothing. The majority of infants are born in the hospital or clinic, and sometimes the umbilical cord is saved. Family provides clean clothing and meals. At home the delivery may be done by a traditional midwife with on-the-job training. Breastfeeding usually continues until about 12 months, and the infant's diet is supplemented at about 3 months, sometimes with bean juice (the soup of beans). Milk formulas may be diluted or the formula prepared with contaminated water.

Death Rites: Unlike many other countries, the Dominican Republic has a higher death rate for females than males; perhaps this is affected by the lower value placed on females in view of the resources available.

Food Practices and Intolerances: Vitamin A deficiency is a public health problem. Rice and red beans are dietary staples, with the amount of beans decreasing as poverty increases. Though fish is abundant, some consider it contaminated and do not eat it. Plantains are common. Meals are taken 2 or 3 times a day. If food is scarce, the working male is less likely to have to cut back nutritionally than the unemployed.

Infant Feeding Practices: Depending on economic standing and time between babies, the duration of breastfeeding varies from 2 months to 1½ years. The first foods, bean broth and plantain broth, are often introduced between 4 and 5 months of age.

Child Rearing Practices: Until age 2 or 3, children have a very permissive upbringing. After that children, especially girls, have to take on a lot of responsibility for cooking, cleaning, and taking care of younger children. Mothers are responsible for everyday discipline; fathers handle larger problems.

National Childhood Immunizations: BCG at birth; DPT at 2, 3, and 4 months; OPV at birth and 2, 3, and 4 months; measles at 9 months.

Other Characteristics: Anise tea is believed to have medicinal qualities.

BIBLIOGRAPHY

Basch CE et al.: Validation of mothers' reports of dietary intake by four to seven-year-old children, *AJPH* 81(11):1314, 1990.

Bittner MJ: Health in the batey Libertad, *Hosp Pract* 17(11):163, 1982.

Curtin A: Intercultural nursing: working in the Dominican Republic, *News Views,* Fall 1994.

de Alvarez JT: The third age in the third world in the third millennium, *Caring* 13(1):8, 1994.

Desjardins J: Post operative pain in Dominicans, unpublished honors thesis, 1996, University of Connecticut.

Estrella J: Contributor.

Geissler EM: Personal observations, 1994-1997.

Gordon AJ: Mixed strategies in health education and community participation: an evaluation of dengue control in the Dominican Republic, *Health Educ Res* 3(4):399, 1988.

Kaiser MA: The Dominican Republic's focus on aging, *Caring* 11(10):80, 1992.

Loaiza E: Sterilization regret in the Dominican Republic: looking for quality-of-care issues, *Stud Fam Plann* 26(1):39, 1995.

Mora JO, Dary O: Vitamin A deficiency and actions for its prevention and control in Latin America and the Caribbean, *Bol Oficina Sanit Panam* 117(6):519, 1994.

Nichols FH: Health status of children in rural areas of the Dominican Republic: policy implications for nursing practice and nursing education in Third World countries, *J Community Health Nurs* 1(2):125, 1984.

Ruiz PM: Dominican concepts of health and illness, *J NY State Nurses Assoc* 21(4):11, 1990.

Tidwell MA et al.: Emergency control of Aedes aegypti in the Dominican Republic using the Scorpion 20 ULV forced-air generator, *J Am Mosquito Assoc* 10(3):403, 1994.

Whiteford LM: Child and maternal health and international economic policies, *Soc Sci Med* 37(11):1391, 1993.

Whitwell J: Teamwork in the Dominican Republic, *Can Nurse,* vol 5, 1988.

Wiarda HJ, Kryzanek MJ: *The Dominican Republic: a Caribbean crucible,* ed 2, Boulder, Colo, 1992, Westview Press.

◆ ECUADOR

MAP PAGE (314)

Location: Ecuador is named for the equator, on which it lies. Two mountain ranges that are part of the Andes—including the tall volcanic peaks (the highest, 20,577 feet [6272 m])—split the country into hot, humid lowlands on the Pacific coast. Temperate highlands are found between the ranges, as well as the mostly unexplored and uninhabited tropical jungle of the Amazon basin. The Galápagos Islands are part of the country.

Major Languages	Ethnic Groups		Major Religions	
Spanish	Mestizo	55%	Catholic	95%
Quechua	Native	25%	Other	5%
English	American			
German	Spanish	10%		
Jivaro	Black	10%		

Predominant Sick Care Practices: Traditional. A traditional healer is called a "brujo." Western medicine is disease oriented and hospital based.

Health Care Beliefs: Some people, for example, diabetics, find it difficult to understand why treatment should be continued when one feels well. Health teaching is not a part of health care.

Ethnic/Race Specific or Endemic Diseases: ACTIVE: Cholera (in 1991); diarrheal disorders; protein-calorie malnutrition in children. ENDEMIC: Yellow fever. RISK: Chloroquine-resistant malaria. The AIDS rate per 100,000 is 0.60.

Families' Role in Hospital Care: Helping with some care is permitted, along with providing food when it is scarce within the hospital.

Dominance Patterns: The family's and an individual's position in society (rather than the family or individual) predominate. Several generations may live together, and the elderly are respected.

Touch Practices: It is acceptable for members of the same sex to touch, and men may greet one another with an embrace.

Perceptions of Time: Siesta time is during the afternoon. Time and punctuality are somewhat relaxed.

Food Practices and Intolerances: The main meal is at noon. Staples include chicken, corn, potatoes, and beans. Fried foods are popular. The discipline of diet therapy does not exist.

National Childhood Immunizations: BCG at birth and 6 years; DPT at 2, 4, 6, and 18 months; DT at 5 years; OPV at birth and 2, 4, 6, and 18 months; measles at 9 months.

BIBLIOGRAPHY

Axtell RE, editor: *Do's and taboos around the world,* ed 2, New York, 1990, John Wiley & Sons.

Finerman RD: A matter of life and death: health care change in an Andean community, *Soc Sci Med* 18(4):329, 1984.

Fitzgerald KA: Nursing in the third world: teaching burn care in Ecuador, *Focus Crit Care* 17(2):142, 1990.

Ruffing KL, Smith HL: Maternal and child health care in Ecuador: obstacles and solutions, *Health Care Women Int* 5(4):195, 1984.

Ruffing KL, Smith HL: Planning for rural community health nursing needs: the experience of Ecuador, *J Adv Nurs* 9(2):136, 1984.

Schmidt KM: Marlene Goertzen, RN: home care nurse in Ecuador, *J Christ Nurs* 11(4):36, 1994.

Stewart EC, Bennett MJ: American cultural patterns: a cross-cultural perspective, rev ed, Yarmouth, Me, 1991, Intercultural Press.

World Monitor TV, April 11, 1991.

◆ EGYPT

MAP PAGE (316)

Location: Egypt occupies the northeast corner of Africa. Most of its citizens reside in the Nile river valley because 97% of Egypt is desert.

Major Languages	Ethnic Groups		Major Religions	
Arabic	Eastern	99%	Sunni Muslim	94%
English	Hamitic		Other	6%
French	Other	1%		

Predominant Sick Care Practices: Biomedical; magico-religious. The "evil eye" and hot/cold disease factors (see Cambodia, p. 41) are beliefs that coexist with Western medical practices.

Health Care Beliefs: Passive role. Injections and intravenous fluids are perceived as more effective than oral medication. The belief that health is dictated by Allah promotes a passive role. Self-medication is practiced. Pharmacists and nurses can prescribe drugs. Amulets inscribed with verses of the Koran, turquoise stones, or a charm of a hand with five fingers enhances protective powers against the evil eye.

Ethnic/Race Specific or Endemic Diseases: ENDEMIC: Chloroquine-sensitive malaria. RISK: Schistosomiasis. The AIDS rate per 100,000 is 0.03.

Health Team Relationships: The reason for asking personal questions during assessment needs to be clarified. Males may refuse care by female physicians or nurse practitioners, especially if the problem is a sexually sensitive one. Sudden termination of a long-term relationship between health care professional and patient is tactless and inconsiderate. Generally it is the physician who does the decision making.

Families' Role in Hospital Care: Culture dictates that family and friends visit the patient as much as possible to ensure that health care personnel care for and attend the patient properly. Some may wish to be present during the patient's interview and examination and may answer questions for the patient. The health care professional should include the eldest family member present in the discussion. Taking individual responsibility for health actions and signing informed consent forms are usually reserved for those with expert knowledge; therefore the patient's signature may not mean that informed permission has been given.

Dominance Patterns: Male dominated. Today women have access to higher education and professional careers. Yet women's walking alone is taboo. Though the law mandating women's wearing a veil was overturned decades ago, many women choose to wear one.

Eye Contact Practices: Observing the eyes at close range (approximately 2 feet) during conversation permits evaluation. The pupil of the eye dilates with interest or contracts with dislike.

Touch Practices: Touch is an important part of communication. It is, however, limited to members of the same sex.

Perceptions of Time: Time is oriented to the present because planning ahead contains the potential for defying God's will.

Pain Reactions: Pain relief is expected to be immediate and may be requested persistently. Therapies requiring exertion are incompatible with belief in energy conservation for recovery. Pain is expressed privately or in the company of close relatives or friends. The exception is during labor and delivery.

Birth Rites: Sugar water is added very early, with introduction of other foods as soon as 40 days after birth. Weaning is occurring earlier than before and can be perceived as a difficult and dangerous transition period. Newborns are swaddled and dressed in a shirt called a "jalabiya," which is made by relatives. The grandmother stays close to the mother during the mother's hospital stay. A celebration that is sponsored by the grandparents is held on the infant's seventh day.

Death Rites: Hope is valued; therefore confronting the patient with a grave diagnosis shatters hope and creates mistrust. The belief is that only God knows the true prognosis, and no one must speak of death. Health care professionals may be asked to shield the patient with a terminal illness from the truth. At death, a Muslim should help the patient recite the Declaration of the Faith: "There is no God but God, and Muhammed is his Messenger." Expressive, vocal wailing is acceptable. The family may prefer to stay in the room with the body to talk to the deceased and reflect on the person's accomplishments. More time is needed with the death of a child so the family can think about what the child might have accomplished. Touching the body is part of the final farewell. Family members wash the body according to Islamic tradition. Muslim belief forbids organ donations or transplants. Muslim physicians may recommend transfusions to save lives. Autopsy is uncommon because the deceased must be buried intact. Cremation is not permitted. For Muslim burial the body is wrapped in special pieces of cloth and buried without a coffin in the ground.

Food Practices and Intolerances: The evening meal is taken at approximately 10 PM. Pork, carrion, and blood are forbidden. Food tends to be spicy. Ramadan fasting is practiced between sunrise and sunset, with exemptions for the sick and children.

National Childhood Immunizations: BCG at birth; DPT at 2, 4, and 6 months, between 18 and 24 months, and at 6 years; OPV at 2, 4, 6, and 9 months and between 18 and 24 months; measles at 9 months; hep B at 2, 4, and 6 months.

Other Characteristics: Female circumcision is viewed as the ultimate proof of virginity, and the practice is widespread in traditional groups or remote areas when a girl is 7 or 8 years old. Menarche may occur later than 15 years of age. Verbal consent is equal to written consent; pressing for written consent suggests mistrust of a verbal contract and is an insult to an individual's honor. Hope, optimism, and the positive advantages of treatment should be stressed when discussing outcomes. Some women retain their surname after marriage.

BIBLIOGRAPHY

Brown Y: Female circumcision, *Can Nurse,* April 1989, p 19.

Davis CF: Culturally responsive nursing management in an international health care setting, *Nurs Adm Q* 16(2):36, 1992.

Gadalla S, McCarthy J, Campbell O: How the number of living sons influences contraceptive use in Menoufia Governorate, Egypt, *Stud Fam Plann* 16(3):164, 1985.

Galanti GA: *Caring for patients from different cultures,* ed 2, Philadelphia, 1997, University of Pennsylvania Press.

Gary R: Nurse development program, *Nurs Adm Q* 16(2):25, 1992.

Govaerts K, Patino E: Attachment behavior of the Egyptian mother, *Int J Nurs Stud* 18:53, 1981.

Green J: Death with dignity: Islam, *Nurs Times* 85(5):56, 1989.

Hall ET: Learning the Arabs' silent language, *Psychol Today,* Aug 1979, p 45.

Harrison GG et al.: Breastfeeding and weaning in a poor urban neighborhood in Cairo, Egypt: maternal beliefs and perceptions, *Soc Sci Med* 36(8):1063, 1993.

Hathout MM: Comment on ethical crises and cultural differences, *West J Med* 139(3):380, 1983.

Lally MM: Last rites and funeral customs of minority groups, *Midwife Health Visit Comm Nurse* 14(7):224, 1978.

Meleis AI: The Arab American in the health care system, *Am J Nurs,* June 1981, p 1180.

Meleis AI, Jonsen AR: Medicine in perspective: ethical crises and cultural differences, *West J Med* 138(6):889, 1983.

Meleis AI, LaFever CW: The Arab American psychiatric care, *Perspect Psychiatr Care* 22(2):72, 1984.

Meleis AI, Sorrell L: Arab American women and their birth experiences, *MCN Am J Matern Child Nurs* 6:171, 1981.

Overfield T: *Biologic variation in health and illness,* Menlo Park, Calif, 1985, Addison-Wesley.

Reizian A, Meleis AI: Arab-Americans' perceptions of and responses to pain, *Crit Care Nurse* 6(6):30, 1986.

Ross HM: Societal/cultural views regarding death and dying, *Top Clin Nurs* 1(1):1, 1981.

Segall ME: Return to Aswan: picking up the threads, *Int Nurs Rev* 32(3):84, 1985.

Segall ME: Return to Aswan: planning the course, *Int Nurs Rev* 32(4):109, 1985.

Stern PN: Editorial: Women of Egypt!, *Health Care Women Int* 15(2):v-vii, 1994.

Stern PN: Editorial: Women of Egypt !!, *Health Care Women Int* 15(3):v-vii, 1994.

Wright J: Female genital mutilation: an overview, *J Adv Nurs* 24:251, 1996.

◆ EL SALVADOR

MAP PAGE (312)

Location: This smallest of the Central American countries is situated on the Pacific coast, and much of the land is a fertile volcanic plateau.

Major Languages	Ethnic Groups		Major Religions	
Spanish	Mestizo	94%	Catholic	75%
Nahua	Native American	5%	Other	25%
	White	1%		

Predominant Sick Care Practices: Biomedical, with less reliance on folk beliefs than some other Latino cultures.

Health Care Beliefs: Fresh air, sleep, and good nutrition are important health practices.

Ethnic/Race Specific or Endemic Diseases: ENDEMIC: Chloroquine-sensitive malaria; no risk in urban areas. The AIDS rate per 100,000 is 6.59.

Health Team Relationships: Physicians and nurses share information, and physicians retain the superior role.

Food Practices and Intolerances: White bread or rolls are unknown. Black beans are served with breakfast and dinner. Rice with tortillas is served at lunch and dinner. Some believe that being thin is unhealthy, and weight control is not equated with good nutrition.

National Childhood Immunizations: BCG at birth; DPT at 2, 4, and 6 months, 1½ years, and between 4 and 5 years; OPV at birth and 2, 4, and 6 months, 1½ years, and between 4 and 5 years; measles at 9 months.

BIBLIOGRAPHY

Andrews MM, Boyle JS: *Transcultural concepts in nursing care,* ed 2, Philadelphia, 1995, Lippincott.

Boyle JS: Constructs of health promotion and wellness in a Salvadoran population, *Pub Health Nurs* 6(3):129, 1989.

Diamond-de La Mata R: Latin American food: more than beans and rice, *Top Clin Nurs* 11(4):57, 1996.

Liveoak V: A Texas RN in El Salvador, *Texas Nurse* 63(6):12, 1989.

Moccia P: We're building peace, *Nurs Health Care* 13(4):180, 1992.

Tigerman NS: Health beliefs, knowledge and health seeking behaviors of recently immigrated Central American mothers in Los Angeles (California), doctoral dissertation, Los Angeles, 1988, University of California.

Umanzor S: Nightmare in El Salvador: a nursing student's story, *J Christ Nurs* 3(2):10, 1986.

Zadel J: Nurse returns after three years in El Salvador, *Chart* 82(10):1, 1985.

◆ EQUATORIAL GUINEA

MAP PAGE (317)

Location: Equatorial Guinea, formerly Spanish Guinea, is located on the western coast of Africa. This nation includes several islands in the Gulf of Guinea.

Major Languages	Ethnic Groups		Major Religions	
Spanish	Fang	83%	Catholic	60%
Pidgin English	Bubi	10%	Indigenous	40%
Fang	Other	7%	and Other	

Ethnic/Race Specific or Endemic Diseases: ENDEMIC: Yellow fever; chloroquine-resistant malaria. RISK: Schistosomiasis. The AIDS rate per 100,000 is 24.38.

National Childhood Immunizations: BCG at birth; DPT at 6, 10, and 14 weeks and 15 months; OPV at birth and 6, 10, and 14 weeks; measles at 9 months.

BIBLIOGRAPHY

No data located.

◆ ERITREA

MAP PAGE (316)

Location: Since Eritrea was formerly the northernmost province of Ethiopia, Eritreans and Ethiopians are essentially the same. Primarily a mountainous country, it has a narrow plain along the Red Sea that is one of Africa's hottest and driest places. There are fertile agricultural valleys in the central highlands.

Major Languages	Ethnic Groups		Major Religions	
Tigrinya	Tigrays	50%	Muslim	50%
Tigre	Tigre	40%	Christian	50%
	and Kunama			
	Afar	4%		
	Other	6%		

Ethnic/Race Specific or Endemic Diseases: Malnutrition, anemia, intestinal parasites, and respiratory disorders are common. The AIDS rate per 100,000 is 20.58.

Birth Rites: There are midwives and traditional birth attendants from within the community.

Child Rearing Practices: There are areas in which most girls have female circumcision, including infibulation.

National Childhood Immunizations: BCG at birth; DPT at 6, 10, and 14 weeks; OPV at birth and 6, 10, and 14 weeks; measles at 9 months.

Other Characteristics: Large numbers of disabled fighters have been produced by 30 years of war. Because of their high status within society, the incidence of posttraumatic stress syndrome and depression is very low.

BIBLIOGRAPHY

Kingham T: War babies, *Nurs Times* 86(30):28, 1990.
Rayner T: Mending lives, *Nurs Times* 89(51):30, 1993.
Wright J: Female genital mutilation: an overview, *J Adv Nurs* 24:251, 1996.

◆ ESTONIA

MAP PAGE (315)

Location: Bordering on the Baltic Sea to its north and west, Estonia is mainly lowland country with numerous lakes.

Major Languages	Ethnic Groups		Major Religion
Estonian	Estonian	62%	Lutheran
Latvian	Russian	30%	
Lithuanian	Other	8%	

Ethnic/Race Specific or Endemic Diseases: Cardiovascular disease is the greatest killer. The AIDS rate per 100,000 is 0.20.

Health Team Relationships: Physician-directed patient care, with no nursing content identifiable in schools or practice.

Birth Rites: One hospital provides 24 hour-per-day care and contact between mother and infant.

Food Practices and Intolerances: Fresh vegetables are very limited in the diet.

National Childhood Immunizations: BCG at between 3 and 5 days and at 7 and 15 years; DPT at 3, 4½, and 6 months and 2 years; OPV at 3, 4½, and 6 months and 2 and 6 years; measles and rubella at 12 months; mumps at 18 months.

BIBLIOGRAPHY

Kalnins I: Pioneers in academia: higher education for nurses in Estonia, Latvia, and Lithuania, *Nurs Outlook* 43(2):84, 1995.

Levin A: The mother-infant unit at Tallinn Children's Hospital, Estonia: a truly baby-friendly unit, *Birth* 21(1):39, 1994.

Puska P: Health promotion challenges for countries of the former Soviet Union: results from collaboration between Estonia, Russian Karelia and Finland, *Health Promot Int* 10(3):219, 1995.

◆ ETHIOPIA

MAP PAGE (316)

Location: Black Africa's oldest state is located in east central Africa and borders the Red Sea on the north. Subsistence farming is severely affected by drought. Ethiopians and Eritreans are similar cultural groups.

Major Languages	Ethnic Groups		Major Religions	
Amharic	Oromo	40%	Muslim	45%
Tigrinya	Amhara and	32%	Ethiopian	35%
Orominga	Tigrean		Orthodox	
Arabic	Sidamo	9%	Animist and	20%
English	Shankella	6%	Other	
	Somali and	13%		
	Other			

Predominant Sick Care Practices: Magico-religious. Some local practices may include wearing amulets for protection against disease and bloodletting to treat malaria.

Ethnic/Race Specific or Endemic Diseases: ACTIVE: Septic abortion the most common cause of maternal death; leprosy. ENDEMIC: Chloroquine-resistant malaria, with the exception of Addis Ababa; yellow fever. RISK: Schistosomiasis; pneumonia; post-measles complications; malnutrition; anemia; intestinal parasites; diarrhea; eye infections; vitamins A and B deficiencies, including night blindness. The AIDS rate per 100,000 is 7.02.

Health Team Relationships: The health care professionals' warmth is more important to patients than their professional appearance. Patients tend to let the physicians decide what needs to be done.

Families' Role in Hospital Care: Families may move into the hospital, help with the patient's physical care, and provide home-cooked meals or supplements to the simple meals that are served. Patients do not want to be left alone, especially if gravely ill. The sick role is passivity and dependency on family and friends.

Dominance Patterns: Women are socialized to be fragile, therefore they should not be given adverse information first.

Eye Contact Practices: Patients may use little eye contact with doctors and nurses as a sign of respect for authority figures.

Touch Practices: Greetings include three or four kisses on the cheeks; hugs between men are common, as are handshakes. Bowing when shaking hands is very common. Spitting on children while remarking on their good looks prevents inadvertently casting the evil eye.

Perceptions of Time: Usually late in both social and business situations.

Pain Reactions: People are stoic and may refuse pain medications even when they are available.

Birth Rites: Pregnancy is a dangerous time because of the potential for the evil eye and sorcery against the fetus. Unfulfilled cravings can cause a miscarriage, malformation, or prematurity. The country does not require registration of births. Delivery is attended by a traditional midwife or older, female family member and is in the lithotomy position. Traditional fathers do not participate in labor or delivery. During the first hours after birth, the mother may turn away from the infant—a symbolic rejection for the pain the infant caused during birth. The mother remains confined for 14 to 40 days. While immunizing children, the opportunity is taken to administer tetanus toxoid boosters to mothers.

Death Rites: The country does not require registration of deaths. Muslim belief forbids organ donations or transplants. Muslim physicians may recommend transfusions to save lives. Autopsy is uncommon because the deceased must be buried intact. Cremation is not permitted. For Muslim burial the body is wrapped in special pieces of cloth and buried without a coffin in the ground. Loud wailing is a normal grief reaction for both men and women.

Food Practices and Intolerances: About 40% of children suffer some level of malnutrition. Some people, considering chicken dirty, do not eat it. Spicy food is preferred. The usual pattern is three meals a day. Drinks should be offered at room temperature and encouraged, as water intake tends to be low. Some religious groups will not eat meat of wild animals, wild fowl, snakes, wild and domestic pigs, dogs, horses, and shellfish. Coptic Christians do not eat meat or dairy products for 200 days of the year.

Infant Feeding Practices: Sugar and water are given instead of colostrum, which is believed to be bad for the newborn. Food and fluids may be withheld from children to treat diarrhea. Breastfeeding occurs for about 2 years.

Child Rearing Practices: Children are kept in a highly protective, indulged atmosphere until they are about 3 years old, when a disciplinary regimen begins. Obedience and politeness are goals of upbringing. Children who are ill may be kept lying in one place until they get better. Female circumcision and excision is widespread among some groups.

National Childhood Immunizations: BCG at birth; DPT at 6, 10, and 14 weeks; OPV at 6, 10, and 14 weeks; measles at 9 months.

BIBLIOGRAPHY

Beyene Y: Ethiopians & Eritreans. In Lipson JG, Dibble SL, Minarik PA: *Culture & nursing care: a pocket guide,* San Francisco, 1996, UCSF Nursing Press.

Galanti GA: *Caring for patients from different cultures,* ed 2, Philadelphia, 1997, University of Pennsylvania Press.

Hartz J: *Children in exile,* March 8, 1992, NBC-TV.

Hughes MR: Life and motherhood in Ethiopia, *Midwives* 108(1287):102, 1995.

Kingham T: War babies, *Nurs Times* 86(3):28, 1990.

Ravid C et al.: Internal body perceptions of Ethiopian Jews who emigrated to Israel, *West J Nurs Res* 17(6):631, 1995.

Ross HM: Societal/cultural views regarding death and dying, *Top Clin Nurs* 1(1):1, 1981.

Stuhr D: Destination Ethiopia, *J Christ Nurs* 3(4):28, 1986.

Trites P: Ethiopian experience, *Can Nurse,* Nov 1985, p 13.

Wallace C: A day in clinic and hospital, *Can Nurse,* Oct 1988, p 36.

Wright J: Female genital mutilation: an overview, *J Adv Nurs* 24:251, 1996.

◆ FIJI

MAP PAGE (311)

Location: More than 500 islands in the southern Pacific (about 2000 miles east of Australia) make up Fiji.

Major Languages	Ethnic Groups		Major Religions	
English	Fijian	49%	Christian	52%
Fijian	East Indian	46%	Hindu	38%
Hindustani	European and	5%	Muslim	8%
	Other		Other	2%

Ethnic/Race Specific or Endemic Diseases: RISK: Dengue fever. The AIDS rate per 100,000 is reported by the country as zero.

National Childhood Immunizations: BCG at birth and between 5 and 6 years; DPT at 2, 3, and 4 months; OPV at birth, 2, 3, and 4 months, and between 5 and 6 years; measles at 9 months; rubella at 11 years for girls; hep B at birth and 2 and 4 months.

Other Characteristics: It is considered impolite to raise the arms while talking to someone. Talking with the arms crossed over the chest is a sign of respect.

BIBLIOGRAPHY

Andy TC: The utilisation of a primary health care centre on an isolated island: Cicia, Fiji, *Cent Afr J Med* 36(10):246, 1990.

◆ FINLAND

MAP PAGE (314)

Location: Finland stretches about 700 miles (1126 km) north and south from the Arctic Circle to the Gulf of Finland, with Russia along its eastern border. It is the second most northern country in the world. Finland has long, cold winters, and it enjoys one of the highest standards of living in the world.

Major Languages	Ethnic Groups		Major Religions	
Finnish	Finnish	94%	Lutheran	89%
Swedish	Swedish, Lapp,	6%	Greek	1%
Lapp	and Other		Orthodox	
Russian			Other	10%

Predominant Sick Care Practices: Biomedical. Legislation provides the right to good health care and related treatments, the right to be informed, and the right to self-determination and participation in health care.

Health Care Beliefs: Active involvement; health promotion important. Illness equates to loss of independence and sense of well-being.

Ethnic/Race Specific or Endemic Diseases: RISK: Congenital nephrosis; generalized amyloidosis syndrome; polycystic liver disease, alcohol abuse; cardiovascular diseases; cancer. Lifestyle diseases are emerging as the most common. The AIDS rate per 100,000 is 0.78.

Health Team Relationships: Clients desire good interactive relationships with nurses.

Dominance Patterns: Males may have slight dominance in some families; however, in making health care decisions for children, husband and wife share responsibility.

Eye Contact Practices: Direct eye contact, but it is held intermittently.

Touch Practices: Most touch infrequently; however, young couples often touch more frequently.

Perceptions of Time: People are usually punctual and may be irritated by tardiness.

Pain Reactions: People are willing to communicate pain; however, they are not expressive.

Birth Rites: A midwife-assisted hospital birth predominates, with one of the lowest infant mortality rates in the world. For the sick infant, parental involvement is encouraged, with open visiting hours for siblings. Kangaroo care is utilized, and breastfeeding is the method of choice. Having one or two children is common.

Death Rites: Relatives desire to be at the bedside of the dying person to pay final respects. Funeral directors provide all postmortem care. Burial in the ground is the common practice and is held several days after the death is announced in newspapers.

Food Practices and Intolerances: Coffee, sandwiches of meat and cheese, and porridge are common for breakfast. Lunch is the main meal. A small meal of coffee and sandwiches is taken after work. Reindeer meat is popular.

Infant Feeding Practices: Breastfeeding is common.

Child Rearing Practices: Mothers get 263 working days of maternity allowance, and fathers get 6 paid days. The mother's job is secure until the child is 3 years old or 7 years old if the mother works only 6 hours a day. Free dental care is provided until age 18, and free health care, from birth to school age. Compulsory military service begins for boys at age 19. Two full meals are offered to children at school.

National Childhood Immunizations: BCG at birth; DPT at 3, 4, and 5 months and between 20 and 24 months; OPV at 6 and 12 months, between 20 and 24 months, at 6 and 11 years, and between 16 and 18 years.

Other Characteristics: Carrying on a conversation with hands in the pockets is impolite. The term *health center* means an organization of services rather than a building.

BIBLIOGRAPHY

Andrews MM, Boyle JS: *Transcultural concepts in nursing care,* ed 2, Philadelphia, 1995, Lippincott.

Callister LC: Cultural meanings of childbirth, *JOGNN* 24(4):327, 1995.

Callister LC: Cultural perceptions of childbirth, *J Holistic Nurs* 14(1):66, 1996.

Carr C: A four-week observation of maternity care in Finland, *J Obstet Gynecol Neonatal Nurs* 18(2):100, 1989.

Forni PR: Health care delivery in Sweden and Finland: a challenge to the American system, *J Prof Nurs* 2(4):234, 1986.

Geissler EM: Personal observations, Aug 5-11, 1992.

Häggman-Laitila A, Astedt-Kurki P: What is expected of the nurse-client interaction and how these expectations are realized in Finnish health care, *Int J Nurs Stud* 31(3):253, 1994.

Häggman-Laitila A, Astedt-Kurki P: Experiential health knowledge from the perspective of Finnish Adults, West J Nurs Res 17(6):614, 1995.

Lammi UK et al.: Functional capacity and associated factors in elderly Finnish men, *Scand J Soc Med* 17(1):67, 1989.

Lauri S et al.: Public health nurses' decision making in Canada, Finland, Norway, and the United States, *West J Nurs Res* 19(2):143, 1997.

Leina-Kilpi H, Kurittu K: Patients' rights in hospital: an empirical investigation in Finland, *Nurs Ethics* 2(2):103, 1995.

Lindquist GJ: Primary health care in four countries, *J Prof Nurs* 2(4):203, 1986.

Mäki K: Neonatal nursing in Finland, *Neonatal Net* 12(3):54, 1993.

Nikkonen M: Changes in psychiatric caring values in Finland, *J Transcultural Nurs* 6(1):12, 1994.

Pietilä A, Hentinen M, Myhrman A: The health behaviour of northern Finnish men in adolescence and adulthood, *Int J Nurs Stud* 32(3):325, 1995.

Pietinen P et al.: Nutrition as a component in community control of cardiovascular disease, *Am J Clin Nutr* 49(Suppl 5):1017, 1989.

Rautava P et al.: The Finnish family competence study: childbearing attitudes in pregnant nulliparae, *Acta Paedopsychiatr* 55(1):3, 1992.

Teperi J, Rimpela M: Menstrual pain, health and behaviour in girls, *Soc Sci Med* 29(2):163, 1989.

Valkama E: Personal communication, Aug 5, 1992.

Virgin C, Jacobsen U: More female warmth and less high technology. Paper presented at the Fifth International Council on Women's Health Issues, 1992, Copenhagen.

◆ FRANCE

MAP PAGE (314)

Location: The second largest European nation, France, is mountainous in the extreme east and consists of river basins and a plateau throughout the rest of the nation.

Major Languages	Ethnic Groups		Major Religions	
French	French	97%	Catholic	90%
Alsatian	Other	3%	Protestant	2%
Breton			Jewish	1%
Corsican			Muslim	1%
Basque			Unaffiliated and Other	6%

Health Care Beliefs: Eating proper food, wearing proper clothing, resting, and taking cod liver oil daily are believed to promote health.

Ethnic/Race Specific or Endemic Diseases: The AIDS rate per 100,000 is 8.41.

Health Team Relationships: When meeting people, protocol is observed and behavior is polite. Titles and status are important. First names should not be used. Engaging in general conversation to establish social contact is acceptable. Often details are not included in communications, and hidden meanings may not be verbalized. Giving logical, sequential reasons for actions is important to ensure the patient's compliance. Rules and regulations may be circumvented to reach a goal.

Eye Contact Practices: Direct eye contact is maintained. The face is expressive, as are gestures.

Touch Practices: The French touch frequently. The southern French prefer closeness during conversation. Handshaking and a kiss on each cheek when greeting or leaving are common.

Perceptions of Time: The present is viewed in the context of French history. Strictly adhering to schedules is not routinely expected; changing plans at the last minute is acceptable.

Death Rites: Chrysanthemums are used exclusively for funerals.

Food Practices and Intolerances: The main meal is usually at noon if that time is compatible with work schedules. A loaf of bread is torn rather than sliced.

National Childhood Immunizations: BCG before 6 and 18 years; DPT at 2, 3, 4, and 18 months; DT/Td at 6, 11, 15, and

18 years; IPV at 2, 3, 4, and 18 months and 6, 11, and 15 years; MMR at 12 months; measles at 9 months.

Other Characteristics: Carrying on a conversation with the hands in the pockets is not received well. Only written formal agreements are considered binding.

BIBLIOGRAPHY

Giger JN, Davidhizar RE: *Transcultural nursing: assessment and intervention,* ed 2, St. Louis, 1995, Mosby.

Hall ET, Hall MR: *Understanding cultural differences: Germans, French and Americans,* Yarmouth, Me, 1990, Intercultural Press.

Prosser MH: *The cultural dialogue,* Washington, DC, 1985, SIETAR.

Samovar LA, Porter RE: *Intercultural communication: a reader,* Belmont, Calif, 1985, Wadsworth.

Spector RE: *Cultural diversity in health & illness,* ed 4, Stamford, Conn, 1996, Appleton & Lange.

Storti C: *The art of crossing cultures,* Yarmouth, Me, 1990, Intercultural Press.

◆ GABON

MAP PAGE (317)

Location: This western African nation sits astride the equator along the Atlantic seaboard. Most of the country is covered by dense tropical forest.

Major Languages	Ethnic Groups		Major Religions	
French	Fang	25%	Christian	60%
Fang	Bapounou	10%	Muslim	1%
Myene	Other	65%	Indigenous and Other	39%

Ethnic/Race Specific or Endemic Diseases: ENDEMIC: Chloroquine-resistant malaria; yellow fever. RISK: Schistosomiasis. The AIDS rate per 100,000 is 25.34.

National Childhood Immunizations: BCG at birth; DPT at 6, 10, and 14 weeks; OPV at 6, 10, and 14 weeks; measles at 9 months; hep B at birth and 1 and 6 months; yellow fever at 12 months.

BIBLIOGRAPHY

No data located.

◆ GAMBIA

MAP PAGE (316)

Location: Referred to as "The Gambia," this smallest country of Africa is located on the Atlantic coast. The country is primarily savanna and is bisected by the wide Gambia River. Most major health care facilities are located on the south side of the river. Many people live at a subsistence level in bush villages.

Major Languages	Ethnic Groups		Major Religions	
English	Mandinka	42%	Muslim	90%
Mandinka	Fula	18%	Christian	9%
Wolof	Wolof	16%	Other	1%
Fula	Jola	10%		
Other	Serahuli and Other	14%		

Predominant Sick Care Practices: Biomedical; magico-religious; traditional.

Health Care Beliefs: Health promotion is important. The country's primary health care plan is considered an excellent model for other developing countries.

Ethnic/Race Specific or Endemic Diseases: ACTIVE: Yellow fever. ENDEMIC: Chloroquine-resistant malaria (including urban areas). RISK: Schistosomiasis and tuberculosis. Most young children are pneumococcus carriers. Infant, child, and maternal mortality rates are high. Hemoglobin levels below 10 g are common. The AIDS rate per 100,000 is 5.55.

Dominance Patterns: Polygamy is practiced. Traditionally the man occupies one house and his one to four wives and their children occupy another house.

Birth Rites: Both squatting and supine positions are used for birthing. Some believe that the father must provide the razor blade used to cut the umbilical cord. A special naming celebration with drums and dancing is held on the eighth day. A witch doctor (maribou) provides small leather pouches containing holy verses to be secured on a string and worn around the infant's neck for protection.

Death Rites: Muslim belief forbids organ donations or transplants. Muslim physicians may recommend transfusions to save lives. Autopsy is uncommon because the deceased must be buried intact. Cremation is not permitted. For Muslim burial the body is wrapped in special pieces of cloth and buried without a coffin in the ground.

Food Practices and Intolerances: Rice is the dietary staple. Groundnuts (peanuts) are grown.

Infant Feeding Practices: The newborn is given only warm water the first day. Breastfeeding is started the second day. Weaning foods such as sanyo, a local millet, tend to be low in energy and protein. Goats are often kept, but their milk is not commonly used in infant food preparation.

Child Rearing Practices: Family planning may not be acceptable. Female circumcision and excision is widespread in some groups.

National Childhood Immunizations: BCG at birth; DPT at 2, 3, and 4 months; OPV at birth and 2, 3, and 4 months; measles and yellow fever at 9 months; hep B at birth and 2 months.

BIBLIOGRAPHY

Campbell H, Byass P, Greenwood BM: Acute lower respiratory infections in Gambian children: maternal perception of illness, *Ann Trop Paediatr* 10(1):45, 1990.

Daly C, Pollard AJ: Traditional birth attendants in The Gambia, *Midwives Chron* 103(1227):104, 1990.

Gudmundsen AM: Building an infrastructure for international health promotion and disease prevention: the Peace Corps fellows program, *J Prof Nurs* 5(4):172, 1989.

Ho E: Midwifery training and practice in The Gambia, *Midwives Chron* 100(1191):109, 1987.

Hoare K: Health visiting in rural Gambia, *Health Visit* 64(1):19, 1991.

Hoare K: Tackling infant malnutrition in The Gambia, *Health Visit* 67(3):102, 1994.

Ross HM: Societal/cultural views regarding death and dying, *Top Clin Nurs* 1(1):1, 1981.

Slack P: Built on tradition, *Nurs Times* 84(47):40, 1988.

Wright J: Female genital mutilation: an overview, *J Adv Nurs* 24:251, 1996.

◆ GEORGIA

MAP PAGE (315)

Location: Formerly part of the Soviet Union, Georgia is located in southwestern Asia on the eastern shore of the Black Sea. It is characterized by snow-capped mountains, dense forests, fertile valleys, and turbulent rivers that provide abundant hydroelectric power.

Major Languages	Ethnic Groups		Major Religions	
Georgian	Georgian	70%	Georgian Orthodox	65%
Russian	Armenian	8%	Muslim	11%
	Russian	6%	Russian Orthodox	10%
	Other	16%	Other	14%

Ethnic/Race Specific or Endemic Diseases: The AIDS rate per 100,000 is 0.02.

National Childhood Immunizations: BCG at birth, between 5 and 6 years, and between 14 and 15 years; DPT at 2, 3, 4, and 18 months; OPV at 2, 3, 4, and 18 months; measles at 1 year; hep B at 2, 3, 4, and 18 months and 12 years.

BIBLIOGRAPHY

No data located.

◆ GERMANY

MAP PAGE (314)

Location: Following World War II, Germany was divided, with East Germany (German Democratic Republic) going to the Soviet Union and West Germany (Federal Republic of Germany) occupied by the United States. Reunification took place on October 3, 1990.

Major Language	Ethnic Groups		Major Religions	
German	German	95%	Protestant	45%
	Other	5%	Catholic	37%
			Other	18%

Predominant Sick Care Practices: Biomedical; magico-religious. Younger people tend to oppose technical medicine and consult herbalists instead. The "evil eye" and God are thought by some to cause illness.

Health Care Beliefs: Active involvement; passive role; health promotion important. Older people tend to take a passive health care role. Former East Germans may demonstrate less responsibility for their health promotion and care than former West Germans do.

Ethnic/Race Specific or Endemic Diseases: RISK: *Bordetella pertussis* (whooping cough) in parts of former West Germany. The AIDS rate per 100,000 is 1.70.

Health Team Relationships: Introductory social conversation is not encouraged; instead getting to the immediate issue is common. Patients often address the health professional by title rather than name. Patients may not ask questions of a health professional because this would be a challenge to that authority. Information may not be shared freely. Only the physician may give information to the patient. Nursing care is primarily technical, with high dependence on physicians.

Dominance Patterns: Males and females share responsibility in decision making; children can be involved. Many married women do not work outside the home.

Eye Contact Practices: Sustained direct eye contact indicates that the person listens, trusts, is somewhat aggressive, or, in some situations, is sexually interested. Looking inside a room is considered the same as entering the room; therefore doors are often kept closed.

Touch Practices: Touch is infrequent. A handshake is common at the beginning and end of an interaction.

Perceptions of Time: Punctuality in all situations is maintained. People are oriented to the present and near future. A strong consciousness of history is exhibited, particularly in the older generation. Business people end work promptly at 5 PM.

Pain Reactions: Strong, stoic behavior is exhibited. If feeling the pain is perceived as part of the healing process, it may be tolerated; otherwise, relief of pain is desired.

Birth Rites: Most deliveries occur in hospitals; the father may choose to be present during birth. High-risk infants are given an IM shot of vitamin K. Courses for natural childbirth, prenatal care, and postnatal care are popular. The birth rate in the former East Germany has dropped since reunification in part because of fewer governmental support systems.

Death Rites: Crying in private is expected. Cremation is becoming popular. A delay of 3 days to a week before burial may occur because of the bureaucratic processing of paperwork. German society tends to put the elderly in long-term care facilities.

Food Practices and Intolerances: Traditionally lunch is the preferred main meal; however, for working families it is dinner. Potatoes, other vegetables, bread, and thick soups are common. Champagne, beer, soft drinks, and meat are popular. Rolls are served only at breakfast, with cheese or ham. Hot coffee or tea is the morning beverage. Mealtime is the time to enjoy discussing political or intellectual issues.

Infant Feeding Practices: Breastfeeding is common, with bottle feeding introduced at 6 months to 1 year.

Child Rearing Practices: Mild discipline is common; reasoning is used to influence behavior.

National Childhood Immunizations: BCG at birth; DPT at 3, 4, and 5 months and 2 years; OPV at 3 and 5 months and 2 and 10 years; MMR at 15 months and 6 years; rubella for girls at 11 and 15 years.

Other Characteristics: Privacy, formality, and social distance are highly valued. With reunification, respect for the former East German sector is important. The thumbs up gesture may mean the number one.

BIBLIOGRAPHY

Anderson N: Different values . . . orthopaedic nursing . . . in France and Germany, *Nurs Times* 91(42):42, 1995.

Bueche MN: Maternal-infant health care: a comparison between the United States and West Germany, *Nurs Forum* 25(4):25, 1990.

Clift JM: Nursing education in Austria, Germany, and Switzerland, *IMAGE: J Nurs Sch* 29(1):89, 1997.

Condon JC, Yousef F: *An introduction to intercultural communication,* New York, 1975, Macmillan.

Davies BJ: Germany: healing the wounds, *Midwives Chron* 107(1276):198, 1994.

Dopson L: Health care in Germany, *Nurs Times* 84(17):33, 1988.

Finger H et al.: The epidemiological situation of pertussis in the Federal Republic of Germany, *Dev Biol Stand* 73:343, 1991.

Galanti GA: *Caring for patients from different cultures,* ed 2, Philadelphia, 1997, University of Pennsylvania Press.

Giger JN, Davidhizar RE: *Transcultural nursing: assessment and intervention,* ed 2, St. Louis, 1995, Mosby.

Goldberg RT: Comparison of the German and American systems of rehabilitation, *J Rehabil* 55(1):59, 1989.

Hall ET, Hall MR: *Understanding cultural differences: Germans, French and Americans,* Yarmouth, Me, 1990, Intercultural Press.

Language Research Center: *German-speaking people of Europe,* Provo, Utah, 1976, Brigham Young University.

Luegenbiehl DL: The birth system in Germany, *J Obstet Gynecol Neonatal Nurs* 14(1):45, 1985.

Prosser MH: *The cultural dialogue,* Washington, DC, 1985, SIETAR.

Rieke HJ: Contributor.

Samovar LA, Porter RE: *Intercultural communication: a reader,* Belmont, Calif, 1985, Wadsworth.

Spector RE: *Cultural diversity in health & illness,* ed 4, Stamford, Conn, 1996, Appleton & Lange.

Stewart EC, Bennett MJ: *American cultural patterns: a cross-cultural perspective,* rev ed, Yarmouth, Me, 1991, Intercultural Press.

Tinsley RL Jr, Woloshin DJ: Approaching German culture: a tentative analysis, reprint from *Die Unterrichtspraxis* 3(1):125, 1974.

van der Zee J et al.: Community nursing in Belgium, Germany and the Netherlands, *J Adv Nurs* 20(5):791, 1994.

Whetstone WR: Perceptions of self-care in East Germany: a cross-cultural empirical investigation, *J Adv Nurs* 12:167, 1987.

Wittich A, Murjahn B, Hartmann A: Solving conflict on the ward, *Nurs Times* 92(2):40, 1996.

◆ GHANA

MAP PAGE (316)

Location: Ghana was formerly the Gold Coast. Its southern border lies along the Gulf of Guinea in western Africa. The majority of people are black Africans with many different languages and a diverse ethnicity.

Major Languages	Ethnic Groups		Major Religions	
English	Akan	44%	Indigenous	38%
Akan	Moshi Dagomba	16%	Beliefs	
Moshi Dagomba	Ewe	13%	Muslim	30%
Ewe	Ga	8%	Christian	24%
Ga	Other	19%	Other	8%

Health Care Beliefs: Traditional healers include fetish priests and priestesses and herbalists. Treatment and information can be gotten from pharmacies and informal drug sellers. The traditional belief is that mental disorders are caused by a witch, sorcerer, or ancestor and can only be cured by a traditional healer.

Ethnic/Race Specific or Endemic Diseases: ACTIVE: Yellow fever. ENDEMIC: Chloroquine-resistant malaria; schistosomiasis; guinea worm disease; Burkitt's lymphoma. The AIDS rate per 100,000 is 14.77.

Health Team Relationships: The patient is expected to submit to the health care provider's plan. Mass media, churches, and religious organizations teach health education, as information flows routinely from the Ministry of Health. A town crier, also known as a "gong man," passes health information along in rural areas.

Families' Role in Hospital Care: In some places only patients with special diets may be provided with meals. Families may wash and cook for the patient. Some believe that hospitals are places to go to die.

Dominance Patterns: It is a polygamous society; however, men do not socialize with their wives. Some tribes are matrilineal. The traditional support for the extended family is decreasing, resulting in the abandonment of increased numbers of elderly.

Eye Contact Practices: Staring is taboo; however, direct eye contact is used in conversations.

Touch Practices: Men and women touch frequently in this culture.

Perceptions of Time: Punctuality is not important. Continuing a social interaction is more important than being punctual at another event.

Pain Reactions: The choice of analgesic for pain may be inappropriate, and people tend to take any analgesic they can get in any quantity.

Birth Rites: Approximately 70% of babies are delivered by untrained birth attendants. Once they are assured the babies are alive and well, mothers may not look at their infants for a while.

Food Practices and Intolerances: The main meal of three is in the evening. The staple food is boiled root crops mixed together. Fruit is eaten, often as a dessert. The right hand is used to eat because the left hand is used to clean oneself after elimination. Malnutrition is found in 30% to 50% of the population, and 50% do not have access to safe drinking water.

Infant Feeding Practices: Breastfeeding is almost universal.

Child Rearing Practices: Female circumcision and excision is widespread among some groups. The population is young, with 45% under 15 years old.

National Childhood Immunizations: BCG at birth; DPT at 6, 10, and 14 weeks; OPV at birth and 6, 10, and 14 months; measles and yellow fever at 9 months.

BIBLIOGRAPHY

Akiwumi A: In search of the 21st century nurse for Ghana, *Int Nurs Rev* 41(4):118, 1994.

Bosompra K: Dissemination of health information among rural dwellers in Africa: a Ghanaian experience, *Soc Sci Med* 29(9):1133, 1989.

Bowditch, Susan: Personal communication, July 24, 1991, Portland, Oregon.

Buckle G: A change for the better, *Nurs Times* 91(25):52, 1995.

Fosu GB: Women's orientation toward help-seeking for mental disorders, *Soc Sci Med* 40(8):1029, 1995.

McGinn T et al.: Private midwives: a new approach to family planning service delivery in Ghana, *Midwifery* 6(3):117, 1990.

Nagelkerk J: Nursing in Ghana, *J Nurs Adm* 24(9):17, 1994.

Osae-Addae M: Pain management of cancer in Ghana, *Cancer Nurs* 14(4):218, 1990.

Winsor C: A volunteer in Ghana, *Nurs Times* 18:8, 1983.

Wright J: Female genital mutilation: an overview, *J Adv Nurs* 24:251, 1996.

◆ GREECE

MAP PAGE (314)

Location: Situated on the Mediterranean Sea, Greece is the southernmost country on the Balkan Peninsula in southern Europe.

Major Languages	Ethnic Groups		Major Religions	
Greek	Greek	98%	Greek Orthodox	98%
English	Turkish	1%	Muslim	1%
French	Other	1%	Other	1%

Predominant Sick Care Practices: Biomedical; magico-religious.

Health Care Beliefs: The "evil eye" is usually cast by witches. Protective blue beads or stone charms are worn. Garlic or onions may be hung in the traditional home or worn on the body to prevent illness.

Ethnic/Race Specific or Endemic Diseases: RISK: Mediterranean-type G6PD deficiency; β-thalassemia; familial Mediterranean fever. The AIDS rate per 100,000 is 1.68.

Health Team Relationships: Nursing is not a valued profession.

Dominance Patterns: Love of family and respect for elders are strong values.

Eye Contact Practices: Staring in public is acceptable.

Touch Practices: Close proximity is maintained during conversation.

Pain Reactions: Passive reactions to pain are practiced.

Birth Rites: Most babies are delivered by physicians in the hospital.

Death Rites: The dying may be physically isolated, and truth of a terminal diagnosis may be withheld. Death at home is important. Folk culture incorporates a dread of death. Death rites serve to maintain a social relationship with the deceased. Children are not excluded from the rituals. Traditionally, a relative or elderly woman washes the body with water or wine. Rituals are not concluded until the body has been exhumed 5 years after death and the bones have been placed in an urn or a vault. For the rest of her life a widow wears dark mourning clothes. The widow's social support systems, providing food, hospitality, and companionship, may span several generations.

Food Practices and Intolerances: The main meal of the day is at noon.

Child Rearing Practices: Parents may be overprotective of daughters. Children depend heavily on the family.

National Childhood Immunizations: BCG at between 5 and 6 years; DPT at 2, 4, 6, and 18 months; DT/Td at between 14 and 16 years; OPV at 2, 4, 6, and 18 months and 4 years; MMR at 15 months and 10 years.

Other Characteristics: The head motions for "yes" and "no" are opposite those used in the United States. Because a man's body hair is linked to manhood, shaving body hair for treatments may be resisted or refused.

BIBLIOGRAPHY

Andrews MM, Boyle JS: *Transcultural concepts in nursing care,* ed 2, Philadelphia, 1995, Lippincott.

Dracopoulou S, Doxiadis S: Care of the dying in Greece: lament for the dead, denial for the dying, *Hastings Center Rep,* Aug 1988, p 15.

Eisenbruch M: Cross-cultural aspects of bereavement, Part 2: Ethnic and cultural variations in the development of bereavement practices, *Cult Med Psychiatry* 8(4):315, 1984.

Ierodiakonou CS: Adolescents' mental health and the Greek family: preventive aspects, *J Adolesc* 11(1):11, 1988.

Irujo S: An introduction to intercultural differences and similarities in nonverbal communication. In Wurzel JS: *Toward multiculturalism,* Yarmouth, Me, 1988, Intercultural Press.

Lofvander M, Papastavrou D: Clinical factors, psycho-social stressors and sick-leave patterns in a group of Swedish and Greek patients, *Scand J Soc Med* 18(2):133, 1990.

Parker G, Lipscombe P: Parental characteristics of Jews and Greeks in Australia, *Aust NZ J Psychiatry* 13(3):225, 1979.

Rosenbaum JN: Cultural care of older Greek Canadian widows within Leininger's theory of culture care, *J Transcultural Nurs* 2(1):37, 1990.

Rosenbaum JN: The health meanings and practices of older Greek-Canadian widows, *J Adv Nurs* 16(11):1320, 1991.

Solomon J: Critical care nursing, *Focus Crit Care* 13(3):10, 1986.

Spector RE: *Cultural diversity in health & illness,* ed 4, Stamford, Conn, 1996, Appleton & Lange.

Taylor R: Relactation in the Peloponnese, *Midwives* 108(1228):152, 1995.

Tripp-Reimer T: Retention of folk-healing practice (Matiasma) among four generations of urban Greek immigrants, *Nurs Res* 32(2):97, 1983.

◆ GRENADA

MAP PAGE (313)

Location: Located 100 miles from the South American coast, Grenada is the southernmost of the Caribbean Windward Islands.

Major Languages	Ethnic Groups		Major Religions	
English	African	99%	Catholic	53%
French Patois	Other	1%	Anglican	14%
			Other	33%

Ethnic/Race Specific or Endemic Diseases: The AIDS rate per 100,000 is 19.57.

National Childhood Immunizations: DPT at 3 weeks, between 4 and 5 weeks, between 5 and 6 weeks, and at 19 months; OPV at 3 weeks, between 4 and 5 weeks, and between 5 and 6 weeks; measles at 1 year; MMR at 12 months.

BIBLIOGRAPHY

DeVooght J, Walker K: Community mental health care in Grenada, *Int Nurs Rev* 36(1):22, 1989.

Walker K, DeVooght J: Invasion—new psychiatric facility: Grenada, *J Psychosoc Nurs Ment Health Serv* 27(1):37, 1989.

◆ GUATEMALA

MAP PAGE (312)

Location: Bordered on the north, west, and east by Mexico, Guatemala is the northernmost of the Central American nations. The cool highlands contain the heaviest population. The lands bordering the Caribbean and Pacific are tropical.

Major Languages	Ethnic Groups		Major Religions	
Spanish	Mestizo	56%	Catholic	88%
Indian Languages	Native American and Other	44%	Mayan and Other	12%

Predominant Sick Care Practices: Traditional herbs are incorporated into some health care. The nervo forza is a popular liquid vitamin taken to promote health. Shots may be preferred over pills. In rural areas health care comes from health promoters and midwives, and in some remote areas witch doctors are important providers.

Health Care Beliefs: Acute sick care only. Measures to cure acute problems are valued and are linked to preventive measures by some health care practitioners.

Ethnic/Race Specific or Endemic Diseases: ENDEMIC: Chloroquine-sensitive malaria; filaria. RISK: Malnutrition; diarrhea; lower respiratory tract infections; measles in young children. Vitamin A deficiency is the most common cause of childhood blindness. The AIDS rate per 100,000 is 0.98.

Health Team Relationships: Attempts to institute primary health care are strongly opposed. Family may care for all personal needs and sleep on mats around the patient's bed.

Perceptions of Time: Punctuality is not valued.

Food Practices and Intolerances: The Mayan dietary staples are corn and beans.

National Childhood Immunizations: BCG at birth; DPT at 3, 5, and 7 months and 5 and 12 years; OPV at birth and 2, 4, and 6 months; measles at 9 months.

BIBLIOGRAPHY

Annel MV: Overview—experience and community participation count in Guatemala, *Public Health Rev* 12(3-4):261, 1984.

Boyle JS: Caring practices in a Guatemalan Colonia. In Leininger MM: *Care: the essence of nursing and health,* Thorofare, NJ, 1984, Slack.

Boyle JS: Ideology and illness experiences of women in Guatemala, *Health Care Women Int* 6(1-3):73, 1985.

Broach J, Newton N: Food and beverages in labor, Part 1: Cross-cultural and historical practices, *Birth* 15(2):81, 1988.

Glittenberg J: Adapting health care to a cultural setting, *Am J Nurs* 74(12):2218, 1974.

Heggenhougen HK: Will primary health care efforts be allowed to succeed? *Soc Sci Med* 19(3):217, 1984.

Krauthahn K, Basarsky L: People of the corn: a nursing student experience in Guatemala, *Alberta Assoc of RNs* 51(4):18, 1995.

Kunkel P: Guatemala Journal: Part II, *Wash Nurse* 15(4):34, 1985.

Kunkel P: Guatemala Journal: Part III, *Wash Nurse* 16(6):10, 1985.

Kunkel P: Guatemala Journal: Part IV, *Wash Nurse* 15(8):9, 1985.

Kunkel P: Guatemala Journal: Part V, *Wash Nurse* 16(4):34, 1987.

Kunkel P: Guatemala Journal: Part VI, *Wash Nurse* 17(5):18, 1987.

Lechtig A et al.: Nutrition, family planning, and health promotion: the Guatemalan program of primary health care, *Birth* 9(2):97, 1982.

Luecke R: *A new dawn in Guatemala,* Prospect Heights, Ill, 1993, Waveland Press.

Richards F et al.: Knowledge, attitudes and perceptions (KAP) of onchocerciasis: a survey among residents in an endemic area in Guatemala, *Soc Sci Med* 32(11):1275, 1991.

Rowell M: Eradication of vitamin A deficiency with 5 cents and a vegetable garden, *J Ophthalmic Nurs Tech* 12(5):217, 1993.

Spector RE: *Cultural diversity in health & illness,* ed 4, Stamford, Conn, 1996, Appleton & Lange.

Stewart EC, Bennett MJ: *American cultural patterns: a cross-cultural perspective,* rev ed, Yarmouth, Me, 1991, Intercultural Press.

◆ GUINEA

MAP PAGE (316)

Location: This western African nation is located on the Atlantic and consists of a coastal plain, a mountainous region, a savanna interior, and a forest in the Guinea highlands.

Major Languages	Ethnic Groups		Major Religions	
French	Peul	40%	Muslim	85%
African Languages	Malinke	30%	Christian	8%
	Soussou	20%	Indigenous	6%
	Other	10%	Beliefs	
			Other	1%

Ethnic/Race Specific or Endemic Diseases: ACTIVE: Cholera; yellow fever. RISK: Chloroquine-resistant malaria; schistosomiasis. The AIDS rate per 100,000 is 9.10.

Death Rites: Muslim belief forbids organ donation or transplants. Muslim physicians may recommend transfusions to save lives. Autopsy is uncommon because the deceased must be buried intact. Cremation is not permitted. For Muslim burial the body is wrapped in special pieces of cloth and buried without a coffin in the ground.

National Childhood Immunizations: BCG at birth; DPT at 6, 10, and 14 weeks; OPV at 6, 10, and 14 weeks; measles at 9 months.

BIBLIOGRAPHY

Ross HM: Societal/cultural views regarding death and dying, *Top Clin Nurs* 1(1):1, 1981.

◆ GUINEA-BISSAU

MAP PAGE (316)

Location: Formerly Portuguese Guinea, Guinea-Bissau is located on the Atlantic coast of western Africa. Most of the country consists of rain forests, swamps, and mangrove-covered wetlands.

Major Languages	Ethnic Groups		Major Religions	
Portuguese	Balanta	30%	Indigenous	65%
Crioulo	Fulani	20%	Beliefs	
Other	Manjaca	14%	Muslim	30%
	Mandinga	13%	Christian	5%
	Papel and	23%		
	Other			

Ethnic/Race Specific or Endemic Diseases: ENDEMIC: Chloroquine-resistant malaria; yellow fever. RISK: Schistosomiasis. The AIDS rate per 100,000 is 7.38.

National Childhood Immunizations: BCG at birth; DPT at 6, 10, and 14 weeks; OPV at 6, 10, and 14 weeks; measles at 9 months.

BIBLIOGRAPHY

No data located.

◆ GUYANA

MAP PAGE (314)

Location: Formerly British Guiana, the country is located on the northern coast of South America. The low coastal areas are inhabited by 90% of the population. Highlands are in the south, and an extensive network of rivers runs from north to south.

Major Languages	Ethnic Groups		Major Religions	
English	East Indian	51%	Christian	57%
Indian Languages	Black and Mixed	43%	Hindu	33%
	Native American	4%	Muslim	9%
	European and Chinese	2%	Other	1%

Ethnic/Race Specific or Endemic Diseases: ENDEMIC: Chloroquine-resistant malaria; yellow fever; filariasis. The AIDS rate per 100,000 is 11.50.

National Childhood Immunizations: BCG at birth; DPT at 3 months, between 4 and 4½ months, between 5 and 5½ months, and at 18 months; OPV at 3 months, between 4 and 4½ months, between 5 and 5½ months, and at 18 months; measles at 9 months.

BIBLIOGRAPHY

Nathan MB, Stroom V: Prevalence of Wuchereria bancrofti in Georgetown, Guyana, *Bull Pan Am Health Organ* 24(3):301, 1990.

◆ HAITI

MAP PAGE (313)

Location: Located in the West Indies of the Caribbean, Haiti occupies the western one third of the island of Hispaniola; Haiti shares it with the Dominican Republic. Much of the mountainous northern soil is denuded. Haiti is known as the poorest nation in the Western Hemisphere.

Major Languages	Ethnic Groups		Major Religions	
French	Black	95%	Catholic	80%
Creole	Mulatto and	5%	Protestant	16%
	European		Other	4%
			Voodoo*	

*Regardless of their religion, as many as 90% of the people believe in voodoo.

Predominant Sick Care Practices: Biomedical; magico-religious. Western medical treatment is sought (including in rural areas) more often than traditional medicine is used. Belief in voodoo is important, as well as the belief in prayer and the healing power and protection of God against misfortune. Illnesses that are perceived to originate supernaturally or magically can be treated with voodoo medicine only. Ethno-medical beliefs about disease are based on maintenance of a hot/cold equilibrium within the body. Herbalists treat common disorders and specialize in the treatment of the "evil eye" (maldyok). Prevention is not a strong concept.

Health Care Beliefs: Passive and somewhat fatalistic role; acute sick care only. Traditional individuals may evaluate their illness according to symptoms previously experienced by close relatives.

Ethnic/Race Specific or Endemic Diseases: ENDEMIC: Chloroquine-sensitive malaria. Vitamin A deficiency is the most common cause of childhood blindness. The AIDS rate per 100,000 was reported by the country as zero for 1995.

Health Team Relationships: The doctor is the primary authority in hospital settings, and nurses are subordinate. If nurses are the only health care professionals available, they are afforded more respect. Patients believe that expert authority should dictate events. Disapproval with a health care professional will not be outwardly expressed, but contact will be severed.

Families' Role in Hospital Care: The family is required to stay with the patient and provide food and basic hygiene. Some may wait to be directed about how they can help.

Dominance Patterns: This is a matriarchal society. The family is a mutual support system; siblings remain close, even after marriage.

Eye Contact Practices: It is customary to hold eye contact with everyone except authority figures and the poor.

Perceptions of Time: Punctuality is not an important value. A formal social system of publishing one starting time exists when, in reality, the real starting time is later. Hope for the future promotes a future-oriented view; however, the society is oriented predominantly to the present.

Pain Reactions: A high tolerance for pain and discomfort exists, although some sources indicate a low threshold. Loud verbal expressions may be heard during labor.

Birth Rites: Some believe that they must continue sexual intercourse during pregnancy to keep the birth canal lubricated or that they must avoid exposing themselves to cold air during that time. Purgatives are regularly taken during pregnancy to cleanse impurities from the insides of the fetus, primarily from its blood and stomach. The child may receive laxatives to foster health and strength. Most babies are delivered at home with the mothers in a squatting or semiseated position. For believers in voodoo, the delivery is performed underneath a sheet because bright light during delivery is feared. Traditionalists may bury the placenta beneath the doorway at the birth site or burn it at a corner of the home. Infants are not named until after the confinement month. If they die during confinement, burial is done without ceremony. Postpartum confinement practices, however, are becoming less common. According to the hot/cold equilibrium theory, postpartum is the hottest state the body reaches, and mothers do not eat foods that are categorized as hot during this time. Nutmeg, castor oil, or spider webs placed on the umbilical cord may contribute to neonatal tetanus. Bellybands are commonly used. Haiti has one of the highest infant mortality rates in the world.

Death Rites: Death is believed to be caused by natural or supernatural circumstances. Relatives and friends expend considerable effort to be present when death nears. The family does not express grief out loud until most of the deceased's possessions have been removed from the home; then wailing and crying begin. People who are knowledgeable in the customs wash and dress the body and place it in a coffin. A priest may be summoned to conduct the burial service. Burial usually takes place within 24 hours, with no embalming. A popular local belief alleges that witch doctors use herbal substances to make people appear dead and bring them back to life later to enslave them. Because of this popular story, doubts exist about whether a person is truly dead or merely appears dead. White clothing represents death. During grieving, some may assume the symptoms of the deceased's last illness. Cremation is not acceptable.

Food Practices and Intolerances: The majority of people usually eat once a day. If they eat more than one meal, the largest is often at lunchtime. Water is taken only after the meal is finished. Women may wish to avoid cold orange juice while menstruating. The diet is spicy, with rice, beans, and plantains as staples. Being plump is considered healthy.

Infant Feeding Practices: Colostrum is not considered good milk. Its use is encouraged as a purgative (instead of castor oil) to rid the infant's body of meconium. Some mothers stop breastfeeding if the infant develops diarrhea; some believe that breast milk causes diarrhea or intestinal parasites. Breastfeeding is more common in rural areas and may be continued for 9 to 18 months. A plantain porridge supplement is given as early as 2 months. The median age for weaning is 6 months. A fat child is believed to be a healthy child.

Child Rearing Practices: It is customary to treat children in a harsh, strict manner and use corporal punishment such as spanking. Children who ask questions or seek information from parents are thought to show disrespect for parental authority. When adults are speaking, children are expected to remain quiet. Bottle-feeding is used as a pacifier to keep children quiet. Many children have multiple caretakers (relatives or friends). In cases of extreme poverty, children work after school to help support the family. Haitians are reluctant to discuss sex education or reproduction with those health care professionals who are not Haitian. Male circumcision is not encouraged. Bladder and bowel control is expected between 3 and 5 years of age. Early independence is promoted; very young children help with daily chores.

National Childhood Immunizations: (No recent data on file with WHO.) DPT-1 at 6 weeks; DPT-2 at 4 months; DPT-3 at 5 months; DPT booster 1 year after DPT-3; OPV-1 between birth and 6 weeks; OPV-2 at 4 months; OPV-3 at 5 months; OPV booster 1 year after OPV-3; measles at 9 months; BCG at birth.

BIBLIOGRAPHY

Adler MW, editor: Statistics from the World Health Organization and the Centers for Disease Control, *AIDS* 6(10):1229, 1992.

Andrews MM, Boyle JS: *Transcultural concepts in nursing care,* ed 2, Philadelphia, 1995, Lippincott.

Berggren GG et al.: Traditional midwives, tetanus immunization, and infant mortality in rural Haiti, *Trop Doct,* April 1983, p 79.

Berggren WL, Ewbank DC, Berggren GG: Reduction of mortality in rural Haiti through a primary health care program, *N Engl J Med* 304:1324, 1981.

Colin JM, Paperwalla G: Haitians. In Lipson JG, Dibble SL, Minarik PA: *Culture & nursing care: a pocket guide,* San Francisco, 1996, UCSF Nursing Press.

Colman RM: *The Haitian immigrant community in Connecticut,* Storrs, 1985, University of Connecticut.

Coreil J: Allocation of family resources for health care in rural Haiti, *Medicine* 17(11):709, 1983.

DeSantis L: Bridging the gap: cultural diversity in nursing, Unpublished manuscript, 1990.

DeSantis L, Tappen RM: Preventive health practices of Haitian immigrants. Paper presented at the West Virginia Nurses Association research symposium, Sulphur Springs, W Va, 1990.

DeSantis L, Thomas JT: Parental attitudes toward adolescent sexuality: transcultural perspectives, *Nurse Pract* 12(8):43, 1987.

DeSantis L, Thomas JT: The immigrant Haitian mother: transcultural nursing perspective on preventive health care for children, *J Transcultural Nurs* 2(1):2, 1990.

DeSantis L, Thomas JT: Health education and the immigrant Haitian mother: cultural insights for community health nurses, *Public Health Nurs* 9(2):87, 1992.

DeSantis L, Thomas JT: Childhood independence: views of Cuban and Haitian immigrant mothers, *J Pediatr Nurs* 9(4):258, 1994.

DeSantis L, Ugarriza DN: Potential for intergenerational conflict in Cuban and Haitian immigrant families, *Arch Psychiatr Nurs* IX(6):354, 1995.

Eisenbruch M: Cross-cultural aspects of bereavement, Part 2: Ethnic and cultural variations in the development of bereavement practices, *Cult Med Psychiatry* 8(4):315, 1984.

Gebrian BM: Contributor.

King KW et al.: Preventive and therapeutic benefits in relation to cost: performance over 10 years of mothercraft centers in Haiti, *J Clin Nutr* 31:679, 1978.

Kirkpatrick S, Cobb A: Health beliefs related to diarrhea in Haitian children: building transcultural nursing knowledge, *J Transcultural Nurs* 1(2):2, 1990.

Li GR: Funeral practices, New York, World Relief, n.d.

Rowell M: Eradication of vitamin A deficiency with 5 cents and a vegetable garden, *J Ophthalmic Nurs* 12(5):217, 1993.

St. Hill PF: Acceptability and use of family planning services by refugee Haitian women in Miami, doctoral dissertation, San Francisco, 1992, University of California, San Francisco.

Scalora S: *Haiti: flesh of politics, spirit of Vodun,* Storrs, 1991, University of Connecticut.

Smith-Campbell B: Haiti: an international nursing experience, *Kansas Nurse,* March 1988, p 4.

Thomas JT, DeSantis L: Feeding and weaning practices of Cuban and Haitian immigrant mothers, *J Transcultural Nurs* 6(2):34, 1995.

United Nations Children's Fund: *The status of the world's children,* 1989, Oxfordshire, United Kingdom, 1989, Oxford University Press.

◆ HONDURAS

MAP PAGE (312)

Location: Honduras is part of the north central section of Central America. Coastlines include the Caribbean Sea and the Pacific Ocean. Although Honduras is primarily mountainous, it also has fertile plateaus, a river valley, and a narrow coastal plain.

Major Languages	Ethnic Groups		Major Religions	
Spanish	Mestizo	90%	Catholic	97%
Indian Languages	Native American	7%	Protestant and Other	3%
	Black	2%		
	White	1%		

Predominant Sick Care Practices: The country has significant resources and traditional knowledge regarding herbal medicine; its combination of herbal and Western medicine is of interest to other countries. Honduras is one of the poorest countries in the Western Hemisphere; health promotion practices are not a high priority to the average person.

Ethnic/Race Specific or Endemic Diseases: ENDEMIC: Chloroquine-sensitive malaria; tuberculosis. RISK: Diarrhea;

malnutrition; respiratory diseases. The AIDS rate per 100,000 is 16.08. One in 10 has tuberculosis.

Dominance Patterns: Males dominate.

Infant Feeding Practices: The 1980s brought a marked increase in breastfeeding. The danger of diarrhea from contaminated food should be considered when determining age of weaning from the breast. Medicinal teas may be given when the infant is ill.

Child Rearing Practices: Approximately one half of the population is under 15 years of age.

National Childhood Immunizations: BCG at birth and 7 and 12 years; DPT at 2, 4, and 6 weeks; OPV at birth and 2, 4, and 6 weeks; measles at 9 months and between 1 and 14 years.

BIBLIOGRAPHY

Adler MW, editor: Statistics from the World Health Organization and the Centers for Disease Control, *AIDS* 6(10):1229, 1992.

Cohen RJ et al.: Effects of age of introduction of complementary foods on infant breast milk intake, total energy intake, and growth: a randomized intervention study in Honduras, *Lancet* 344(8918):288, 1994.

Educational News Service: Tuberculosis, octava causa de muerte en Honduras, *El Puente* 1(7):4, 1997.

Holmes P: Diary from Honduras, *Nurs Times* 83(50):24, 1987.

Levine ML: Teaching the peasant midwife, *Midwives Chron* 104(1240):142, 1991.

Markatos JL: Mission to Honduras, *Nurs Health Care* 16(3):132, 1995.

Popkin BM et al.: An evaluation of a national breast-feeding promotion programme in Honduras, *J Biosoc Sci* 23(1):5, 1991.

Quillian JP: Community health workers and primary health care in Honduras, *J Am Acad Nurse Pract* 5(5):219, 1993.

◆ HUNGARY

MAP PAGE (314)

Location: Hungary is a country of fertile, rolling plains that is located in central Europe.

Major Languages	Ethnic Groups		Major Religions	
Hungarian	Hungarian	97%	Catholic	68%
Other	German	2%	Calvinist	20%
	Gypsy and	1%	Lutheran"	5%
	Other		Other	7%

Predominant Sick Care Practices: Biomedical.

Health Care Beliefs: People are attempting to strengthen health promotion and primary care.

Ethnic/Race Specific or Endemic Diseases: RISK: Heart and lung diseases such as cancer and tuberculosis. The AIDS rate per 100,000 is 0.31.

Health Team Relationships: Nurses are subordinate to physicians. The pharmaceutical industry has always been highly developed. Illegal and corrupting gratuities for services are rampant.

Families' Role in Hospital Care: Some hospitals are letting mothers stay with their hospitalized babies.

Birth Rites: Pregnant women are required to see a state physician four times to be eligible for their confinement grant. Though physicians must be present, many deliveries are done by midwives. Hospital stay is 4 to 7 days long, and there is minimal contact beyond breastfeeding between mother and infant because of the hospital schedule. A health visitor is required to make a home visit within 24 hours after discharge. Visiting nurses help the family with baby care.

Food Practices and Intolerances: A heavy diet is traditional and is rich in carbohydrates. Breakfast includes buttered bread, cold cuts, and sausages, and recently cereals have been eaten. Lunch consists mostly of soups heavy in starch, broiled vegetables with meat, and sweet pastries. Common drinks are coffee and alcoholic beverages.

Infant Feeding Practices: Breastfeeding is encouraged, and gradual introduction to fresh fruit juice begins at 2 weeks. At 6 months the infant is introduced to mashed vegetables and cow's milk that is thinned with boiled water.

Child Rearing Practices: Children's health is monitored by health visitors until age 14; yearly vision and dental checkups are required.

National Childhood Immunizations: BCG between 3 and 42 days, between 10 and 11 years, at 16 and 18 years, and between 18 and 30 years; DPT at 3, 4, 5, and 36 months and 6 years; OPV at 4, 5, and 36 months and 6 years; IPV at 3 months; MMR at 15 months; measles at 11 years.

BIBLIOGRAPHY

Arrindell WA et al.: Cross-national generalizability of dimensions of perceived parental rearing practices: Hungary and the Netherlands: a correction and repetition with healthy adolescents, *Psychol Rep* 65(3 Part 2):1079, 1989.

Charles J: Hungary for change, *Nurs Times* 88(9):36, 1992.

Magyar EK: Personal communication, Sept 1997.

Mucha K et al.: The status of nursing administrators in Hungary, *Int Nurs Rev* 38(4):115, 1991.2

Porcsin I, Suranyi S: The hundred years of midwifery education in Debrecen, Part 2: Today's practice, future tasks (Hungarian), *Nover* 7(6):16, 1994.

Roemer MJ: Recent health system development in Poland and Hungary, *J Community Health* 19(3):153, 1994.

Salvage J: Health in Hungary, *Senior Nurse* 5(1):27, 1986.

Solomon J: Critical care nursing, *Focus Crit Care* 13(3):10, 1986.

Trevelyan J: Taking the waters: natural thermal springs to treat a wide variety of ailments, *Nurs Times* 86(40):38, 1990.

◆ ICELAND

MAP PAGE (314)

Location: This relatively isolated northern Atlantic island is Europe's most western point; it touches on the Arctic Circle. More than 13% is covered with snowfields and glaciers; it is one of the most volcanic regions in the world.

Major Language	Ethnic Groups		Major Religions	
Icelandic	Icelandish	99%	Lutheran	96%
	Other	1%	Unaffiliated and Other	4%

Ethnic/Race Specific or Endemic Diseases: Phenylketonuria. The AIDS rate per 100,000 is 1.21.

Health Team Relationships: Very little private health care exists. Physicians, nurses, and patients call each other by their first name, and health care professionals work collaboratively. Basic care is provided, but family can assist if desired and appropriate.

Dominance Patterns: Decision making is cooperative between parents; mothers are more influential, however, in the arena of child rearing. Living geographically close fosters a large extended family orientation.

Eye Contact Practices: Comfortable with direct eye contact.

Touch Practices: Low touch, but hand holding between nurse and patient appreciated as a supportive measure.

Pain Reactions: Patients don't complain; therefore pain is probably severe when medication is given. Often they won't ask for pain medication rather than bother the nurse.

Birth Rites: Almost all births occur in the hospital. Hospital stays range from 1 to 4 days. The semisitting position is common. The father and supportive individuals may be present. Normal deliveries are handled by midwives. A shower may be desired soon after delivery. Health visitors are available for home follow-up if desired.

Death Rites: Burial is in the ground 5 to 7 days after death; cremation is also practiced.

Food Practices and Intolerances: Daily cod liver oil is common during childhood and with some adults.

Infant Feeding Practices: Breastfeeding is very common and continues for at least 6 months.

Child Rearing Practices: Child rearing is permissive. During hospitalization of their children, parents have indicated the need for trust in the health care professional and the need for information; the need for support and guidance has been rated the lowest.

National Childhood Immunizations: DPT at 3, 4, 6, and 14 months and between 6 and 7 years; IPV at 6, 7, and 14 months and 4, 9, and 14 years; MMR at 18 months and 7 years.

Other Characteristics: Each member of a four-person nuclear family can have a different last name. For example, female child uses father's first name with "dóttir" added as her last name; male child uses father's first name with "son" added, mother keeps her own maiden name, and father has his own last name.

BIBLIOGRAPHY

Andrews MM, Boyle JS: *Transcultural concepts in nursing care,* ed 2, Philadelphia, 1995, Lippincott.

Einarsdóttir ES: Midwifery education in Iceland, *J Nurse Midwifery* 28(6):31, 1983.

Geissler EM: Personal observations, June 18-29, 1995.

Halldórsdóttir E: Personal communication, June 22, 1995.

Haraldsdóttir R: Quality issues and nursing education, *Nurs Standard* 9(2):6, 1994.

Kristjansdóttir G: Perceived importance of needs expressed by parents of hospitalized two to six year olds, *Scand J Caring Sci* 9(2):95, 1995.

Paine LL, Palsdóttir B: An American look at midwifery in Iceland, *J Nurse Midwifery* 32(5):319, 1987.

◆ INDIA

MAP PAGE (320)

Location: The world's most populous democracy extends from the Bay of Bengal on the east to the Arabian Sea on the west. India's three great river systems, the Ganges, Indus, and Brahmaputra, all have extensive deltas.

Major Languages	Ethnic Groups		Major Religions	
Hindi	Indo-Aryan	72%	Hindu	80%
English	Dravidian	25%	Muslim	14%
Other	Mongol and Other	3%	Christian	2%
			Sikh	2%
			Buddhist and Other	2%

Predominant Sick Care Practices: Those biomedical and traditional (Ayurveda) practices whose focus is on prevention of disease. Spiritual values permeate most aspects of life and death. Allopathic medicine may be used in almost all rural communities. The poorer use more informal or traditional systems of medicine.

Health Care Beliefs: Generally acute sick care is practiced; however, traditional medicine employs several principles of primary health care. Yoga is also practiced. Diseases are believed to be caused by an upset in body balance.

Ethnic/Race Specific or Endemic Diseases: ACTIVE: Cholera. ENDEMIC: Chloroquine-resistant malaria. Anemia in women. RISK: Japanese encephalitis; schistosomiasis. Vitamin A deficiency is the most common cause of childhood blindness. Overpopulation is the basis for many health problems. The AIDS rate per 100,000 is 0.12.

Health Team Relationships: Some women object to being examined by a male physician. Health care professionals do not discuss terminal illness with the patient; however, it may be discussed with the patient's relatives. Adults will not enter into the decision-making process if elderly parents are present. Nurses may not be able to influence health care decisions of patients and may work under medical or nontechnical personnel.

Dominance Patterns: Built on hierarchies within the family of age, sex, ordinal position, and kinship relationships or within the community based on caste, lineage, learning, wealth, occupation, and relationship with the ruling power. Unquestioned obedience to elders is expected. A male child is especially desired. The husband's ownership of his wife is quite pervasive and may permit violence and death without sanction under some circumstances. Women are dependent on men at every stage of life in traditional families; however, increased education and decision-making for some women are reported.

Touch Practices: Men may shake hands with other men but not with women. Instead, the man places his palms together and bows slightly. Bare upper arms or shoulders are considered indecent.

Perceptions of Time: Minimal future time perspective is demonstrated. People are more oriented to the past. The concept of time is closely allied with an infinite universe of unending cycles that extend beyond birth, life, and death.

Pain Reactions: The patient has a quiet acceptance of pain and will accept some relief measures.

Birth Rites: Voluntary sterilization in males is encouraged, with monetary incentives and prizes. Amniocentesis may be used to determine the sex of the fetus, and abortion is possible for a female. Cravings during pregnancy are satisfied because they are thought to be those of the fetus. Celebration of the birth of a son may include the beating of drums or blowing of conch shells. The midwife is paid a reward.

Death Rites: Hindu patients, often accepting God's will, may make indirect references to their own deaths. The patient's desire to be clearheaded as death approaches must be assessed in planning medical treatment. Provision of time and place for prayer is essential for the family members and patient; prayer helps them deal with anxiety and conflict. The Hindu priest or anyone present may read from the Holy Sanskrit books. Some priests tie strings (signifying a blessing) around the neck or wrist and, after death, pour water into the mouth of the deceased. Families may prefer that non-Hindus not touch the body and may wash the body themselves. Blood transfusions, organ transplants, and autopsies are permitted. Cremation is preferred. Reincarnation is a Hindu belief.

Food Practices and Intolerances: Beef is not eaten.

Infant Feeding Practices: Breastfeeding on demand is the norm, and supplementing with other foods starts between 6 months and 1 year; breastfeeding may continue up to 3 years.

Child Rearing Practices: The predominant theme in child rearing is protective nurturing. The child is indulged, cuddled, and held and remains intimately and strongly attached to its mother until age 3 or 4. The toddler is not pushed into toilet training. The female's childhood is shorter than the male's because domestic responsibilities occur early. Discipline in late childhood includes scolding and light spanking. Children are rarely praised for doing what is expected of them; praise may bring on the "evil eye."

National Childhood Immunizations: BCG at birth; DPT at 1½, 2½, and 3½ months and between 16 and 24 months; OPV at 1½, 2½, and 3½ months and between 16 and 24 months; measles between 9 and 11 months.

Other Characteristics: More male children receive immunizations than female children. Mortality statistics are higher for women than men, possibly because males receive preferential treatment. The Sikh religion forbids cutting or shaving any body hair. Older women enjoy a heightened social prestige. No expression for "thanks" exists; a social act is a fulfillment of an obligation or duty that requires no verbal acknowledgment. The motions of the head for "yes" and "no" are opposite those in the United States. Modern youngsters often follow the "Western" style rather than traditional customs regarding things such as premarital sex, establishing nuclear families, and choosing their own partners.

BIBLIOGRAPHY

Ahmad WI: Patients' choice of general practitioner: intolerance of patients' fluency in English and the ethnicity and sex of the doctor, *J R Coll Gen Pract* 39(321):153, 1989.

Basu AM: Cultural influences on health care use: two regional groups in India, *Stud Fam Plann* 21(5):275, 1990.

Becktell PJ: Endemic stress: environmental determinants of women's health in India, *Health Care Women Int* 15(2):111, 1994.

Clark MJ: *Nursing in the community,* Norwalk, Conn, 1992, Appleton & Lange.

Condon JC, Yousef F: *An introduction to intercultural communication,* New York, 1975, Macmillan.

Davis CF: Culturally responsive nursing management in an international health care setting, *Nurs Adm Q* 16(2):36, 1992.

Dickson GL: The metalanguage of menopause research, *IMAGE: J Nurs Sch* 22(3):168, 1990.

Discovery Channel: *A planet for the taking,* March 15, 1989.

Fisher P: Chinese population crises, Unpublished paper, SOC 107W, University of Connecticut, 1989.

Francis MR: Concerns of terminally ill adult Hindu cancer patients, *Cancer Nurs* 9(4):164, 1986.

Galanti GA: *Caring for patients from different cultures,* ed 2, Philadelphia, 1997, University of Pennsylvania Press.

Ghai S, Ghai CM: Health for all by 2000 ad: the role of Ayurveda, *Nurs J India* 85(6):122, 1994.

Green J: Hinduism, *Nurs Times* 85(6):50, 1989.

Irujo S: An introduction to intercultural differences and similarities in nonverbal communication. In Wurzel JS, editor: *Toward multiculturalism,* Yarmouth, Me, 1988, Intercultural Press.

Izhar N: Patient origins and usage of a Unani clinic in Aligarh Town, India, *Soc Sci Med* 30(10):1139, 1990.

Kakar S: The child in India. In Wurzel JS, editor: *Toward multiculturalism,* Yarmouth, Me, 1988, Intercultural Press.

Lally MM: Last rites and funeral customs of minority groups, *Midwife Health Visit Comm Nurse* 14(7):224, 1978.

Marchione J, Stearns SJ: Ethnic power perspectives for nursing, *Nurs Health Care* 11(6):296, 1990.

Meade RD: Future time perspectives of Americans and subcultures in India, *J Cross-cult Psychol* 3(1):93, 1972.

Patel NR: Nursing in India, *Nurs Adm Q* 16(2):72, 1992.

Pethe S: Changing socio-cultural value impact on family, *Nurs J India* LXXXVI(2):39, 1995.

Ramachandran H, Shastri GS: Movement for medical treatment: a study in contact patterns of a rural population, *Soc Sci Med* 17(3):177, 1983.

Rowell M: Eradication of vitamin A deficiency with 5 cents and a vegetable garden, *J Ophthalmic Nurs Tech* 12(5):217, 1993.

Samovar LA, Porter RE: *Intercultural communication: a reader,* Belmont, Calif, 1985, Wadsworth.

Sleed J: Manners abroad need study, Newhouse News Service, n.p., n.d.

Stewart EC, Bennett MJ: *American cultural patterns: a cross-cultural perspective,* rev ed, Yarmouth, Me, 1991, Intercultural Press.

Storti C: *The art of crossing cultures,* Yarmouth, Me, 1990, Intercultural Press.

Ullrich ME: A study of change and depression among Havik Brahmin women in a south Indian village, *Cult Med Psychiatry* 11(3):261, 1987.

Weisfeld GE: Sociobiological patterns of Arab culture, *Ethnol Sociobiol* 11:23, 1990.

◆ INDONESIA

MAP PAGE (321)

Location: Part of the Malay Archipelago along the equator in southeastern Asia, Indonesia consists of 13,677 islands; approximately 6000 are inhabited. The mountains and plateaus in the major islands have a cooler climate than the tropical lowlands.

Major Languages	Ethnic Groups		Major Religions	
Indonesian	Javanese	45%	Muslim	87%
English	Sundanese	14%	Protestant	6%
Dutch	Madurese	8%	Catholic	3%
Javanese	Malay	8%	Hindu	2%
	Other	25%	Other	2%

Predominant Sick Care Practices: Magico-religious. Belief in ancestor spirits, who are engaged in all aspects of life, is widespread. The adat (the way of the ancestors) governs rituals performed at births and funerals, as well as many other aspects of behavior.

Ethnic/Race Specific or Endemic Diseases: ACTIVE: Cholera. ENDEMIC: Chloroquine-resistant malaria, with no risk in major cities. RISK: Japanese encephalitis; schistosomiasis. Vitamin A deficiency is the most common cause of childhood blindness. The AIDS rate per 100,000 is 0.01.

Health Team Relationships: Clients may consider titles more important than names.

Dominance Patterns: The roles of men and women are defined in the Koran; women have limited possibilities.

Eye Contact Practices: Looking someone in the eye, especially for a woman, is improper and disrespectful.

Birth Rites: Having many children is valued. Children are the support of and a source of security for their parents in old age. Free birth control methods are available from the government and are distributed through health stations and in small shops.

Death Rites: Muslim belief forbids organ donations or transplants. Muslim physicians may recommend transfusions to save lives. Autopsy is uncommon because the deceased must be buried intact. Cremation is not permitted. For Muslim burial the body is wrapped in special pieces of cloth and buried without a coffin in the ground.

Food Practices and Intolerances: Pork, carrion, and blood are forbidden. During Ramadan, the Islamic month of fasting, breakfast has to be eaten before dawn; this is followed by a ritual washing to prepare for morning prayer, which must coincide with sunrise. During the day, eating or drinking is forbidden, with exceptions for children, the elderly, and the sick. At dusk, after the fourth ritual prayer of the day, the time for fasting is concluded.

Infant Feeding Practices: Breastfeeding is believed best for 18 months or longer, and about one third of the people question the value of feeding colostrum.

National Childhood Immunizations: BCG at birth; DPT at 2, 3, and 4 months and at admission to school; OPV at birth and 2, 3, 4, and 9 months; measles at 9 months; hep B at birth and 4 and 11 months.

Other Characteristics: Many Indonesians use only one name professionally and socially. Men are allowed to have up to four wives at the same time. Carrying on a conversation with hands in the pockets is not received well; hands on the hips is perceived as defiance. The gesture of curling the index finger inward is used to call animals only.

BIBLIOGRAPHY

Associated Press: Quake, tidal wave kills at least 10 in New Guinea, Hartford Courant, Feb 18, 1996, p A17.

Hamke K, Kievelitz U: *Climbing the intercultural ladder: the gradual adaptation process to a village culture in Indonesia,* New York, 1986, AFS International/Intercultural Programs.

Hull V, Thapa S, Pratomo H: Breast feeding in the modern health sector in Indonesia: the mother's perspective, *Soc Sci Med* 30(5):625, 1990.

Lickiss JN: Indonesia: status of cancer pain and palliative care, *J Pain Symptom Manage* 8(6):423, 1993.

Paige RM: Formal education and psychosocial modernity in East Java, Indonesia, *Int J Intercult Relations* 3:333, 1979.

Ross HM: Societal/cultural views regarding death and dying, *Top Clin Nurs* 1(1):1, 1981.

Rowell M: Eradication of vitamin A deficiency with 5 cents and a vegetable garden, *J Ophthalmic Nurs Tech* 12(5):217, 1993.

Samovar LA, Porter RE: *Intercultural communication: a reader,* Belmont, Calif, 1985, Wadsworth.

U.S. Agency for International Development: Indonesia lowers infant mortality, *Front Lines* 31(10):16, 1991.

Wikan U: Bereavement and loss in two Muslim communities: Egypt and Bali compared, *Soc Sci Med* 27(5):451, 1988.

◆ IRAN

MAP PAGE (318)

Location: This ancient land of Persia is an Islamic republic in the oil-rich Middle East. Although much is desert, there are oases, maritime lowlands along the Persian Gulf, and the Caspian Sea and mountains in the north. The populated areas are in the north and northwest. Iranians are stereotyped as Arabs; however, the Iranian language and culture are similar in some areas but different in others.

Major Languages	Ethnic Groups		Major Religions	
Farsi	Persian	51%	Shi'a Muslim	93%
Turkish	Azerbaijani	24%	Sunni Muslim	4%
Kurdish	Kurdish	7%	Baha'i and	3%
Arabic	Arab and	18%	Other	
English	Other			

Predominant Sick Care Practices: Biomedical; magico-religious. Various beliefs in the causes of disease, such as the hot/cold humoral theory and the "evil eye," coexist. A physically robust person is considered healthier. Emotional distress, especially fear, anger, and grief, with irregular cardiac rate may be expressed as "heart distress."

Health Care Beliefs: Acute sick care only. Medications by injection may be preferred. Patients who do not receive a written prescription may believe that the physician did not properly treat them.

Ethnic/Race Specific or Endemic Diseases: ENDEMIC: Chloroquine-resistant malaria, with no risk in urban areas. RISK: Schistosomiasis. The AIDS rate per 100,000 is 0.01.

Health Team Relationships: The physician's authority is not questioned; the patient and family may not ask questions or give any information that might be construed as disrespectful. The reason for personal questions during assessment needs to be made clear to the patient. Males may refuse care by female physicians and nurses. Aggressiveness, toughness, and even pushiness are acceptable behaviors for ensuring good care. The patient may agree with health care professionals to avoid embarrassment.

Families' Role in Hospital Care: Being a patient means assuming a passive role. Bad news is usually kept from the patient. A patient may be accompanied by one or more persons who wish to be present during examination and answer questions for the patient. The eldest person present must be included in the discussion. The family role is fulfilled by demanding behavior and extreme concern and attention. Repetition in communication is commonly used for emphasis and to indicate the importance of the matter.

Dominance Patterns: It is a patriarchal society. Children are expected to submit to the authority of the father. The family and its position in society predominate, rather than the individual.

Eye Contact Practices: Eye contact is accepted between equals. A woman's making direct eye contact with a man implies promiscuity and an interest in dating.

Touch Practices: Touch is frequent, as are closeness and embracing on arrival and departure. The personal space desired between two people is relatively small.

Perceptions of Time: Punctuality is not important; establishing a relationship before talking business is more important. On-time demands in business arenas, however, are usually observed.

Pain Reactions: Pain is usually expressed. The Iranian woman may yell throughout labor. The custom is to compensate a woman for her suffering during childbirth by giving her gifts.

Birth Rites: Restrictions do not exist during pregnancy. A suspected pregnancy may not be announced, even to the father. Women may shave their bodies in preparation for childbirth. Birth occurs at home, especially in rural villages. The husband is not present but may be nearby. Males are circumcised anytime after birth until age 5. Dietary restrictions for the mother may be in effect for 40 days after the birth.

Death Rites: Impending death is concealed from the patient by any means possible. Muslim belief forbids organ donations or transplants. Muslim physicians may recommend transfusions to save lives. A Holy Iman does not have to be present at death. A Muslim should recite the Declaration of the Faith or help the patient to recite it; it is as follows: "There is no God but God, and Muhammed is his Messenger." Grief is not permitted in the dying person's presence. After death, family members wash the body, according to Islamic tradition, before the funeral. Once death has occurred, mourning is loud, obvious, and expressive. Autopsy is uncommon because the deceased must be buried intact, without embalming or a casket. Cremation is not permitted.

Food Practices and Intolerances: The main meal is at midday. Islamic law does not permit the consumption of pork, alcohol, or meat that has not been slaughtered according to the Islamic code. In poorer families the male may receive the most nutritious food. Ramadan fasting is observed between sunrise and sunset, with exemptions for children and the sick. Rice, wheat bread, and dairy products are common, along with fruit as a dessert.

Infant Feeding Practices: Pacifiers are acceptable. Weaning may be abrupt at age 2. Supplementary foods are given beginning at 4 to 5 months.

Child Rearing Practices: Fathers have greater control of resources and have the authoritarian power, whereas mothers exert greater control in child nurturing and value transmission. Belief dictates that excessive praise of a child may cast the evil eye. Toilet training may begin as early as 3 months. Traditional girls wear the veil at age 7 or earlier. Girls are taught to look straight ahead and never to look at men when they are outside. Boys and girls no longer play together after age 5. Discipline of male children is limited. Male circumcision is practiced.

National Childhood Immunizations: BCG at birth; DPT at 1½, 3, 4½, and 15 months and between 4 and 6 years; OPV at birth, 1½, 3, 4½, and 15 months, and between 4 and 6 years; measles at 9 and 15 months; hep B at birth and 1½ and 9 months.

Other Characteristics: The U.S. finger gestures for thumbs up and the V are insulting. Close distance is kept during conversation.

BIBLIOGRAPHY

Andrews MM, Boyle JS: *Transcultural concepts in nursing care,* ed 2, Philadelphia, 1995, Lippincott.

Galanti GA: *Caring for patients from different cultures,* ed 2, Philadelphia, 1997, University of Pennsylvania Press.

Green J: Death with dignity: Islam, *Nurs Times* 85(5):56, 1989.

Hafizi H: Iranians. In Lipson JG, Dibble SL, Minarik PA: *Culture & nursing care: a pocket guide,* San Francisco, 1996, UCSF Nursing Press.

Kendall K: Maternal and child care in an Iranian village, *J Transcultural Nurs* 3(1):29, 1992.

Lally MM: Last rites and funeral customs of minority groups, *Midwife Health Visit Comm Nurse* 14(7):224, 1978.

Lipson JG, Meleis AI: Issues in health care of Middle Eastern patients, *West J Med* 139(6):854, 1983.

Luna LJ: Transcultural nursing: care of Arab Muslims, *J Transcultural Nurs* 1(1):22, 1989.

Meleis AI, LaFever CW: The Arab American psychiatric care, *Perspect Psychiatr Care* 22(2):72, 1984.

Pari M, Mura A: Cyclical evolution of nursing education and profession in Iran: religious, cultural, and political influences, *J Prof Nurs* 11(1):58, 1995.

Ross HM: Societal/cultural views regarding death and dying, *Top Clin Nurs* 1(1):1, 1981.

Spector RE: *Cultural diversity in health & illness,* ed 4, Stamford, Conn, 1996, Appleton & Lange.

Stewart EC, Bennett MJ: *American cultural patterns: a cross-cultural perspective,* rev ed, Yarmouth, Me, 1991, Intercultural Press.

Tashakkori A, Thompson VD: Effects of family configuration variables on reported indices of parental power among Iranian adolescents, *Soc Biol* 35(1-2):82, 1988.

◆ IRAQ

MAP PAGE (318)

Location: Iraq occupies the valley between the Tigris and Euphrates rivers. Mountains are located in the north, and desert is found in the southwest; marshland lies along the Persian Gulf.

Major Languages	Ethnic Groups		Major Religions	
Arabic	Arab	75%	Shi'a Muslim	62%
Kurdish	Kurdish	17%	Sunni Muslim	35%
Assyrian	Other	8%	Christian and Other	3%
Armenian				

Ethnic/Race Specific or Endemic Diseases: ENDEMIC: Chloroquine-sensitive malaria. RISK: Schistosomiasis. The AIDS rate per 100,000 is 0.03.

Health Team Relationships: The reason for asking the patient personal questions during assessment needs to be made clear. Males may refuse care by female physicians and nurse practitioners. Nursing is a female profession with a low status and negative image.

Families' Role in Hospital Care: A patient may be accompanied by one or more persons who wish to be present during examination and answer questions for the patient. The eldest person present expects to be included in the discussion. The family role is fulfilled through demanding behavior and extreme concern and attention.

Dominance Patterns: It is a patriarchal society. Sexual inequities are part of the legal system that relegates women to an inferior status. However, women exercise power in the domestic arena.

Touch Practices: Touch, closeness, and embracing on arrival and departure are common.

Perceptions of Time: The society is oriented to the present because planning ahead may defy God's will. Punctuality is not important; establishing a relationship before talking business is more important.

Pain Reactions: Pain relief is expected to be immediate and may be requested persistently. Therapies requiring exertion contraindicate the people's belief in energy conservation for recovery. Pain is usually expressed privately or only with close relatives and friends. However, during labor and delivery, pain may be expressed vehemently.

Death Rites: Muslim belief forbids organ donations or transplants. Muslim physicians may recommend transfusions to save lives. Autopsy is uncommon because the deceased must be buried intact. Cremation is not permitted. For Muslim burial the body is wrapped in special pieces of cloth and buried without a coffin in the ground.

Food Practices and Intolerances: Pork, carrion, and blood are forbidden. Food tends to be spicy. Ramadan fasting is practiced between sunrise and sunset, with exemptions for children and the sick.

Child Rearing Practices: A government-sponsored fertility campaign encourages families to have at least five children.

National Childhood Immunizations: BCG at birth; DPT at 2, 4, and 6 months; OPV at birth and 2, 4, and 6 months; measles at 9 and 15 months; hep B at birth and 1½ and 9 months.

Other Characteristics: Hope, optimism, and the positive advantages of treatment need to be stressed. Negative effects and outcomes should be minimized.

BIBLIOGRAPHY

Andrews MM, Boyle JS: *Transcultural concepts in nursing care,* ed 2, Philadelphia, 1995, Lippincott.

Carlisle D: Sanctioned to starve: how Iraq's children pay the price of the international blockade, *Nurs Times* 92(2):16, 1996.

Green J: Death with dignity: Islam, *Nurs Times* 85(5):56, 1989.

Meleis AI, LaFever CW: The Arab American and psychiatric care, *Perspect Psychiatr Care* 22(2):72, 1984.

Meleis AI, Sorrell L: Arab American women and their birth experiences, *MCN Am J Matern Child Nurs* 6:171, 1981.

Reizian A, Meleis AI: Arab-Americans' perceptions of and responses to pain, *Crit Care Nurse* 6(6):30, 1986.

Ross HM: Societal/cultural views regarding death and dying, *Top Clin Nurs* 1(1):1, 1981.

◆ IRELAND

MAP PAGE (314)

Location: Ireland, an island country in the Atlantic Ocean, is separated from Britain by the Irish Sea. The country is generally bowl shaped; a central plain is surrounded by low mountains. The highest peak is 3415 feet (1041 m).

Major Languages	Ethnic Groups		Major Religions	
Irish (Gaelic)	Irish	99%	Catholic	93%
English	Other	1%	Anglican	3%
			Other	4%

Health Care Beliefs: There is a major shift toward primary health care.

Ethnic/Race Specific or Endemic Diseases: RISK: Phenyl-ketonuria; neural tube defects; high mortality from coronary heart disease. The AIDS rate per 100,000 is 1.21.

Health Team Relationships: Nurses' professional views may not be taken into account.

Pain Reactions: The Irish are typically inexpressive and stoic; they do not vocalize pain and are less apt to describe pain as intense. They prefer company but will try to hide pain from family and friends. The desire to be alone after freely admitting pain is also possible.

Death Rites: The practice of watching or "waking" the dead originates from keeping vigil to keep evil spirits away from the deceased; it has become a religious ritual.

National Childhood Immunizations: BCG at birth and 12 years; DPT at 2, 3, and 4 months and 5 years; OPV at 2, 3, and 4 months and 5 years; MMR at 15 months and 12 years.

BIBLIOGRAPHY

Andrews MM, Boyle JS: *Transcultural concepts in nursing care,* ed 2, Philadelphia, 1995, Lippincott.

Broach J, Newton N: Food and beverages in labor, Part 1: Cross-cultural and historical practices, *Birth* 15(2):81, 1988.

Chavasses J: Shaping a healthier future in the Republic of Ireland, *Br J Nurs* 3(14):700, 1994.

Craughwell K: Letter from Ireland, *Nurs Times* 91(16):145, 1995.

Galanti GA: *Caring for patients from different cultures,* ed 2, Philadelphia, 1997, University of Pennsylvania Press.

Lipton JA, Marbach JJ: Ethnicity and the pain experience, *Soc Sci Med* 19(12):1279, 1984.

Martinelli AM: Pain and ethnicity: how people of different cultures experience pain, *AORN J* 46(2):273, 1987.

Shelley E et al.: The Kilkenny Health Project: a community research and demonstration cardiovascular health programme, *Ir J Med Sci Suppl* 160(9):10, 1991.

Spector RE: *Cultural diversity in health & illness,* ed 4, Stamford, Conn, 1996, Appleton & Lange.

Stone FA: *The Irish in their homeland, in America, in Connecticut,* Storrs, 1975, World Education Project, School of Education, University of Connecticut.

◆ ISRAEL

MAP PAGE (318)

Location: Formerly Palestine, Israel is located at the eastern end of the Mediterranean Sea. The coastal plain is fertile, and the southern region is primarily desert.

Major Languages	Ethnic Groups		Major Religions	
Hebrew	Jewish	82%	Jewish	82%
Arabic	Arab and	18%	Muslim	14%
English	Other		Christian	2%
French			Druze	2%

Predominant Sick Care Practices: Curative, preventive, and promotive care.

Health Care Beliefs: Passive role. A tendency toward passivity exists, and health self-care is not prevalent. Religion is part of daily life. Orthodox Jews may prefer not to travel, write, or turn on electrical appliances on the Sabbath.

Ethnic/Race Specific or Endemic Diseases: RISK: Infantile Tay-Sachs disease; infantile Niemann-Pick disease; adult Gaucher's disease; Mediterranean fever; diabetes; atherosclerosis; hypertension. The AIDS rate per 100,000 is 0.96.

Health Team Relationships: Assertiveness and toughness are acceptable behaviors.

Touch Practices: Touching is demonstrative.

Perceptions of Time: Orientation toward the present is continuous, whereas future orientation decreases with age and past orientation increases.

Pain Reactions: Descriptive adjectives may be used, and overt suffering may be a way to get help and sympathy.

Birth Rites: Orthodox Jews do not allow the husband to touch his laboring wife or be present at the birth. His support comes from praying and reading Psalms. Traditionally, the newborn is believed to be susceptible to evil influences during the first week of life. Circumcision is performed on the eighth day of life.

Death Rites: In the Orthodox custom a relative remains with the dying person to ensure that the soul does not leave the body when the dying person is alone. It would also be a sign of disrespect to leave the body alone. Rituals may start before death has occurred. Embalming and the use of cosmetics are not part of traditional practice. Autopsy is forbidden unless reasons for death are suspicious. Organ donation is permitted but only to other Jews. Burial in the ground (within 24 hours but delayed by the Sabbath) is part of Jewish law; some more liberal people use cremation. The eyes of the deceased should be closed at death, and the body should be left covered and untouched until a family member or a Jewish undertaker is contacted for ritual proceedings.

Food Practices and Intolerances: Pig, rabbit, and shellfish are not eaten by Orthodox Jews. Milk and meat are not taken at the same meal. If kosher meat is not available, a vegetarian diet is acceptable.

Child Rearing Practices: At age 13 the male celebrates becoming an adult with a ceremony of bar mitzvah.

National Childhood Immunizations: BCG at 13 years; DPT at 2, 4, 6, and 12 months and 8 years; OPV at 4, 6, and 12 months and 6 years; IPV at 2, 4, and 12 months; MMR at 15 months; measles at 6 and 14 years; hep B at birth and 1 and 6 months.

BIBLIOGRAPHY

Andrews MM, Boyle JS: *Transcultural concepts in nursing care,* ed 2, Philadelphia, 1995, Lippincott.

Callister LC: Cultural meanings of childbirth, *J Obstet Gynecol Neonatal Nurs* 24(4):327, 1995.

Ellencweig AY, Grafstein O: Inequity in health: a case study, *Eur J Epidemiol* 5(2):244, 1989.

Galanti GA: *Caring for patients from different cultures,* ed 2, Philadelphia, 1997, University of Pennsylvania Press.

Green J: Death with dignity: Judaism, *Nurs Times* 85(8):64, 1989.

Lomranz J et al.: The meaning of time-related concepts across the life-span: an Israeli sample, *Int J Aging Hum Dev* 21(2):87, 1985.

Martinelli AM: Pain and ethnicity: how people of different cultures experience pain, *AORN J* 46(2):273, 1987.

Musgrave C: Rituals of death and dying in Israeli Jewish culture, *Eur J Palliat Care* 2(1):83, 1995.

Dominance Patterns: The trend is matrifocal—for women to have independence. Having a lifetime partner is not important; therefore several different fathers may visit with their children in one household.

Perceptions of Time: Rewards for current activity are preferred over delayed gratification.

Birth Rites: Traditional practices may include smelling the perspiration on the father's shirt to speed labor.

Food Practices and Intolerances: A national dish is ackee and saltfish. Among the poor, coconut oil is used for cooking because it is less expensive; lack of electricity and refrigeration promotes salting to preserve food. Both these factors contribute to hypertension.

Infant Feeding Practices: Even though the rate of infant mortality caused by malnutrition is high, breastfeeding is declining, especially after age 3 months. Carbohydrate gruels, porridge, fruit juices, and herbal teas are bottle-fed at an early age. Mothers from urban middle-income groups terminate breastfeeding earlier than lower-income mothers.

Child Rearing Practices: Mothers often live in an extended family or alone with their children. Infants are often carried and can suckle on demand. Control over aggressive behavior is encouraged.

National Childhood Immunizations: BCG at birth and 3 months; first dose of DPT between 6 and 12 weeks, with 2 more doses at 4-to-8 week intervals and at 18 months and 7 years; first dose of OPV between 6 and 12 weeks, with 2 more doses at 4-to-8 week intervals and at 18 months; MMR at 10 months.

Other Characteristics: Diarrhea is called "runny belly," and vitamins are referred to as "tonic." A love of music and dance is a deep cultural value and may be used as a vehicle for conveying health concepts.

BIBLIOGRAPHY

Bailey KM: Cross cultural experience in Jamaica, *Maine Nurse* 75(20):6, 1989.

Bates B, Turner AN: Imagery and symbolism in the birth practices of traditional cultures, *Birth* 12(1):29, 1985.

Brinday J et al.: Chemical burns as assault injuries in Jamaica, *J Psychol* 22(2):154, 1996.

Cunningham WC, Segree W: Breast feeding promotion in an urban and a rural Jamaican hospital, *Soc Sci Med* 30(3):341, 1990.

Dechesnay M: Jamaican family structure: the paradox of normalcy, *Fam Process* 25:293, 1986.

Giugliani ERJ, Lovel H, Ebrahim GJ: Attitudes, practices and knowledge of health professionals on breast feeding in Kingston, Jamaica, *J Trop Pediatr* 34(4):169, 1988.

Grant M, Hezekiah J: Knowledge and beliefs about hypertension among Jamaican female clients, *Int J Nurs Stud* 33(1):58, 1996.

Green HB: Temporal attitudes in four Negro subcultures, *Studium Generale* 23(6):571, 1970.

Lambert MC, Weisz JR, Knight F: Over- and undercontrolled clinic referral problems of Jamaican and American children and adolescents: the culture general and the culture specific, *J Consult Clin Psychol* 57(4):467, 1989.

Mason C: Women as mothers in Northern Ireland and Jamaica: a critique of the transcultural nursing movement, *Int J Nurs Stud* 27(4):367, 1990.

Sobo EJ: Abortion traditions in rural Jamaica, *Soc Sci Med* 42(4):495, 1996.

Standard KL, Minott OD: A song and a dance, *World Health,* Apr-May 1983, p 5.

Stewart EC, Bennett MJ: *American cultural patterns: a cross-cultural perspective,* rev ed, Yarmouth, Me, 1991, Intercultural Press.

◆ JAPAN

MAP PAGE (319)

Location: A Pacific Ocean archipelago, Japan extends 1744 miles (2790 km) north to south and is separated from the east coast of Asia by the Sea of Japan. The main islands have mountains that are separated by narrow fissures and valleys.

Major Language	Ethnic Groups		Major Religions	
Japanese	Japanese	99%	Shinto Buddhist	84%
	Korean	1%	Other	16%

Predominant Sick Care Practices: Magico-religious. Consultation with priests to seek luck and avoid evil may precede important activities or decisions.

Health Care Beliefs: Physical diseases are placed in the context of the patient's social relations.

Ethnic/Race Specific or Endemic Diseases: RISK: Japanese encephalitis; schistosomiasis; acatalasemia; cleft lip or palate; Oguchi's disease. The AIDS rate per 100,000 is 0.21.

Health Team Relationships: Respect for social rank is pervasive. The physician is expected to know best and use good judgment; consent forms are not generally used. Deference to caregivers' authority results in few questions. People who ask questions involving a "no" answer often fail to get an accurate answer or needed information. "I'll do my best" is a polite way of declining. Titles are important; they may be used rather than the names of caregivers. Patterns of thought are expressed indirectly; the listener is expected to get the point without being explicitly told. Asking the question "What?" is preferred. Increasingly refined details will be uncovered with each question. The patient may divert the subject away from an embarrassing topic or avoid direct confrontation. Patient complaints may be made by a third-party mediator or may be indirectly indicated by the patient. Individual verbal agreement does not mean compliance. The family is consulted before medical decisions are made.

Families' Role in Hospital Care: Family interdependence takes precedence over independence; therefore self-care is not an important concept. Family participation in care is expected. The patient's mother or someone else gives personal care 24 hours a day.

Dominance Patterns: Women are traditionally passive and domesticated. The woman has power in rearing children, in family budgeting, and in achieving success in school. Parents expect their children to care for them in their old age. Many of these traditional patterns are changing, however, in today's Japan.

Eye Contact Practices: Direct eye contact is considered a lack of respect and a personal affront. Preference is for the "lighthouse" sweep or shifting or downcast eyes.

Touch Practices: Handshakes are acceptable; however, a pat on the back is not. A kiss may show deference to superiors.

Perceptions of Time: Promptness is valued.

Pain Reactions: Patients stoically withstand discomfort.

Birth Rites: Japan has one of the lowest infant mortality rates in the industrialized world. Premature birth weight is suggested at 2300 g. The people comply with prenatal care and health promotion readily. Midwives are available. Women labor in silence and eat more food during labor. After delivery, long periods of rest and recuperation are practiced. The mother may remain in the hospital up to 7 days and indoors for as long as 100 days; she may not wish to bathe or wash her hair for a week.

Death Rites: A smile that expresses the desire not to have others worry about a personal bereavement may accompany the announcement or discussion of the death of a family member. The Japanese tend to control public expression of grief.

Food Practices and Intolerances: Raw fish is eaten.

Infant Feeding Practices: Although early breastfeeding is almost universal, only half of babies are breastfed after 1 month. Colostrum is not fed to the newborn.

Child Rearing Practices: The mother-child relationship is strong. The mother may sleep with her child or watch vigilantly while the child sleeps. Respect for authority figures and collaborative decision making are taught. Boys may be socialized to be assertive and successful in their achievements. Girls are taught to enjoy life and suppress ideas. Students spend long hours preparing for university entrance examinations. This period is highly stressful in the child's life.

National Childhood Immunizations: BCG at 3 months; DPT at 3, 4, and 5 months and 6 years; OPV at 3 and 4½ months; measles at 12 months; rubella for girls between 13 and 14 years.

Other Characteristics: Fever is treated by sweating it out, using warm blankets, and drinking hot drinks. As a sign of social politeness, the Japanese hiss by breathing inward suddenly. Laughter is a common sign of embarrassment that also masks bereavement and conceals rage; happiness is masked with a straight face. The Japanese do not rinse themselves in the same water in which they have bathed. Bathing usually occurs just before bedtime; however, it is suspended during times of illness. The lower and longer the greeting bow, with the head and eyes lowered, the more respect shown.

BIBLIOGRAPHY

Anders RL: An American's view of nursing education in Japan, *IMAGE: J Nurs Sch* 26(3):227, 1994.

Anders RL, Kanai-Pak M: Karoshi: death from overwork, *Nurs Health Care* 13(4):186, 1992.

Andrews MM, Boyle JS: *Transcultural concepts in nursing care,* ed 2, Philadelphia, 1995, Lippincott.

Bennett MJ: Towards ethnorelativism: a developmental model of intercultural sensitivity. In Paige RM: *Cross-cultural orientation: new conceptualizations and applications,* Lanham, Md, 1986, University Press of America.

Condon JC, Yousef F: *An introduction to intercultural communication,* New York, 1975, Macmillan.

Connor JW, Kankei J: A key concept for an understanding of Japanese-American achievement, *Psychiatry* 39(3):266, 1976.

Eisenbruch M: Cross-cultural aspects of bereavement, II, Ethnic and cultural variations in the development of bereavement practices, *Cult Med Psychiatry* 8(4):315, 1984.

Engel NS: An American experience of pregnancy and childbirth in Japan, *Birth* 16(2):81, 1989.

Galanti GA: *Caring for patients from different cultures,* ed 2, Philadelphia, 1997, University of Pennsylvania Press.

Grove CL: *Communications across cultures,* Washington, DC, 1976, National Education Association.

Kagawa-Singer M: Ethnic perspectives of cancer nursing: Hispanics and Japanese-Americans, *Cancer Nurs Perspect* 14(3):59, 1987.

Kobayashi M: Promoting breast-feeding: a successful regional project in Japan, *Acta Paediatr Jpn* 31(4):404, 1989.

Lally MM: Last rites and funeral customs of minority groups, *Midwife Health Visit Comm Nurse* 14(7):224, 1978.

Lock MM: Scars of experience: the art of moxibustion in Japanese medicine and society, *Cult Med Psychiatry* 2(2):151, 1978.

Myano Y: Personal communication, July 25, 1991.

Overfield T: *Biologic variation in health and illness,* Menlo Park, Calif, 1985, Addison-Wesley.

Prosser MH: *The cultural dialogue,* Washington, DC, 1985, SIETAR.

Pusch MD, editor: *Multicultural education,* Yarmouth, Me, 1981, Intercultural Press.

Shand N: Culture's influence in Japanese and American maternal role perception and confidence, *Psychiatry* 48(1):52, 1985.

Sikkema M, Niyekawa A: *Design for cross-cultural learning,* Yarmouth, Me, 1987, Intercultural Press.

Sleed J: Manners abroad need study, Newhouse News Service, n.p., n.d.

Stewart EC, Bennett MJ: *American cultural patterns: a cross-cultural perspective,* rev ed, Yarmouth, Me, 1991, Intercultural Press.

Stewart EC, Danielian J, Foster RJ: Stimulating intercultural communication through role-playing, Portland, Ore, 1991, seminar handout, SIIC.

Storti C: *The art of crossing cultures,* Yarmouth, Me, 1990, Intercultural Press.

Trommsdorff G: Value change in Japan, *Int J Intercult Relations* 7:337, 1983.

Yamamoto J et al.: Mourning in Japan, *Am J Psychiatry* 125(12):1660, 1969.

Yoshikawa M: Some Japanese and American cultural characteristics. In Prosser MH: *The cultural dialogue,* Washington, DC, 1985, SIETAR.

◆ JORDAN

MAP PAGE (318)

Location: Formerly Transjordan, Jordan is located in the Middle East. It is an arid country, with fertile areas only in the west.

Major Languages	Ethnic Groups		Major Religions	
Arabic	Arab	98%	Sunni Muslim	92%
English	Circassian	1%	Christian	8%
	Armenian	1%		

Predominant Sick Care Practices: Biomedical; magico-religious.

Health Care Beliefs: Acute sick care only. Health means the ability to function. Islam forbids the use of illicit drugs and alcohol and suicide, whereas smoking is considered strongly reprehensible.

Ethnic/Race Specific or Endemic Diseases: The AIDS rate per 100,000 is 0.04.

Health Team Relationships: The patient needs to know the reason for personal questions during assessment. Lying may be viewed as kindness, and sensitive areas such as reproductive health and stress may be too personal to be assessed. Males may refuse care by female physicians or nurse practitioners. Approximately half of the country's nurses are male. Societal roles regarding female behavior discourage nursing as a career. There is little communication between physicians and nurses. The patient's role is generally passive, dependent, and uninvolved. Prestige and influence bring special favors.

Families' Role in Hospital Care: A patient may be accompanied by one or many family members who wish to be present during examination and may answer questions for the patient. Families may sleep and cook in the patient's room. The health care professional should include the eldest person who is present in discussions with the patient. The family may exhibit demanding behavior and show extreme concern toward and attention to the patient.

Dominance Patterns: It is a patriarchal society; women maintain close ties with their kin and promote the position of the family in the community.

Eye Contact Practices: Direct eye contact is practiced in conversation; the listener frequently looks to the side.

Touch Practices: Handshaking is common; however, a traditionally dressed female may not shake hands with or touch a male. Hand holding is practiced among members of the same sex.

Perceptions of Time: Generally, this society is oriented in the present because planning ahead implies defying God's will. Punctuality is not as important as taking time to establish a relationship before talking business.

Pain Reactions: Pain relief is expected immediately and may be requested persistently. Therapies requiring exertion contraindicate the belief in energy conservation for recovery. Pain is expressed privately or in the company of close relatives or friends. During labor and delivery, pain is expressed loudly.

Birth Rites: The mother may have a 40-day lying-in period after birth. Her mother or sisters care for the infant. Males are circumcised. Male infants are more valued than female infants. Traditionally, infants are rubbed with salt and oil and swaddled immediately after delivery. Well-trained midwives are available.

Death Rites: Muslim belief forbids organ donations or transplants. Muslim physicians may recommend transfusions to save lives. Autopsy is uncommon because the deceased must be buried intact. For Muslim burial the body is wrapped in special pieces of cloth and buried without a coffin in the ground. Cremation is not permitted.

Food Practices and Intolerances: Chicken and lamb are widely consumed. Pork, carrion, and blood are forbidden. Food tends to be spicy. Ramadan fasting is practiced between sunrise and sunset, with exemptions for the sick and children.

Child Rearing Practices: Parenting involves attempts to avoid loss of honor and bad reputations.

National Childhood Immunizations: DPT at 2, 3, 4, and 18 months and between 3½ and 4 years; OPV at 2, 3, 4, 9, and 18 months and 6 years; measles at 9 months; hep B at 2, 3, and 9 months.

Other Characteristics: Some very traditional women wear veils, whereas others cover only their hair; still others wear casual Western dress. A close conversational distance (about 18 inches to 2 feet) is practiced. Hope, optimism, and the positive advantages of treatment should be stressed when discussing outcomes.

BIBLIOGRAPHY

AbuGharbieh P: Culture shock: cultural norms influencing nursing in Jordan, *Nurs Health Care* 14(10):534, 1993.

Ahmad SW: Personal perceptions of health: a transcultural study of Jordanian and south western U.S. senior nursing students. Paper presented at the Second Annual Middle East Nursing Conference, Irbid, Jordan, April 1992.

Beardslee C et al.: Nursing care of children in developing countries: issues in Thailand, Botswana and Jordan, *Recent Adv Nurs* 16:31, 1987.

Geissler EM: Personal observations, April 23 to May 4, 1992.

Green J: Death with dignity: Islam, *Nurs Times* 85(5):56, 1989.

Hattar-Pollara M, Meleis AI: Parenting their adolescents: the experiences of Jordanian immigrant women in California, *Health Care Women Int* 16(3):195, 1995.

Hattar-Pollara M, Meleis AI: The stress of immigration and the daily lived experiences of Jordanian immigrant women in the United States, *West J Nurs Res* 17(5):521, 1995.

Jafar E: Personal communication, April 28, 1992, Irbid, Jordan.

Khalaf IA: The relationship between the type of the child's death whether anticipated or unexpected and the Jordanian mother's grief responses, doctoral dissertation, New York, 1989, New York University.

Lawson ED, Smadi OM, Tel SA: Values in Jordanian university students: a test of Osgood's cultural universals, *Int J Intercult Relations* 10:35, 1986.

Meleis AI, LaFever CW: The Arab American psychiatric care, *Perspect Psychiatr Care* 22(2):72, 1984.

Meleis AI, Sorrell L: Arab American women and their birth experiences, *MCN Am J Matern Child Nurs* 6:171, 1981.

Reizian A, Meleis AI: Arab-Americans' perceptions of and responses to pain, *Crit Care Nurse* 6(6):30, 1986.

Ross HM: Societal/cultural views regarding death and dying, *Top Clin Nurs* 1(1):1, 1981.

Sandford V: Nursing in the Middle East: a Jordan experience, *NZ Nurs J* 78(3):8, 1985.

Ziadeh SM, Sunna EI: Decreased Cesarean birth rates and improved perinatal outcome: a seven-year study, *Birth* 22(3):144, 1995.

◆ KAZAKHSTAN

MAP PAGE (315)

Location: This republic, part of the former Soviet Union, lies in central Asia with Russia on the north and China to the east. It has an extensive coastline on the Caspian Sea. Kazakhstan, the second largest of the Commonwealth of Independent States, has vast often deserted steppes and barren mountains. Horses and sheep are common pastoral animals.

Major Languages	Ethnic Groups		Major Religions	
Kazak	Kazak	42%	Muslim	47%
Russian	Russian	37%	Russian Orthodox	44%
	Ukrainian	5%	Other	9%
	German	5%		
	Other	11%		

Ethnic/Race Specific or Endemic Diseases: ENDEMIC: Contaminated water supplies and environment from earlier nuclear testing. **RISK:** Incidence of congenital abnormalities and cancers is 30% to 50% higher than Western rates. The AIDS rate per 100,000 is reported by the country as zero.

Health Team Relationships: Nurses have a dependent role that does not include making independent decisions.

National Childhood Immunizations: BCG at birth and 6, 12, and 17 years; DPT at 2, 3, and 4 months, between 18 and 24 months, and at 9 and 15 years; OPV at birth, 2, 3, and 4 years, between 18 and 24 years, and at 7 years; measles at 8 months.

BIBLIOGRAPHY
Sawyer D: Tucson nurses making a difference in Kazakhstan, *Ariz Nurse* 48(4):5, 1995.

◆ KENYA

MAP PAGE (317)

Location: Kenya is located on the equator on the east coast of Africa. Part of its border is on the Indian Ocean. Kenya is arid in the north. In the southwestern corner lies the fertile Lake Victoria Basin. The Great Rift Valley, flanked by high mountains, extends north to south.

Major Languages	Ethnic Groups		Major Religions	
English	Kikuyu	22%	Protestant	38%
Swahili	Luhya	14%	Catholic	28%
Other	Luo	13%	Indigenous Beliefs	26%
	Kalenjin	12%	Muslim	8%
	Kamba	11%		
	Other	28%		

Predominant Sick Care Practices: Biomedical; traditional. Herbalists often boil ingredients into tea.

Ethnic/Race Specific or Endemic Diseases: ACTIVE: Cholera. ENDEMIC: Yellow fever; chloroquine-resistant malaria. RISK: Schistosomiasis. The AIDS rate per 100,000 is 29.13.

Dominance Patterns: This culture is male dominated. Polygamy is traditional but changing.

Pain Reactions: Pain relief measures are not common. Some believe that pain is necessary to become well again.

Child Rearing Practices: Female circumcision and excision is widespread in some groups. The economic value of girls predisposes one tribe to practice somewhat preferential treatment in medical care and nutritional resources for girls.

National Childhood Immunizations: BCG at birth; DPT at 6, 10, and 14 weeks; OPV at birth and 6, 10, and 14 weeks; measles at 9 months. Some do not understand the preventive nature of immunizations.

Other Characteristics: Nairobi women hold positions in business and, although not at high levels, in government offices. Birth control is strongly encouraged. Urban women place high value on maintaining a small family unit. Injections are preferred over tablets, and rectal medications may not be tolerated because the rectum is a taboo area of the body.

BIBLIOGRAPHY

Blair J: Health teaching in the context of culture: nursing in East Africa, *Kansas Nurse* 66(4):4, 1991.

Cronk L: Parental favoritism toward daughters, *Am Scientist* 81:272, 1993.

Dean NR: A community study of child spacing, fertility and contraception in West Pokot district, Kenya, *Soc Sci Med* 38(11):1575, 1994.

deVries MW, deVries MR: Cultural relativity of toilet training readiness: a perspective from East Africa, *Pediatrics* 60(2):170, 1977.

Jackson M, Morris S: An African adventure, *Nurs J Clin Pract Educ Manage* 4(21):28, 1990.

McInerney TG: Cross-cultural nursing: a perioperative experience in Kenya, *AORN J* 45(4):1000, 1987.

Mpoke S, Johnson KE: Baseline survey of pregnancy practices among Kenyan Massai, *West J Nurs Res* 15(3):298, 1993.

Wolfson E: Health care in Nairobi, Kenya, *Minn Nurs Accent* 65(5):13, 1993.

Wright J: Female genital mutilation: an overview, *J Adv Nurs* 24:251, 1996.

◆ KIRIBATI

MAP PAGE (311)

Location: Kiribati, formerly the Gilbert Islands, now includes sixteen Gilbert Islands, eight Phoenix Islands, eight Line Islands, and Banaba. Located in the mid-Pacific, it is the largest atoll state in the world. Most islands are low lying with erratic rainfall.

Major Languages	Ethnic Groups		Major Religions	
English	Micronesian	99%	Catholic	53%
Gilbertese	Other	1%	Protestant	41%
			Other	6%

Ethnic/Race Specific or Endemic Diseases: RISK: Dengue fever; cholera. Vitamin A deficiency is a public health problem. Impaired glucose tolerance is found among males. The AIDS rate per 100,000 is reported by the country as zero.

Dominance Patterns: In this egalitarian society, boasting or elevating oneself above another is not acceptable.

Perceptions of Time: Life moves at a slow and deliberate pace.

Food Practices and Intolerances: Breadfruit boiled or fried in butter is a staple. A great variety of fish is eaten.

National Childhood Immunizations: BCG at birth; DPT at 6, 10, and 14 weeks; OPV at birth and 6, 10, and 14 weeks; measles at 9 months.

Other Characteristics: People are friendly and inquisitive about others; they may appear embarrassingly bold. People squat to defecate; indoor toilet facilities are not readily available.

BIBLIOGRAPHY

King H, Rewers M: Global estimates for prevalence of diabetes mellitus and impaired glucose tolerance in adults, *Diabetes Care* 16(1):157, 1993.

Schaumberg DA et al.: Vitamin A deficiency in the South Pacific, *Public Health* 109(5):311, 1995.

Stanley D: *Micronesia handbook: guide to an American lake,* Chico, Calif, 1985, Moon.

◆ KOREA (NORTH)

MAP PAGE (319)

Location: The Democratic People's Republic of Korea occupies the northern part of the 600-mile (966 km) Korean peninsula off eastern Asia. Most of the country is covered with hills and north-to-south mountains; narrow valleys and small plains lie in between the mountains.

Major Language	Ethnic Groups		Major Religions	
Korean	Korean	99%	Atheist and	95%
	Other	1%	Unaffiliated	
			Buddhist and	5%
			Confucianism	

Health Team Relationships: A person's status and position are respected.

Families' Role in Hospital Care: Family interdependence takes precedence over independence, so self-care is not an important concept.

Touch Practices: Hand holding and touching between friends of the same sex are accepted.

Perceptions of Time: Continuing a social interaction is more important than being on time for another engagement.

Death Rites: Confucian funerals are elaborate rituals. After death and before burial, breakfast and supper are ceremoniously served to the deceased. A chief mourner and the relatives who are present weep.

Food Practices and Intolerances: In traditional families the father, using chopsticks or a spoon, may dine alone. After meals, which usually consist of rice, fish, soup, and vegetables, conversation ensues.

National Childhood Immunizations: BCG at 1 week; DPT at 6 and 10 weeks and between 6 and 12 months; OPV at birth, 6, 10, and 14 weeks, and 2, 3, and 7 years; measles at 1, 7, and 17 years.

Other Characteristics: Both hands are used to transfer something to another person. The legs are not crossed during prayer and song at religious ceremonies. Sunglasses are removed when speaking with others. Males who urinate at the side of the road and children who run around without clothes are displaying acceptable behaviors. Names are placed in the following order: the family name first, generation name second, and personal or first name last. A woman does not change her name when she marries.

BIBLIOGRAPHY

Refer also to South Korea.

Galanti GA: *Caring for patients from different cultures,* ed 2, Philadelphia, 1997, University of Pennsylvania Press.

◆ KOREA (SOUTH)

MAP PAGE (319)

Location: The Republic of Korea (South Korea) is located below the 38th parallel on a peninsula jutting from Manchuria and China off eastern Asia. Eastern Korea is mountainous. The west and south have many mainland harbors and off-shore islands.

Major Languages	Ethnic Groups		Major Religions	
Korean	Korean	99%	Buddhist	47%
English	Other	1%	Christian	49%
			Other	4%

Predominant Sick Care Practices: Biomedical; holistic; traditional. The body is thought to be the property of ancestors; the individual has an obligation to take care of the body. Acupuncture, herbal medicines, moxibustion, and cupping are treatments that are used often. Western and traditional treatments may be sought. Herbal therapies are widely used. Eastern and Western medicine may be used simultaneously.

Health Care Beliefs: Active involvement; health promotion important. Mental illness is feared, is thought to be inherited, and is manifested as somatic complaints. The cause of illness is related to disturbance of the body's vital energies; symptoms may be based on psychosocial determinants. Improvement is evaluated in terms of functional ability. Belief that illness needs to be drawn out of the body is practiced through coin rubbing. A heated coin or one smeared with oil is vigorously rubbed over the body; this produces red welts.

Ethnic/Race Specific or Endemic Diseases: RISK: Japanese encephalitis.

Health Team Relationships: Physicians and nurses are viewed as authority figures and treated with great respect; people generally do not disagree with them. The response "no" might upset another person's peace of mind or mood; therefore "yes" is often the answer given, regardless of the truth.

Families' Role in Hospital Care: The family performs personal care, which can get to the point where ambulation and basic self-care are inhibited.

Dominance Patterns: Father-son relationships are more highly regarded than are husband-wife relationships. The eldest son inherits the patriarchal position. The father makes decisions for all family members, including decisions involving health and medical care. Women have no legal rights to their children; children belong to the husband's family. Status as an elder and retirement are earned at age 60. In the less traditional family, decision making is more family focused but the dominant male may have the final decision.

Eye Contact Practices: Status determines whether direct eye contact is avoided or maintained for a brief time. When looking away, the eyes are turned to the side; they are not turned up or down.

Touch Practices: Physical touching is considered an affront, particularly with the elderly. Touching among good friends of the same sex is acceptable. Physical contact with members of the opposite sex is not proper.

Perceptions of Time: Punctuality is flexible; a 30-minute leeway for keeping appointments is acceptable. Rushing to be on time is considered undignified.

Pain Reactions: People tend toward stoicism. It is proper to display no facial expression.

Birth Rites: The father is not present during birth. Immediately after birth, bowls of clear water and rice may be placed in the delivery room to give thanks to the spirit who guards childbirth. Mothers avoid exposure to cold, including air conditioning, and take no iced drinks; they may wish to eat warm foods only. A son's birth is celebrated but not a daughter's.

Death Rites: Buddhist influence accepts death as birth into another life. Family members are summoned to observe the dying person's last breath and may respond with loud wailing and displays of intense emotion. Organ donation may be refused.

Food Practices and Intolerances: The Korean diet is essentially a healthy one, with the exception of high sodium intake. Lactose intolerance is common. Rice is a basic food; fruit is dessert. Many meals include kimchi, which is a pickled cabbage. Fruit snacks are frequently eaten. Chopsticks and a large spoon are used to eat. Cold fluids are often not preferred.

Child Rearing Practices: Infants are not allowed to cry for long and are breastfed (on demand) until they are approximately 2 years old. Children may sleep with parents until age 4. The mother cares for the child in a permissive, affectionate atmosphere until age 7; then the father, who tends to be more demanding, takes over supervision; he often does not hug, caress, or kiss the child. Children are expected to be humble and obedient.

National Childhood Immunizations: BCG at 4 weeks and 12 years; DPT at 2, 4, 6, and 12 months; OPV at 2, 4, and 6 months; measles at 9 months; hep B at birth, 1 month, and between 2 and 6 months.

Other Characteristics: The Korean has three names; the family name is written first, the generational name is second, and the given name is last. The given name is used by family and intimate friends only. A woman does not change her name when she marries. Food or drink, when first offered, will be refused out of politeness, no matter how much it is desired. The offer must be repeated. Bowel and urine elimination is done by squatting over a receptacle on the floor. Toilets with seats may be a safety hazard to people who are unfamiliar with them. Bedpans may be preferred on the floor. It is rude to show the sole of the shoe or foot to another person.

BIBLIOGRAPHY

Brigham Young University Language Research Center: Building bridges of understanding: Koreans, Provo, Utah, 1976, Brigham Young University Press.

Choi EC: Unique aspects of Korean-American mothers, *J Obstet Gynecol Neonatal Nurs* 15(5):394, 1986.

Choi EC: A contrast of mothering behaviors in women from Korea and the United States, *J Obstet Gynecol Neonatal Nurs* 24(4):363, 1995.

Galanti GA: *Caring for patients from different cultures,* ed 2, Philadelphia, 1997, University of Pennsylvania Press.

Inglis M, Gudykunst WB: Institutional completeness and communication acculturation: a comparison of Korean immigrants in Chicago and Hartford, *J Intercult Relations* 6:251, 1982.

Langer C: Contributor.

Merchant JJ: Korean interpersonal patterns: implications for Korean/ American intercultural communication, term paper, Ashland, Ore, Southern Oregon State College, n.d.

National Association for Foreign Student Affairs: The Republic of Korea: an educational exchange profile, Washington, DC, 1988, The Association.

Pang KY: The practice of traditional Korean medicine in Washington, DC, *Soc Sci Med* 28(8):875, 1989.

Park JH: Nursing administration in Korea, *Nurs Adm Q* 16(2):78, 1992.

Reardon T: Koreans. In Lipson JG, Dibble SL, Minarik PA: *Culture & nursing care,* San Francisco, 1996, UCSF Nursing Press.

◆ KUWAIT

MAP PAGE (318)

Location: Located on the northwestern shore of the Persian Gulf, Kuwait is flat; it has a wide temperature range and high humidity. Most people live in cities and, to escape summer heat and humidity, are extensive travelers.

Major Languages	Ethnic Groups		Major Religions	
Arabic	Kuwaiti	45%	Sunni Muslim	45%
English	Other Arab	35%	Shi'a Muslim	30%
	South Asian	9%	Other Muslim	10%
	Iranian	4%	Christian and	15%
	Other	7%	Other	

Predominant Sick Care Practices: Biomedical; magico-religious. Belief in the "evil eye" exists.

Health Care Beliefs: Active involvement; health promotion important. Intrusive procedures such as injections and intravenous fluids are perceived as more effective. Males tend to view illness as the inability to function; females define illness in terms of signs, symptoms, and pain. Pharmacists and nurses have the right to prescribe drugs; self-medication is practiced.

Ethnic/Race Specific or Endemic Diseases: The AIDS rate per 100,000 is 0.26.

Health Team Relationships: Patients shop around continually for the ideal physician with a common ethnic background. Health history questions relating to personal or family health, business, or social status may not be answered. Medicine is male dominated; nursing is a low-esteem woman's job that is marked by compliance and by following physicians' orders.

Families' Role in Hospital Care: Family and friends expect to be with the patient as much as possible and are demanding with health care personnel to ensure that the patient receives care and attention.

Dominance Patterns: By law, men and women are not equal. Passive-aggressive behaviors, rather than confrontational behaviors, are used (especially by women) to solve problems.

Eye Contact Practices: Approximately 2 feet separate conversation participants. Closeness permits evaluation of pupil responses. Pupils dilate with interest and contract with dislike.

Touch Practices: Touching is limited to members of the same sex; it is important in communication between men.

Pain Reactions: Pain relief is expected immediately and may be persistently requested. However, large numbers of hospitalized patients believe that pain medication should not be requested. The belief in conserving energy for recovery is in conflict with therapies that require exertion. Pain is expressed only privately or with close relatives and friends. However, pain is expressed during labor and delivery.

Death Rites: Hope is valued. God is believed to know the true prognosis; therefore death or a bad prognosis is discussed with extreme reluctance. Muslim belief forbids organ donations or transplants. Muslim physicians may recommend transfusions to save lives. Autopsy is uncommon because the deceased must be buried intact. For Muslim burial the body is wrapped in special pieces of cloth and buried without a coffin in the ground. Cremation is not permitted.

Food Practices and Intolerances: Pork, carrion, and blood are forbidden to Muslims. Food tends to be spicy. Ramadan fasting is practiced, with exemptions for the sick and children.

Infant Feeding Practices: Breastfeeding, which has a duration of 16 months, is practiced by 50% of the mothers.

Child Rearing Practices: Formal school education of children begins at 4 years. Public denigration of children is preferred over praise for fear of the evil eye.

National Childhood Immunizations: BCG between 3½ and 4 years; DPT at 3, 4, 5, and 18 months and between 3½ and 4 years; DT at 10 years; OPV at birth, 3, 4, 5, 6, and 18 months, 2½ years, between 3½ and 4 years, and between 4½ and 5½ years; measles at 12 and 15 months; rubella at 12 years; hep B at birth and 3 and 6 months. A very large percentage of children are immunized.

Other Characteristics: Hope, optimism, and the positive advantages of treatment should be stressed.

BIBLIOGRAPHY

Dalayon A: Nursing in Kuwait: problems and prospects, *Nurs Manage* 21(9):129, 1990.

Dalayon AP: Components of preoperative patient teaching in Kuwait, *J Adv Nurs* 19(3):537, 1994.

Green J: Death with dignity: Islam, *Nurs Times* 85(5):56, 1989.

Hall ET: Learning the Arabs' silent language, *Psychol Today,* Aug 1979, p 45.

Harrison A: Comparing nurses' and patients' pain evaluations: a study of hospitalized patients in Kuwait, *Soc Sci Med* 36(5):683, 1993.

Hathout MM: Comment on ethical crises and cultural differences, *West J Med* 139(3):380, 1983.

Meleis AI: The health care system of Kuwait: the social paradoxes, *Soc Sci Med* 13A:743, 1979.

Meleis AI: The Arab American in the health care system, *Am J Nurs,* June 1981, p 1180.

Meleis AI, Jonsen AR: Medicine in perspective: ethical crises and cultural differences, *West J Med* 138(6):889, 1983.

Miller K: *NBC News,* July 31, 1992.

Reizian A, Meleis AI: Arab-Americans' perceptions of and responses to pain, *Crit Care Nurse* 6(6):30, 1986.

Ross HM: Societal/cultural views regarding death and dying, *Top Clin Nurs* 1(1):1, 1981.

Shah MA, Shah NM, Yunis MK: Allied health manpower in Kuwait: issues and answers, *J Allied Health* 19(2):117, 1990.

Shah NM, Shah MA: Socioeconomic and health care determinants of child survival in Kuwait, *J Biosoc Sci* 22(2):239, 1990.

◆ KYRGYZSTAN

MAP PAGE (315)

Location: Formerly Kirghizia, part of the former Soviet Union, the republic became part of the Commonwealth of Independent States with the dissolution of the Soviet Union. Kyrgyzstan is located in central Asia; 95% of the territory comprises the Tien Shan mountain range, which is covered with perennial snow and glaciers.

Major Languages	Ethnic Groups		Major Religions	
Kyrgyz	Kyrgyz	52%	Muslim	70%
Russian	Russian	22%	Other	30%
	Uzbek	13%		
	Other	13%		

Ethnic/Race Specific or Endemic Diseases: The AIDS rate per 100,000 as reported by the country is zero.

National Childhood Immunizations: BCG at 3 to 4 days, 7 years, between 11 and 12 years, and between 16 and 17 years; DPT at 2, 3, and 4½ months, between 2 and 3 years, at 9 years, and between 16 and 17 years; OPV at 3 to 4 days, 2 months, between 3 and 4 months, and at 5, 16, and 18 months; measles at 12 months.

BIBLIOGRAPHY

No data located.

◆ LAOS

MAP PAGE (321)

Location: Laos is located in southeastern Asia in the northeastern part of the Indochinese peninsula. The land is mountainous (especially in the north) with dense forests and jungle.

Major Languages	Ethnic Groups		Major Religions	
Lao	Lao (Lao Lum)	68%	Buddhist	85%
French	Tribal Thai	22%	Animist and	15%
English	(Lao Tung)		Other	
	Lao Soung	9%		
	Other	1%		

Laos has approximately 67 different ethnic groups.

Predominant Sick Care Practices: Biomedical; magico-religious; traditional. Traditional health practices are closely linked with religious traditions. The Lao believe that 32 spirits inhabit the body and govern its functioning. Herbal medicine is an important traditional practice. The medicines are classified as cool, whereas most Western medicines are considered hot. Traditionally illness is handled with self-care and self-medication.

Health Care Beliefs: Acute sick care only. Unhealthy air currents or bad winds are thought to cause illness. Pinching or scratching the area and producing marks or red lines let the bad winds out of the body and restore health. Wrist strings around the neck, ankles, or waist prevent soul loss, which is thought to cause illness.

Ethnic/Race Specific or Endemic Diseases: ENDEMIC: Chloroquine-resistant malaria. RISK: Japanese encephalitis; schistosomiasis in the southern regions; dengue fever; iodine deficiency in the mountainous regions. The AIDS rate per 100,000 is 0.08.

Health Team Relationships: In traditional families the oldest male makes health care decisions and may answer questions directed toward the female patient. Physicians are thought to be authority figures and experts; therefore patients are told little about their conditions, the medicines, or the diagnostic procedures. As a result patients may be poor historians.

Families' Role in Hospital Care: Many family members may accompany the patient to the hospital and remain with the patient for the duration of the stay.

Dominance Patterns: The basic family unit often has three or four generations living together. Decision making is influenced by the astrologic and lunar calendars. Women defer to men's decisions in most matters of the outside world; however, women frequently control the home and the community economy.

Eye Contact Practices: Looking steadily into the eyes of someone who is respected is not proper.

Touch Practices: Because many believe that the head is the seat of life, it is revered and invasive procedures are frightening. Only parents are permitted to touch the heads of their children. The female's breast is accepted dispassionately as the means of infant feeding, whereas the female's lower torso is extremely private. Women cover the area between the waist and knees, even in private. Females who sit with crossed legs are behaving offensively. Handshaking has gained wide acceptance among men; however, it is not acceptable among women. Touching or kissing between brother and sister is not allowed. Waving the hand with the palm up is not acceptable.

Perceptions of Time: Emphasis is not placed on the urgency of getting a task done. Punctuality is reserved for important circumstances.

Pain Reactions: Pain may be severe before relief is requested.

Birth Rites: Abandoned or relatives' children who are incorporated into the family may be inadvertently included in an obstetrical history. The husband may or may not be welcomed in the delivery room but may play a major role in traditional home births. The preferred delivery position is squatting. Some may consider vernix to be accumulated sperm. Circumcision is generally unknown. Newborns are not given compliments so that they will not be captured by evil spirits. Traditionally the woman must remain inside the home for 1 month after delivery. Traditional mothers may lie near or sit over a smoldering fire for several days after delivery to help dry up the womb. The newborn's age is considered to be 1 year at birth.

Death Rites: The preference is quality of life over quantity of life because of the belief in reincarnation and the expectation of less suffering in the next life. Death at home is preferred. Cremation and burial are practiced. People who die in hospitals or from accidents, however, are not cremated but are taken directly from the hospital or scene of the accident to the temple and buried quickly. After death the body is cleaned and dressed in good clothes, and the face is washed with coconut water. White flowers and candles may be put into the deceased's hands. In some areas jewels or money (a wealthier family) and rice (a poorer family) will be put in the mouth of the deceased in the belief that these objects will help the soul encounter gods and devils.

Food Practices and Intolerances: Glutinous rice, a salad made of green papaya known as "tam mahoun," and hot chilies are the main foods. Lop (raw or cooked meat pounded together with herbs and spices) is eaten at celebrations. Laolao, a form of locally prepared rice liquor, is particularly enjoyed by the men daily. Soup made of rice and water is a popular food for the sick.

Infant Feeding Practices: Newborns are not allowed to breastfeed until the mother has a full milk supply. The colostrum is considered poisonous and may give the infant diarrhea. Rice paste or boiled sugar water is substituted during this time. For several days postpartum (weeks in the case of the first child) the mother will eat large amounts of salt and fat. During this time she does not eat red meats, fruits, or vegetables. Small amounts of chicken may be eaten.

Child Rearing Practices: A fat infant is a healthy one. Methods for calculating the age of an infant may vary by as much as 2 years. At approximately age 6 strict upbringing begins, independence is discouraged, and parents demand obedience. The oldest child (boy or girl) is responsible for younger siblings if the parents are dead, old, or ill. Segregation of females is common.

National Childhood Immunizations: BCG at birth; DPT at 6, 10, and 14 weeks; OPV at birth and 6, 10, and 14 weeks; measles at 9 months.

Other Characteristics: Because of stigma against mental illness, emotional disturbances may be manifested somatically. The family name is written first and followed by the given name. Married women officially use their husbands' last name. Given names are used almost exclusively. Family names are used only for formal occasions or on written documents.

BIBLIOGRAPHY

D'Avanzo C: Bridging the cultural gap with southeast Asians, *MCN Am J Matern Child Nurs* 17:204, 1992.

Galanti GA: *Caring for patients from different cultures,* ed 2, Philadelphia, 1997, University of Pennsylvania Press.

Kurtz JR: Contributor.

Lawson LV: Culturally sensitive support for grieving parents, *MCN Am J Matern Child Nurs* 15:76, 1990.

Li GR: Funeral practices, New York, World Relief, n.d.

Muecke MA: Caring for Southeast Asian refugee patients in the USA, *Am J Public Health* 73(4):431, 1983.

Nguyen A, Bounthinh T, Mum S: *Folk medicine, folk nutrition, superstitions,* Washington, DC, 1980, Team Associates.

Schreiner D: S.E. Asian folk healing practices/child abuse? Paper presented at the Indochinese Health Care Conference, Eugene, Ore, 1981.

Shadick KM: Development of a transcultural health education program for the Hmong, *Clin Nurse Spec* 7(2):48, 1993.

Shellenberger J: Contributor.

Stewart EC, Bennett MJ: *American cultural patterns: a cross-cultural perspective,* rev ed, Yarmouth, Me, 1991, Intercultural Press.

Storti C: *The art of crossing cultures,* Yarmouth, Me, 1990, Intercultural Press.

Uland E, Smith S: Southeast Asian mental health issues, Unpublished paper, 1984.

U.S. Department of Health, Education, and Welfare Social Security Administration Office of Family Assistance SSA. A guide to two cultures: Indochinese, Washington, DC#77-21013, n.d.

Vandeusen J et al.: Southeast Asian social and cultural customs: similarities and differences, *J Refugee Resettlement* 1:20, 1980.

◆ LATVIA

MAP PAGE (315)

Location: Latvia, one of the three Baltic states, regained its independence with the dissolution of the Soviet Union. The eastern part of the country, a fertile lowland, has lakes and hills.

Major Languages	Ethnic Groups		Major Religions
Latvian	Latvian	52%	Lutheran
Russian	Russian	34%	Russian Orthodox
	Other	14%	

Ethnic/Race Specific or Endemic Diseases: Because of the poor quality of the industrial air, childhood asthma is a problem. The AIDS rate per 100,000 is 0.12.

Health Team Relationships: Before Latvia broke away from the Soviet bloc, the word "nursing" had no meaning, physicians directed all activities and were not questioned, and people could not differentiate between what is medicine and what is nursing. Patients still, however, receive almost no explanations, and consent is not a recognized concept. Bribes to physicians may result in commodities otherwise not available. Health care professionals have been socialized to be concerned about self more than about patients. Some changes are presently occurring, but basic survival needs to be addressed before health care reform.

Families' Role in Hospital Care: Caring for hospitalized family is not a cultural phenomenon; it is needed to survive a hospital stay. Little food is provided. Patients must obtain their medications elsewhere. During a lengthy hospital stay, patients return home to take a bath on Saturdays.

Pain Reactions: The terminally ill may not be provided with pain medications because of the scarcity of supplies.

National Childhood Immunizations: BCG at birth; DPT at 3, 4½, 6, and 18 months, 9 years, and between 16 and 17 years; OPV at 3, 4½, 6, and 18 months and 6 years; MMR at between 15 and 18 months and at 12 years.

BIBLIOGRAPHY

Kalnins I: Pioneers in academia: higher education for nurses in Estonia, Latvia, and Lithuania, *Nurs Outlook* 43(2):84, 1995.

Kalnins ZGP: Nursing in Latvia from the perspective of oppressed theory, *J Transcultural Nurs* 3(1):11, 1992.

Priede-Kalnins Z: Latvia: nursing reborn, *Nurs Health Care* 16(3):148, 1995.

Priede-Kalnins Z: Oppression's influence on behavior: first hand impressions, *J Cult Diversity* 2(3):83, 1995.

◆ LEBANON

MAP PAGE (318)

Location: Located on the eastern end of the Mediterranean Sea, Lebanon has two mountain ranges that run from north to south and the fertile agricultural Bekáa Valley in between.

Major Languages	Ethnic Groups		Major Religions	
Arabic	Arab	95%	Muslim	70%
French	Armenian	4%	Christian and	30%
Armenian	Other	1%	Other	
English				

Health Care Beliefs: Acute sick care only.

Ethnic/Race Specific or Endemic Diseases: RISK: Dyggve-Melchoir-Clausen syndrome. Stress may be somatized. The AIDS rate per 100,000 is 0.27.

Families' Role in Hospital Care: The patient is usually accompanied by one or more family members or close friends who expect to participate in care or at least take on a vigilant supervisory role.

Dominance Patterns: This is a male-dominated culture with different responsibilities with regard to gender-based roles.

Perceptions of Time: Planning ahead has the potential of defying God's will.

Pain Reactions: Immediate pain relief is expected and may be persistently requested. The belief in conserving energy for recovery is in conflict with therapies that require exertion. Pain tends to be expressed only privately or with close relatives and friends. During labor and delivery, pain may be very expressive.

Birth Rites: Male children are preferred. Contraception is contrary to religious values.

Death Rites: Muslim belief forbids organ donations or transplants. Muslim physicians may recommend transfusions to save lives. Autopsy is uncommon because the deceased must be buried intact. Cremation is not permitted. For Muslim burial the body is wrapped in special pieces of cloth and buried without a coffin in the ground.

Food Practices and Intolerances: The national dish is mansaf, which is made of stewed lamb and cooked yogurt sauce served over rice. Pork, carrion, and blood are forbidden. Food tends to be spicy. Ramadan fasting is practiced, with exemptions for the sick and children.

National Childhood Immunizations: DPT at 3, 4, 5, and 18 months; OPV at 3, 4, 5, and 18 months; measles at 9 and 15 months.

Other Characteristics: Hope, optimism, and the positive advantages of treatment should be stressed.

BIBLIOGRAPHY

Andrews MM, Boyle JS: *Transcultural concepts in nursing care,* ed 2, Philadelphia, 1995, Lippincott.

Farhood L et al.: The impact of war on the physical and mental health of the family: the Lebanese experience, *Soc Sci Med* 36(12):1555, 1993.

Green J: Death with dignity: Islam, *Nurs Times* 85(5):56, 1989.

Kronfol NM, Bashshur R: Lebanon's health care policy: a case study in the evolution of a health system under stress, *J Public Health Policy* 10(3):377, 1989.

Luna L: Care and cultural context of Lebanese Muslims in an urban U.S. community: an ethnographic and ethnonursing study conceptualized within Leininger's theory, doctoral dissertation, Detroit, 1989, Wayne State University.

Luna L: Care and cultural context of Lebanese Muslim immigrants using Leininger's theory, *J Transcultural Nurs* 5(2):12, 1994.

Meleis AI, Sorrell L: Arab American women and their birth experiences, *MCN Am J Matern Child Nurs* 6:171, 1981.

Reizian A, Meleis AI: Arab-Americans' perceptions of and responses to pain, *Crit Care Nurse* 6(6):30, 1986.

Ross HM: Societal/cultural views regarding death and dying, *Top Clin Nurs* 1(1):1, 1981.

Sadler C: Dealing with disaster, *Nurs Mirror,* March 1983, p 22.

◆ LESOTHO

MAP PAGE (317)

Location: Lesotho (formerly Basutoland) is landlocked and almost completely surrounded by the eastern region of the Republic of South Africa. The country consists primarily of mountains and rocky tableland; the weather seasons are cold and severe. The majority of the people live in rural areas, and some can be reached only on horseback or by airplane.

Major Languages	Ethnic Groups		Major Religions	
English	Sotho	99%	Christian	80%
Sesotho	Other	1%	Indigenous	20%
Zulu			Beliefs	
Xhosa				

Predominant Sick Care Practices: Biomedical; magico-religious; traditional.

Health Care Beliefs: Acute sick care only; health promotion important. Curative care is practiced; however, the government encourages primary health care.

Ethnic/Race Specific or Endemic Diseases: ENDEMIC: Waterborne diseases; typhoid; gastroenteritis. In children: acute respiratory infections, pneumonia. RISK: Gastroenteritis among children; gonorrhea; measles; mumps; whooping cough; typhoid; schistosomiasis; tuberculosis. The AIDS rate per 100,000 is 16.64.

Health Team Relationships: In the rural areas the village chief is the leader and helps people make health care changes and decisions. Nursing care is performed primarily by aides in hospitals.

Families' Role in Hospital Care: They are required by hospitals to participate in childcare. Traditional birth attendants are available. Mothers have 60 days of maternity leave.

Infant Feeding Practices: Mothers prefer to use powdered milk; therefore the breastfeeding period may be short. At work the mother is given 1 hour a day for 1 year for breastfeeding.

Child Rearing Practices: Almost half of the population is 14 years old or younger.

National Childhood Immunizations: BCG at birth; DPT at 6, 10, and 14 weeks; OPV at 6, 10, and 14 weeks; measles at 9 months.

BIBLIOGRAPHY

Andriessen PP, van der Endt RP, Gotink MH: The village health worker project in Lesotho: an evaluation, *Trop Doct* 20(3):111, 1990.

Hollifield M et al.: Anxiety and depression in a village in Lesotho, Africa, *Br J Psychiatry* 156:343, 1990.

Jones S, Makoae M, Thulo F: Health care in Lesotho, *Nurs Times* 84(41):39, 1988.

Moiloa T, Wilson ME: Child health and pediatric nursing in the Kingdom of Lesotho, *J Pediatr Nurs* 10(6):393, 1995.

Mpeta AM: The private sector's contribution to primary health care in Lesotho, *Int Nurs Rev* 29(6):187, 1982.

Touchette P et al.: An analysis of home-based oral rehydration therapy in the Kingdom of Lesotho, *Soc Sci Med* 39(3):425, 1994.

◆ LIBERIA

MAP PAGE (316)

Location: Liberia is located on the Atlantic coast of south-western Africa. Much of the country is covered with dense tropical forests that experience a heavy annual rainfall.

Major Languages	Ethnic Groups		Major Religions	
English	African	95%	Traditional	70%
African	Americo-	5%	Muslim	20%
Languages	Liberian		Christian	10%

Health Care Beliefs: Acute sick care.

Ethnic/Race Specific or Endemic Diseases: ACTIVE: Cholera. ENDEMIC: Malaria; dysentery; pneumonia; meningitis. RISK: Schistosomiasis. The AIDS rate per 100,000 is 2.21.

Families' Role in Hospital Care: Tradition dictates that the family accompany the patient to the hospital and take care of cooking and laundry; however, central hospital services are the current trend.

Birth Rites: The traditional midwife is valued and active in rural Liberia.

Food Practices and Intolerances: Food shortages have been critical since the 1989 civil war began.

Infant Feeding Practices: Some parents may hold the strong belief that Western medicine's tablets or injections can cure severe malnutrition in children.

Child Rearing Practices: Female circumcision and excision is widespread among some groups.

National Childhood Immunizations: BCG at birth; DPT at 6, 10, and 14 weeks; OPV at birth and 6, 10, and 14 weeks; measles at 9 months.

BIBLIOGRAPHY

Etzel RA: Liberian obstetrics, the birth and development of midwifery. Paper submitted in partial fulfillment of the requirements of the Student Project for Amity Among Nations, Minneapolis, 1975, University of Minnesota.
Long N: Meals distributed in Liberia, *Front Lines* 32(5):7, 1992.
Rosemergy I, Robinson J: Suffer the little ones, *NZ Nurs J* 84(4):18, 1991.
Weeks RM: A perspective on controlling vaccine-preventable diseases among children in Liberia, *Infect Control Hosp Epidemiol* 5(11):538, 1984.
Wright J: Female genital mutilation: an overview, *J Adv Nurs* 24:251, 1996.

◆ LIBYA

MAP PAGE (316)

Location: Libya is officially named the Socialist People's Libyan Arab Jamahiriya. The country is 92% desert and semidesert. Topography includes some mountains in the north and south and a narrow Mediterranean coastline in northeastern Africa.

Major Languages	Ethnic Groups		Major Religions	
Arabic	Arab Berber	97%	Sunni Muslim	97%
Italian	Other	3%	Other	3%
English				

Ethnic/Race Specific or Endemic Diseases: ENDEMIC: Chloroquine-sensitive malaria (no risk in urban areas). RISK: Schistosomiasis; cystinuria. The AIDS rate per 100,000 is 0.04.

Families' Role in Hospital Care: Family members or close friends accompany the patient and expect to participate in care or at least take on a vigilant supervisory role.

Dominance Patterns: Sociocultural and religious traditions strongly favor male dominance; however, attitudes are changing among educated young males.

Pain Reactions: Immediate pain relief is expected and may be persistently requested. The belief in conserving energy for recovery is in conflict with therapies that require exertion. Pain is expressed only privately or with close relatives and friends. However, during labor and delivery, pain is very expressive.

Death Rites: Muslim belief forbids organ donations or transplants. Muslim physicians may recommend transfusions to save lives. Autopsy is uncommon because the deceased must be buried intact. Cremation is not permitted. For Muslim burial the body is wrapped in special pieces of cloth and buried without a coffin in the ground.

Food Practices and Intolerances: Pork, carrion, and blood are forbidden. Food tends to be spicy. Ramadan fasting is practiced, with exemptions for the sick and children.

National Childhood Immunizations: BCG at birth; DPT at 6, 10, and 14 weeks and 18 months; DT at 6 years; OPV at birth, 6, 10, and 14 weeks, and 18 months; measles at 8 and 18 months; hep B at birth and 1½ and 8 months.

Other Characteristics: Hope, optimism, and the positive advantages of treatment should be stressed.

BIBLIOGRAPHY

Andrews MM, Boyle JS: *Transcultural concepts in nursing care,* ed 2, Philadelphia, 1995, Lippincott.

Biri EW et al.: Correlates of men's attitudes toward women's roles in Libya, *Int J Intercult Relations* 11(3):295, 1987.

Green J: Death with dignity: Islam, *Nurs Times* 85(5):56, 1989.

Reizian A, Meleis AI: Arab-Americans' perceptions of and responses to pain, *Crit Care Nurse* 6(6):30, 1986.

Ross HM: Societal/cultural views regarding death and dying, *Top Clin Nurs* 1(1):1, 1981.

◆ LIECHTENSTEIN

MAP PAGE (314)

Location: The tiny country of Liechtenstein is located between Austria and Switzerland; the topography consists of a part of the Rhine Valley and the Alps.

Major Languages	Ethnic Groups		Major Religions	
German	Alemannic	95%	Catholic	87%
Alemannic	Italian and Other	5%	Protestant	8%
			Other	5%

BIBLIOGRAPHY

No data located. WHO does not have immunization schedule for country.

◆ LITHUANIA

MAP PAGE (315)

Location: Lithuania is located in Eastern Europe on the eastern shore of the Baltic Sea. The land is characterized by gentle rolling hills, forests, lakes, and rivers.

Major Languages	Ethnic Groups		Major Religions	
Lithuanian	Lithuanian	80%	Catholic	89%
Russian	Russian	9%	Other	11%
Polish	Polish	8%		
	Other	3%		

Predominant Sick Care Practices: Biomedical; holistic; traditional; magico-religious. Older persons are more likely to consult folk healers. For protection or to overcome illness, some believe in the "evil eye" and in prayer.

Health Care Beliefs: Health promotion is important and is emphasized in maternal-child care. Younger people take a more active role. Free universal care is provided primarily in health care facilities rather than in community settings; however, payment is expected for some treatments.

Ethnic/Race Specific or Endemic Diseases: RISK: Phenylketonuria; tuberculosis; nutritional deficiencies; hepatitis; influenza; cardiac disease; thyroid disorders. The AIDS rate per 100,000 is 0.08.

Health Team Relationships: Nurses and physicians are predominantly female, and nurses follow doctors' orders. Nursing reflects 50 years of Soviet influence. A significant percentage of people do not select nursing as a career but are directed into it. Introductory social conversation is not common. Expression of feelings may not be encouraged by professional caregivers. Asking questions of the health care provider is considered a challenge to authority; therefore information may not be shared freely. Patients address the health care professional by title rather than by name. Patients may offer gifts to health care providers to ensure quality care.

Families' Role in Hospital Care: Family members may assist with bathing, feeding, comforting, and elimination needs.

Dominance Patterns: Traditionally the male assumes a slightly more dominant role; however, the male and the female share responsibility in decision making. Decisions are usually not made quickly but debated at length. The female is usually responsible for the household, food shopping, and food preparation.

Eye Contact Practices: They vary; direct eye contact may shift during conversation.

Touch Practices: Touch is infrequent even within families. A handshake between males is common at the beginning and end of an interaction and for both sexes in professional situations.

Perceptions of Time: Present-oriented crisis management in health care. Past traditions, including how an elder healed illnesses, are important. Little emphasis is placed on health promotion or prevention. If a patient is not present and prompt when called, the health care provider calls the next patient.

Pain Reactions: Pain tolerance is valued though pain relief is both desired and requested. Verbal expression would signify more severe pain. During labor women are encouraged to keep silent and be stoic. Because of short supplies, pain medications may be limited or unavailable in the hospital.

Birth Rites: Almost all deliveries occur in hospitals and are done by midwives, who may or may not be nurses, and a physician, who is legally required to be present. The father may choose to be present during delivery but is not permitted to coach labor. Courses for natural childbirth and prenatal and postpartum care are becoming more popular. The semi-sitting position is common for delivery. Circumcision is not practiced.

Death Rites: If an illness is fatal, the family is told first and they decide if the patient should be told. The dying person should not be left alone without family present. After death an open coffin permits viewing of the body for up to 3 days. Burial occurs on the third afternoon and may be followed by a church service. Cremation is not practiced. Grief may be verbally expressed, and crying in private is expected.

Food Practices and Intolerances: The preferred main meal is at midday. Potatoes, seasonal vegetables, bread, meat, and soups are common. Great quantities of milk, other dairy products, tea, and coffee are consumed.

Infant Feeding Practices: Breastfeeding is encouraged over bottle-feeding. Foods are introduced at 4 to 5 months.

Child Rearing Practices: Children are cooperative and reared using disciplinary styles ranging from logical reasoning to authoritarian rule. The grandmother may have a valued position in child rearing, especially in single-parent families or if both parents work. Sharing of possessions is verbally encouraged but may not be enforced. Some children may have chores to do at home or be taught to rely more on their parents. Women are entitled maternity leave at 32 weeks gestation; it continues until the child is 3 years old.

National Childhood Immunizations: BCG on first day after birth, repeated at 11 months if there is no evidence of a scar; DPT at 3, 4½, 6, and 18 months; DT at between 15 and 16 years; OPV at 3, 4½, and 18 months and between 6 and 7 years; measles at between 15 and 16½ months; rubella at 12 years.

BIBLIOGRAPHY

The Baltic states: a reference book—Estonia, Latvia, and Lithuania, Tallinn, Riga, Vilnius, 1991, Encyclopedia.

Birutis AL: The facts, needs and prospects; Lithuania. Nursing in the world, Tokyo, 1992, International Nursing Foundation of Japan.

Birutis AL: Guidelines for the development and reconstruction of nursing profession in Lithuania, Amsterdam, 1992, The European Nursing Congress.

Birutis AL: Country nursing-midwifery profile: Lithuania. Paper presented at the Third Meeting of European Chief Governmental Nursing Officers, Bucharest, 1993.

Birutis AL: Nursing in Lithuania. Paper presented at the Second Meeting of Selected Nursing Leaders, WHO Regional Office for Europe, Copenhagen, 1993.

Highlights on health in Lithuania, WHO Regional Office for Europe, Copenhagen, 1992.

Kalnins I: Pioneers in academia: higher education for nurses in Estonia, Latvia, and Lithuania, *Nurs Outlook* 43(2):84, 1995.

Karosas L: Nurse practitioner revisits Lithuania, *Npnews* 2(1):3, 1994.

Karosas L: Nursing in Lithuania as perceived by Lithuanian nurses, *Nurs Outlook* 43(4):153, 1995.

Lithuania: health sectors review report, *EUROHEALTH,* WHO Regional Office for Europe, Copenhagen, 1991.

Stuttle C: Midwifery in Lithuania, *Midwives Chron Nurs Notes* 107(1275):144, 1994.

Vasyliunas R: Where's home? *J Multicult Nurs Health* 1(3):30, 1995.

◆ LUXEMBOURG

MAP PAGE (314)

Location: Luxembourg is located in western Europe and has heavy forests in the north and low, open plateaus in the south.

Major Languages	Ethnic Groups		Major Religions	
Luxembourgish	French-German	99%	Catholic	97%
German	Other	1%	Other	3%
French				
English				

Ethnic/Race Specific or Endemic Diseases: The AIDS rate per 100,000 is 3.69.

National Childhood Immunizations: BCG at birth; DPT at 2, 3, 4, and 18 months and 5 and 15 years; OPV at 3, 4, 10, and 18 months and 3 years; MMR at 15 months.

BIBLIOGRAPHY

Kuffer C: Towards quality in Luxembourg, *Nurs Standard* 9(2):7, 1994.

◆ MACEDONIA

MAP PAGE (314)

Location: Formerly part of Yugoslavia, Macedonia is a land-locked republic in the heart of the Balkans. A mountainous country, it has areas of agricultural land linked by rivers.

Major Languages	Ethnic Groups		Major Religions	
Macedonian	Macedonian	65%	Eastern Orthodox	67%
Albanian	Albanian	22%	Muslim	30%
Turkish	Other	13%	Other	3%
Serbo-Croatian				

Ethnic/Race Specific or Endemic Diseases: The AIDS rate per 100,000 is 0.83.

BIBLIOGRAPHY

No data located.

◆ MADAGASCAR

MAP PAGE (317)

Location: Madagascar, the fourth largest island in the world, is situated in the Indian Ocean across the Mozambique Channel from southeastern Africa. The island contains a central plateau and low-lying coastal areas.

Major Languages	Ethnic Groups		Major Religions	
French	Malayo-	98%	Indigenous	52%
Malagasy	Indonesian		Beliefs	
	European and	2%	Christian	41%
	Other		Muslim	7%

Predominant Sick Care Practices: Biomedical; holistic; magico-religious (dominant).

Health Care Beliefs: Passive role; acute sick care only.

Ethnic/Race Specific or Endemic Diseases: ENDEMIC: Chloroquine-resistant malaria. RISK: Schistosomiasis. The AIDS rate per 100,000 is 0.04.

Families' Role in Hospital Care: Family members attend the patient in the hospital.

Dominance Patterns: The extended family is important. Elders and ancestors are respected and honored. Ancestor worship is practiced.

Eye Contact Practices: Eye contact is avoided when confronting people in authority.

Touch Practices: Young boys and girls, as well as husbands and wives, avoid contact in public. Handshaking is the form of greeting. Parents are affectionate with their children.

Pain Reactions: Pain is shown and expressed.

Death Rites: A second funeral is conducted with exhumation after 5 to 7 years.

Food Practices and Intolerances: Rice is the staple food.

Infant Feeding Practices: Breastfeeding is practiced for 2 years or longer.

Child Rearing Practices: Special rites are conducted for boys' circumcision, for Christians' baptism, and for the first haircut.

National Childhood Immunizations: BCG at birth; DPT at 6, 10, and 14 weeks; OPV at 6, 10, and 14 weeks; measles at 9 months.

BIBLIOGRAPHY

Dahl O: Contributor.

◆ MALAWI

MAP PAGE (317)

Location: Malawi (formerly Nyasaland) is a landlocked country in southeastern Africa. The north-to-south Great Rift Valley is flanked with high plateaus and mountains. Lake Malawi, located in the Great Rift Valley, occupies one fifth of the country.

Major Languages	Ethnic Groups		Major Religions	
English	Chewa	80%	Protestant	55%
Chichewa	Other	20%	Catholic	20%
Tombuka			Muslim	20%
			Other	5%

Predominant Sick Care Practices: Traditional. Some diseases such as epilepsy are thought to be best treated by traditional healers.

Health Care Beliefs: Acute sick care only; health promotion important. Traditional healers are important providers to very large numbers of people.

Ethnic/Race Specific or Endemic Diseases: ENDEMIC: Chloroquine-resistant malaria. RISK: Cholera; malnutrition; diarrhea; schistosomiasis. The AIDS rate per 100,000 is 47.27.

Health Team Relationships: Nurses are predominantly female and have a low status.

Dominance Patterns: Women are submissive in this patriarchal society. Grandmothers may hold a dominant family position and decide treatment of children, even if the decisions are in conflict with those of the mother. The eldest son assumes decision making when his father dies.

Birth Rites: Inadequate prenatal care is a factor contributing to the high maternal mortality rate. The use of traditional birth attendants is common. Mothers remain ambulatory during labor. Finding the fetal head engaged in the pelvis before the beginning of labor is uncommon because of the smaller diameter of the pelvis. Household objects that are not sterile may be used to cut the umbilical cord, and local remedies including cow dung may be placed on the umbilical cord.

Death Rites: Open expression of grief with wailing is practiced.

Food Practices and Intolerances: Maize, cassava, and rice are staples. Men and young children receive family preference for available food.

Infant Feeding Practices: Breastfeeding is almost universal. In some areas a sweet liquid made from maize called Thobwa is given to infants.

Child Rearing Practices: The young child, who is tied to the back of the mother or to another female relative, maintains frequent close contact with the mother and at night often sleeps in the mother's bed or on the floor beside her bed. The expression of personal feelings and opinions is suppressed. Housework, obedience, and politeness are encouraged in girls. Boldness and participation in outside activities are encouraged in boys.

National Childhood Immunizations: BCG at birth; DPT at 6, 10, and 14 weeks; OPV at 6, 10, and 14 weeks; measles at 9 months.

Other Characteristics: Almost half of Malawi's population is under 15 years of age, and females outnumber males. More than half the population has had no formal education, and approximately 90% resides in rural areas.

BIBLIOGRAPHY

Adler MW, editor: Statistics from the World Health Organization and the Centers for Disease Control, *AIDS* 6(10):1229, 1992.

Banda EE: A study of family life education experiences among Chewa grandmothers, mothers, and daughters in Malawi, doctoral dissertation, Baltimore, 1991, University of Maryland.

French NV: Some aspects of midwifery practice in Malawi, *Midwives Chron Nurs Notes* 100(1191):98, 1987.

Macaulay C: Neonatal tetanus, *Nurs Times* 13:32, 1985.

Mahat G, Phiri M: Promoting assertive behaviours in traditional societies, *Int Nurs Rev* 38(5):153, 1991.

Mbweza E: Bridging the gap between hospital and home for premature infants in Malawi, *Int Nurs Rev* 43(2):53, 1996.

Namate DE: Nursing in Malawi: challenges to nurses in leadership positions, *Nurs Adm Q* 16(2):24, 1992.

Pauley J: *NBC News,* June 22, 1992.

Phoya AMM: An exploration of the factors that influence early prenatal care enrollment and compliance behavior among rural Malawian pregnant women, doctoral dissertation, Washington DC, 1993, Catholic University of America.

Smit JJM: Traditional birth attendants in Malawi, *Curationis* 17(2):25, 1994.

Speirs J: Midwifery education in Malawi, *Midwifery* 1(3):146, 1985.

Watts AE: A model for managing epilepsy in a rural community in Africa, *BMJ* 298(6676):805, 1989.

◆ MALAYSIA

MAP PAGE (321)

Location: Malaysia has two separate land masses. Western Malaysia is the southern part of the Malay Peninsula of southeastern Asia. It is covered with tropical jungle, which is also a characteristic of its north-to-south mountain range. Eastern Malaysia includes Sabah and Sarawak on the island of Borneo.

Major Languages	Ethnic Groups		Major Religions	
Malay	Malay	59%	Muslim	58%
Chinese	Chinese	32%	Buddhist	30%
English	East Indian	9%	Hindu	8%
Tamil			Christian and Other	4%

Predominant Sick Care Practices: Biomedical; magico-religious; traditional. Traditional systems are firmly established, along with an increase in the practice of modern medicine. Magical practices and belief in animism provide rationalizations for biomedical practices.

Ethnic/Race Specific or Endemic Diseases: ENDEMIC: Seasonal (peak in July/August) dengue hemorrhagic fever in some states. Chloroquine-resistant malaria, with no risk present in urban areas. RISK: Cholera; schistosomiasis. The AIDS rate per 100,000 is 0.71.

Birth Rites: During childbirth the mother's autonomy and control are not questioned. She may eat and drink whatever she wishes. Traditional beliefs include numerous birth taboos, which, if broken, are thought to affect the fetus adversely during pregnancy.

Death Rites: Muslim belief forbids organ donations or transplants. Muslim physicians may recommend transfusions to save lives. Autopsy is uncommon because the deceased must be buried intact. Cremation is not permitted. For Muslim burial the body is wrapped in special pieces of cloth and buried without a coffin in the ground.

Infant Feeding Practices: Breastfeeding and bottle-feeding are practiced.

Child Rearing Practices: Male circumcision takes place between ages 6 and 20. Taboos for menstruating women are quite common, and the Malay word for menstruation means dirt. Cleanliness is valued, and baths are taken several times a day by all age groups. Children's dislikes are generally accepted; therefore the mother finds it stressful to administer medicine to the sick child. Children sleep with the mother for the first few years, and they are toilet trained when they can communicate their needs verbally.

National Childhood Immunizations: BCG at birth and 12 years; DPT at 3, 4, and 5 months; OPV at 3, 4, 5, and 18 months and 7 years; measles at 9 months; hep B at birth and 1 and 5 months.

Other Characteristics: In communication "I'll try" means "I will not consider it," and "Maybe" means "No commitment." People's names are an integral part of their personality. Some patients may not give their names to the health care professional or permit photographs because they equate such actions with giving others power over their souls.

BIBLIOGRAPHY

Althens G: Personal communication, July 24, 1991.

Banks E: Temperament and individuality: a study of Malay children, *Am J Orthopsychiatry* 59(3):390, 1989.

Chen PC: Traditional and modern medicine in Malaysia, *Am J Chin Med* 7(3):259, 1979.

Horn BM: Cultural concepts and postpartal care, *Nurs Health Care* 2(9):516, 1981.

Laderman C: Commentary: cross-cultural perspectives on birth practices, *Birth* 15(2):86, 1988.

Lonergan S, Vansickle T: Relationship between water quality and human health: a case study of the Linggi River Basin in Malaysia, *Soc Sci Med* 33(8):937, 1991.

Peng TT: Item of interest, ostomy care in Malaysia: a cultural view, *World Counc Enterostom Ther J* 16(1):30, 1996.

Ross HM: Societal/cultural views regarding death and dying, *Top Clin Nurs* 1(1):1, 1981.

Teoh JI: Taboo and Malay tradition, *Aust NZ J Psychiatry* 10(1A):105, 1976.

WHO Epidemiological Report Summary 71(26), 1996.

◆ MALDIVES

MAP PAGE (320)

Location: Formerly the Maldive Islands, the country is made up of atolls; it has over 1000 islands. No island's area is greater than 5 square miles, and all areas are flat. The Maldives are located in the Indian Ocean southwest of India. Inhabitants are primarily Islamic seafaring people. The Maldives constitute one of the world's poorest countries.

Major Languages	Ethnic Groups		Major Religions	
Divehi	Sinhalese	40%	Sunni Muslim	90%
English	Dravidian	30%	Other	10%
	Arab and	30%		
	Black			

Ethnic/Race Specific or Endemic Diseases: Chloroquine-sensitive malaria. The AIDS rate per 100,000 is reported by the country as zero.

Death Rites: Muslim belief forbids organ donations or transplants. Muslim physicians may recommend transfusions to save lives. Autopsy is uncommon because the deceased must be buried intact. Cremation is not permitted. For Muslim burial the body is wrapped in special pieces of cloth and buried without a coffin in the ground.

National Childhood Immunizations: BCG at birth and 3 years; DPT at 6, 10, and 14 weeks; DT at 5 years; OPV at birth and 4, 8, 12, and 16 weeks; measles at 9 months; hep B at birth and 1 and 4 months.

BIBLIOGRAPHY

Bose R: Primary health care: experiences of the Maldives and Singapore, *Nurs J India* 76(4):83, 1985.

Ross HM: Societal/cultural views regarding death and dying, *Top Clin Nurs* 1(1):1, 1981.

◆ MALI

MAP PAGE (316)

Location: Mali was the French Sudan until 1920, and then it was called the Sudanese Republic until 1960. It is a land-locked country in western Africa. The only fertile area is located in the south. The northern part of the country extends into the Sahara. The literacy rate is estimated at approximately 10%.

Major Languages	Ethnic Groups		Major Religions	
French	Mande	50%	Muslim	90%
Bambara	Peul	17%	Indigenous Beliefs	9%
	Voltaic	12%	Christian	1%
	Songhai	6%		
	Other	15%		

Health Care Beliefs: Although hot-cold balance is known to most, following it in practice is much less common.

Ethnic/Race Specific or Endemic Diseases: ACTIVE: Cholera; yellow fever. ENDEMIC: Chloroquine-resistant malaria. RISK: Schistosomiasis. The AIDS rate per 100,000 is 4.21.

Death Rites: Muslim belief forbids organ donations or transplants. Muslim physicians may recommend transfusions to save lives. Autopsy is uncommon because the deceased must be buried intact. Cremation is not permitted. For Muslim burial the body is wrapped in special pieces of cloth and buried without a coffin in the ground.

Child Rearing Practices: As high as one third of rural children may be moved within and between households in a uni-directional fashion from lower-status biological mothers to higher-status foster mothers. Economic factors are not associated with this transfer. Female circumcision and excision is widespread within some groups.

National Childhood Immunizations: BCG at birth; DPT at 6, 10, and 14 weeks; OPV at birth and 6, 10, and 14 weeks; measles at 9 months.

BIBLIOGRAPHY

Castle SE: Child fostering and children's nutritional outcomes in rural Mali: the role of female status in directing child transfers, *Soc Sci Med* 40(5):679, 1995.

Randall SC: Blood is hotter than water: popular use of hot and cold in Kel Tamasheq illness management, *Soc Sci Med* 36(5):673, 1993.

Ross HM: Societal/cultural views regarding death and dying, *Top Clin Nurs* 1(1):1, 1981.

Wright J: Female genital mutilation: an overview, *J Adv Nurs* 24:251, 1996.

◆ MALTA

MAP PAGE (314)

Location: Malta consists of five islands in the center of the Mediterranean Sea. The islands have low hills in the interior and heavily indented coastlines.

Major Languages	Ethnic Groups		Major Religions	
Maltese	Italian	80%	Catholic	98%
English	Arab and Other	20%	Other	2%
Italian				

Ethnic/Race Specific or Endemic Diseases: The AIDS rate per 100,000 is 0.81.

Birth Rites: A flower bud may be placed in the delivery room because the belief holds that when the bud opens, the birth will occur.

National Childhood Immunizations: BCG at 12 years; DPT at 3, 4, and 5 months and 4 and 15 years; OPV at 3, 4, and 5 months and 4 years; MMR at 15 months and 11 years.

BIBLIOGRAPHY

Bates B, Turner AN: Imagery and symbolism in the birth practices of traditional cultures, *Birth* 12(1):29, 1985.

McMillan I: Island reforms, Malta, mental health workers are struggling to reform, *Nurs Times* 91(21):20, 1995.

◆ MAURITANIA

MAP PAGE (316)

Location: This northwestern African country has approximately 350 miles (592 km) of coastline along the Atlantic. The north is arid and extends into the Sahara. The Senegal River valley in the south is fertile; however, famines have occurred in the past decade.

Major Languages	Ethnic Groups		Major Religions	
Hasaniya Arabic	Mixed Moor/	40%	Muslim	99%
Wolof	Black		Other	1%
French	Moor	30%		
	Black	30%		

Ethnic/Race Specific or Endemic Diseases: ACTIVE: Cholera. **ENDEMIC:** Yellow fever; chloroquine-resistant malaria. **RISK:** Schistosomiasis. In the capital city more than one third do not have direct access to water. The AIDS rate per 100,000 is 1.45.

Death Rites: Muslim belief forbids organ donations or transplants. Muslim physicians may recommend transfusions to save lives. Autopsy is uncommon because the deceased must be buried intact. For Muslim burial the body is wrapped in special pieces of cloth and buried without a coffin in the ground. Cremation is not permitted.

Child Rearing Practices: Female circumcision and excision is widespread within some groups.

National Childhood Immunizations: BCG at birth; DPT at 6, 10, and 14 weeks; OPV at 6, 10, and 14 weeks; measles at 9 months.

BIBLIOGRAPHY

Perspectiva 8(7):13, 1996.
Ross HM: Societal/cultural views regarding death and dying, *Top Clin Nurs* 1(1):1, 1981.
Wright J: Female genital mutilation: an overview, *J Adv Nurs* 24:251, 1996.

◆ MAURITIUS

MAP PAGE (317)

Location: The island nation Mauritius is located in the Indian Ocean east of Madagascar. It is a volcanic island surrounded by coral reefs. A central plateau is encircled by mountain peaks.

Major Languages	Ethnic Groups		Major Religions	
English	Indo-Mauritian	68%	Hindu	52%
Creole	Creole	27%	Christian	28%
French	Sino-Mauritian	3%	Muslim	17%
Hindi	Franco-Mauritian	2%	Other	3%
Urdu				

The above data are uncertain because the government avoids compilation of statistics on ethnic lines.

Ethnic/Race Specific or Endemic Diseases: RISK: Respiratory system diseases; infectious and parasitic diseases. The AIDS rate per 100,000 is 0.63.

National Childhood Immunizations: BCG at birth; DPT at 3, 4, and 5 months; OPV at 3, 4, and 5 months; measles at 9 months.

BIBLIOGRAPHY

Kalla AC: The inequalities of morbidity and mortality in Mauritius: its ethnic and geographic dimension, *Soc Sci Med* 36(10):1273, 1993.
Subratty AH, Fakim N: Major inhalant allergens in Mauritius, *Ann Allergy Asthma Immunol* 74(6):489, 1995.

◆ MEXICO

MAP PAGE (312)

Location: Located between the United States and Central America, central Mexico is a high plateau with mountain chains on the east and west and oceanfront lowlands.

Major Language	Ethnic Groups		Major Religions	
Spanish	Mestizo	60%	Catholic	89%
	Native American	30%	Protestant	6%
	White	9%	Other	5%
	Other	1%		

Predominant Sick Care Practices: Biomedical, focusing on curative more than preventive; magico-religious; traditional. Common beliefs include mal ojo ("evil eye"), empacho (bolus of food stuck to stomach wall or blocking the intestine), caida de mollera (fallen fontanel), susto (result of a fright or a traumatic emotional experience), and mal puesto (hex or illness imposed by another). Common folk healers include curandero/a (healers), yerbero/a (herbalists), and sobador/a (masseuses), as well as homeopathic medicine, naturopathy, and spiritism. Advice and drugs can be obtained from pharmacists.

Health Care Beliefs: Passive role; acute sick care only. People of all socioeconomic and educational levels use biomedical and folk health systems, sometimes concurrently. Health is believed to be a matter of chance or God's will. Disease conditions are influenced by hot and cold imbalances. Males are perceived as being healthier than females or children, and good health in males is part of appearing macho. Severity of the patient's illness may be determined in part by pain or the appearance of blood. Some call stomachaches and headaches illnesses.

Ethnic/Race Specific or Endemic Diseases: ENDEMIC: Chloroquine-sensitive malaria, with no risk in urban areas. RISK: Obesity; diabetes; tuberculosis; dengue fever; higher hemoglobin and hematocrit levels; gastroenteritis. The AIDS rate per 100,000 is 4.60.

Health Team Relationships: The health care system is physician driven, and the government has incorporated traditional healers into the system. The practitioner is viewed as an outsider. Family interdependence takes precedence over independence, so self-care is not an important concept. Personal matters are discussed and handled within the family. The curandero or folk healer is a member of the nuclear or extended family network. Valued behaviors by health care practitioners are being informal and friendly, including family members in interaction, giving careful and concrete explanations, sharing experiences, taking time to listen, and inquiring about the patient's health. Health care practitioners should be the same sex as their patients.

Families' Role in Hospital Care: Family members are expected to be involved in care. The male should be consulted before health care decisions are made and should be included in any counseling sessions. Culturally, a mother is not allowed the authority to give consent for her child's treatment, and family decisions supersede decisions made by health care providers. Female health care providers and family members, with the exception of one's spouse, may not give care at home if that care involves touching adult male genitalia.

Dominance Patterns: The family structure is patriarchal; a slight move toward more democratic gender roles, however, is appearing. The mother is in charge of running the household and decides when health care will be sought. Deference is given to elders, fathers, and grandfathers. The collective needs of the family, be it extended or nuclear, take precedence over those of the individual.

Eye Contact Practices: Sustained direct contact is rude, immodest, or dangerous for some. Mal ojo is the result of excessive admiration. Women and children are thought to be more susceptible to mal ojo; therefore children may avoid direct eye contact.

Touch Practices: Touch is used often. Touching people while complimenting them neutralizes the power of the evil eye in believers. Closeness and physical contact are valued in familiar situations.

Perceptions of Time: The tendency is to focus on the present and be relatively unconcerned about the future. The concept of time is a relaxed one. Mañana may or may not mean tomorrow.

Pain Reactions: Emotional self-restraint and stoic inhibition of strong feelings and emotional expression are seen. Expression of pain may be a self-help relief mechanism. Pain relief might be refused as a means for atonement. During labor the loud verbal repetition of "Aye, yie, yie" requires long, slow breaths; thus it is becoming a culturally and medically appropriate method of pain relief.

Birth Rites: Beliefs about pregnancy may include sleeping flat on the back to protect the baby, keeping active to ensure a small baby and an easy delivery, avoiding cold air, and continuing sexual intercourse to lubricate the birth canal. Folk beliefs include antojos (food cravings that can cause the infant to have a characteristic such as strawberry spots if the cravings are not satisfied) and cuarentena (40-day lying-in period during which time the woman rests, stays warm, avoids bathing and exercise, and eats special foods that promote warmth). It is inappropriate for the husband to be with his wife during delivery; he is not expected to see his wife or child until both have been cleaned and dressed. The request for the woman's mother and/or sister to be present during delivery may be made.

Death Rites: Small children may be shielded from dying and death rituals. Family members take turns staying around the clock with the dying person in the hospital. Grief can be expressive; for example, el ataque consists of hyperkinetic or seizure-type behavior patterns that serve to release emotions. For many it may be a day of music, dancing, and rejoicing, especially after the death of a child. All Souls' Day is a major celebration of the day that souls travel home to the living and they are remembered.

Food Practices and Intolerances: Lactose intolerance is seen. Prenatal vitamins are thought to be a hot food and are not to be taken during pregnancy. Dietary staples such as rice, corn, and beans provide complete proteins. Pineapples, pumpkins, peanuts, sweet potatoes, squashes, avocados, papayas, and mangos are native to Mexico.

Infant Feeding Practices: Colostrum may be perceived as bad milk; therefore bottle-feeding may be used until the breasts fill.

Child Rearing Practices: A coin is strapped firmly to the infant's navel to make the navel attractive. Most mothers are willing to wipe the coin with alcohol before putting it in place. Birth control methods other than rhythm are not popular in the Catholic population. Children are expected to respect and obey their parents and elders. The elderly often help with child raising. Older male children may discipline younger siblings.

National Childhood Immunizations: BCG at birth and 6 years; DPT at 2, 4, and 6 months and 2 and 4 years; OPV at 2, 4, and 6 months; measles at 9 months and 6 years.

Other Characteristics: It is believed that a high body temperature may be broken by using warm blankets and hot drinks. The sale of drugs—except for narcotics, barbiturates, and other addictive drugs—is uncontrolled, and self-medication is widely practiced. Intravenous solutions (sueros) are also available and may be infused at home by family members or folk healers. The first surname is the mother's, and the second is the father's. A married woman adds "de" before the husband's surname. Human beings are measured with the palm open and held vertical to the ground at the correct height.

BIBLIOGRAPHY

Adams-McDarty K: Perceptions of health and illness in Mexico, *J Multicult Nurs Health* 2(2):18, 1996.

Andrews MM, Boyle JS: *Transcultural concepts in nursing care,* ed 2, Philadelphia, 1995, Lippincott.

Anthony-Tkach C: Care of the Mexican-American patient, *Nurs Health Care* 2(8):424, 1981.

Baca JE: Some health beliefs of the Spanish speaking, *Am J Nurs* 69(10):2172, 1969.

Burk ME, Wieser PC, Keegan L: Cultural beliefs and health behaviors of pregnant Mexican-American women: implications for primary care, *Adv Nurs Sci* 17(4):37, 1995.

Calatrello RL: The Hispanic concept of illness: an obstacle to effective health care management? *Behav Med* 7(11):23, 1980.

Callister LC: Cultural meanings of childbirth, *J Obstet Gynecol Neonatal Nurs* 24(4):327, 1995.

Calvillo ER, Flaskerud JH: Review of literature on culture and pain of adults with focus on Mexican-Americans, *J Transcultural Nurs* 2(2):16, 1991.

Condon JC, Yousef F: *An introduction to intercultural communication,* New York, 1975, Macmillan.

Day D: A day with the dead, *Nat History,* Oct 1990, p 67.

Diamond de la Mata R: Latin American food: more than beans and rice, *Top Clin Nurs* 11(4):57, 1996.

Douglas MK et al.: The work of auxiliary nurses in Mexico: stressors, satisfiers and coping strategies, *Int J Nurs Stud* 33(5):495, 1996.

Eisenbruch M: Cross-cultural aspects of bereavement. II. Ethnic and cultural variations in the development of bereavement practices, *Cult Med Psychiatry* 8(4):315, 1984.

Embry D, Russell N: Silver strands of Mexico: support systems for the elderly, *J Multicult Nurs Health* 2(2):34, 1996.

Galanti GA: *Caring for patients from different cultures,* ed 2, Philadelphia, 1997, University of Pennsylvania Press.

Giger JN, Davidhizar RE: *Transcultural nursing: assessment and intervention,* ed 2, St. Louis, 1995, Mosby.

Gonzalez HH: Health beliefs of some Mexican-Americans. In *Becoming aware of cultural differences in nursing,* Kansas City, Mo, 1972, American Nurses Association.

Gonzalez-Swafford MJ, Gutierrez MG: Ethno-medical beliefs and practices of Mexican-Americans, *Nurse Pract* 8(10):29, 1983.

Hays C, Mitchell J, Harding J: Death and the Day of the Dead: a Mexican fiesta, *J Multicult Nurs Health* 2(2):29, 1996.

Horn BM: Cultural concepts and postpartal care, *Nurs Health Care* 2(9):516, 1981.

Jones ME, Bond ML: The Mexican health care system: implications for nurses in the United States, *J Multicult Nurs Health* 2(2):12, 1996.

Kay M: Anthropologist of domestic care. In Barbee EL, editor: *The anthropology of nurse anthropologists,* San Francisco, 1991, Council on Nursing and Anthropology.

Keegan L: Use of alternative therapies among Mexican Americans in the Texas Rio Grande valley, *J Holistic Nurs* 14(4):277, 1996.

Lawson LV: Culturally sensitive support for grieving parents, *MCN Am J Matern Child Nurs* 15:76, 1990.

Leininger MM: *Transcultural nursing: concepts, theories, and practices,* New York, 1978, John Wiley & Sons.

Lipton JA, Marbach JJ: Pain differences, similarities found, *Sci News* 118:182, 1980.

Martinelli AM: Pain and ethnicity: how people of different cultures experience pain, *AORN J* 46(2):273, 1987.

Martinez C, Martin HW: Folk diseases among urban Mexican-Americans: etiology, symptoms, and treatments, *JAMA* 196(2):147, 1966.

Massey JG: Decision making: traditional Mexican health practices, *J Multicult Nurs Health* 2(2):39, 1996.

McKenna M: Twice in need of care: a transcultural nursing analysis of elderly Mexican-Americans, *J Transcultural Nurs* 1(1):46, 1989.

Olmos EJ, narrator: The Mexicans: through their eyes, producers Livingston W, Rawlings J, *The World of National Geographic,* Sept 8, 1996, UPN.

Ross HM: Societal/cultural views regarding death and dying, *Top Clin Nurs* 1(1):1, 1981.

Shellenberger JM: A practice model for culturally appropriate nursing care in a primary health care setting for Mexican-American persons, doctoral dissertation, Austin, 1987, University of Texas.

Spector RE: *Cultural diversity in health and illness,* ed 3, Norwalk, Conn, 1991, Appleton & Lange.

Stewart EC, Bennett MJ: *American cultural patterns: a cross-cultural perspective,* rev ed, Yarmouth, Me, 1991, Intercultural Press.

Taylor VL, editor: *Culturgrams: the nations around us,* Provo, Utah, 1987, Brigham Young University, David M Kennedy Center for International Studies.

◆ MOLDOVA

MAP PAGE (315)

Location: Formerly Moldavia and located in the southwestern part of the former Soviet Union, the country is three quarters rich, black, fertile soil of hilly plains.

Major Languages	Ethnic Groups		Major Religions	
Moldovan	Moldovan/	65%	Eastern	99%
Russian	Romanian		Orthodox	
	Ukrainian	14%	Other	1%
	Russian	13%		
	Other	8%		

Ethnic/Race Specific or Endemic Diseases: The AIDS rate per 100,000 is 0.05.

National Childhood Immunizations: No data on file with WHO.

BIBLIOGRAPHY

AACN-News: Minneapolis and Moldova link to advance healthcare in the former Soviet Union, *AACN-News,* Aug 1995, p 9.

◆ MONACO

MAP PAGE (314)

Location: Monaco is a tiny (0.6 square mile), hilly wedge of coastal land on the French Mediterranean.

Major Languages	Ethnic Groups		Major Religions	
French	French	47%	Catholic	95%
English	Monegasque	16%	Other	5%
Italian	Italian	16%		
Monegasque	Other	21%		

Ethnic/Race Specific or Endemic Diseases: The AIDS rate per 100,000 is 9.38.

BIBLIOGRAPHY

No data located, including no immunization schedule with WHO.

◆ MONGOLIA

MAP PAGE (319)

Location: Mongolia (formerly Outer Mongolia) is one of the oldest countries in the world. It is located in east central Asia. Most of the country consists of high plateaus; mountains, salt lakes, and vast grasslands can be found, as well. Much of the Gobi Desert is in southern Mongolia.

Major Languages	Ethnic Groups		Major Religions	
Khalkha Mongol	Mongol	90%	Tibetan Buddhist	95%
Turkish	Kazak	4%	Muslim	4%
Russian	Chinese	2%	Other	1%
Chinese	Russian	2%		
	Other	2%		

Ethnic/Race Specific or Endemic Diseases: ENDEMIC: Infectious and parasitic diseases. The AIDS rate per 100,000 is reported by the country as zero.

Health Team Relationships: The feldsher is a midlevel primary health care worker.

National Childhood Immunizations: BCG between 5 and 7 days and at 8, 13, and 18 years; DPT at 3, 4, and 5 months and 2 years; DT at 6 and 11 years; DPT at 3, 4, and 5 months and 2, 3, 5, and 18 years; measles between 9 and 15 months; hep B at birth and 1 and 6 months.

BIBLIOGRAPHY
Bolormaa D: Mongolia's national drug policy, *World Health* 2:28, 1995.
Davidson I: The wealth of Khan, *American Way,* July 15, 1991.

◆ MOROCCO

MAP PAGE (316)

Location: Morocco is located on the northwestern coast of Africa just south of Spain, across the Strait of Gibraltar. The Atlantic coast has fertile plains, whereas the Mediterranean coast is mountainous.

Major Languages	Ethnic Groups		Major Religions	
Arabic	Arab Berber	99%	Sunni Muslim	99%
Berber	Other	1%	Other	1%
French				

Ethnic/Race Specific or Endemic Diseases: ENDEMIC: Chloroquine-sensitive malaria (no risk in urban areas). RISK: Schistosomiasis; ataxia-telangiectasia; glycogen storage disease type III. The AIDS rate per 100,000 is 0.21.

Families' Role in Hospital Care: Family members or close friends accompany the patient and expect to participate in care or take on a vigilant, supervisory role.

Dominance Patterns: Men and women have contrasting social roles. The father has authority but uses it with some flexibility.

Touch Practices: It is customary for men to walk hand-in-hand in public.

Pain Reactions: Immediate pain relief is expected and may be persistently requested. The belief in conserving energy for recovery is in conflict with therapies that require exertion. Pain is expressed only privately or with close relatives and friends. During labor and delivery, pain is more expressive.

Death Rites: Muslim belief forbids organ donations or transplants. Muslim physicians may recommend transfusions to save lives. Autopsy is uncommon because the deceased must be buried intact. Cremation is not permitted. For Muslim burial the body is wrapped in special pieces of cloth and buried without a coffin in the ground.

Food Practices and Intolerances: Taking only the food that is being served or has been served is preferable to reaching for food. Pork, carrion, and blood are forbidden. Food tends to be spicy. Ramadan fasting is practiced, with exemptions for the sick and children.

National Childhood Immunizations: BCG at birth; DPT at 6, 10, and 14 weeks; OPV at birth and 6, 10, and 14 weeks; measles at 9 months.

Other Characteristics: Hope, optimism, and the positive advantages of treatment should be stressed.

BIBLIOGRAPHY

Andrews MM, Boyle JS: *Transcultural concepts in nursing care,* ed 2, Philadelphia, 1995, Lippincott.
Green J: Death with dignity: Islam, *Nurs Times* 85(5):56, 1989.
Laaziri Z: Morocco: the big day, *World Health,* Dec 1984, p 27.
Murphy EJ: *Tradition and change in modern Morocco, World Education Project,* Storrs, 1974, University of Connecticut, School of Education.
Reizian A, Meleis AI: Arab-Americans' perceptions of and responses to pain, *Crit Care Nurse* 6(6):30, 1986.
Ross HM: Societal/cultural views regarding death and dying, *Top Clin Nurs* 1(1):1, 1981.
Storti C: *The art of crossing cultures,* Yarmouth, Me, 1990, Intercultural Press.

◆ MOZAMBIQUE

MAP PAGE (317)

Location: Mozambique stretches along the southeastern coast of Africa. Coastal lowlands cover nearly one half of the country. The population has suffered from civil war, severe drought, and famine. Crops have failed in some areas. All of these circumstances contribute to Mozambique's standing among the world's poorest countries.

Major Languages	Ethnic Groups		Major Religions	
Portuguese	Bantu Tribes	85%	Indigenous	60%
African Languages	Other	15%	Beliefs	
			Christian	30%
			Muslim	10%

Predominant Sick Care Practices: Traditional medicine men practice.

Health Care Beliefs: Health care is nationalized and includes a policy of primary health care.

Ethnic/Race Specific or Endemic Diseases: ENDEMIC: Chloroquine-resistant malaria. RISK: Schistosomiasis; common diarrheal and respiratory diseases; kwashiorkor; hookworm; multifactorial anemia. African tick fever, Tumba fly infestation, and larva migrans may be seen. The AIDS rate per 100,000 is 7.37.

Birth Rites: The majority of infants are born at home. A traditional birth attendant or a relative is present. Rural infants who are born at home may be delivered onto the ground and are left untouched until the placenta is delivered. High value is placed on having a large number of children; however, couples are encouraged to space the births of their children.

Food Practices and Intolerances: Sorghum and beans are common. Oil is used sparingly in cooking.

Infant Feeding Practices: Breastfeeding is encouraged until the infant is 18 months old. One out of four babies will not live to her/his 5th birthday.

National Childhood Immunizations: BCG at birth; DPT at 6, 10, and 14 weeks; OPV at 6, 10, and 14 weeks; measles at 9 months.

BIBLIOGRAPHY

Farrell M: The price of war, *Nurs Health Care* 13(8):414, 1992.

Galvin M: Medicine men and monkey bites: a trip to northern Mozambique, *NPnews* 3(6):3, 1995.

Mondlane RP, deGraca AMP, Ebrahim GJ: Skin-to-skin contact as a method of body warmth for infants of low birth weight, *J Trop Pediatr* 35:321, 1989.

Pauley J: *NBC News,* June 22, 1992.

Powell M: Beating disease in the bush, *Nurs Times* 26:19, 1984.

Raisler J: Nurse-midwifery in a developing country: maternal and child health in Mozambique, *J Nurse Midwife* 29(6):399, 1984.

Segall M, Marzagão C: Drug revolution in Mozambique, *World Health,* July 1984.

◆ MYANMAR (BURMA)

MAP PAGE (321)

Location: Myanmar occupies the northwestern portion of the Indochinese peninsula, with India to the northwest and China to the northeast. The former Burma consists of a narrow mountain range, a plateau, and a flat fertile delta.

Major Languages	Ethnic Groups		Major Religions	
Burmese	Burman	68%	Buddhist	89%
Shan	Shan	9%	Christian	4%
Karen	Karen	7%	Muslim	4%
	Raljome	4%	Other	3%
	Chinese and Other	12%		

Predominant Sick Care Practices: Biomedical; traditional.

Ethnic/Race Specific or Endemic Diseases: ENDEMIC: Chloroquine-resistant malaria. RISK: Hemoglobin E disease; Japanese encephalitis; leprosy; tuberculosis; goiter; malnutrition; diarrhea; infectious diseases. Intestinal worms are frequently a cause for intestinal surgery in children. The AIDS rate per 100,000 is 1.33.

Health Team Relationships: A direct "no" answer to a question is avoided.

Families' Role in Hospital Care: Families stay with the patient in the hospital, perform basic care, and provide meals and clean linen. Medicines are purchased by the family and brought to the hospital.

Perceptions of Time: Punctuality is not stressed.

Birth Rites: Family planning is contrary to government policy. Cesarean sections may be performed to avoid the birth of a male child on Saturdays or other inauspicious days. After delivery, the mother remains in the hospital bed for 24 hours; if she delivers at home, she remains in the room where she gave birth for 7 days. She does no work during that time. The mother drinks only boiled water for 45 days after delivery. Traditional birth attendants and trained auxiliary midwives provide care.

Death Rites: Preference is for quality of life rather than quantity because Buddhists believe in reincarnation and less suffering in the next life. The dying are helped to recall past good deeds; this enables them to achieve a fit mental state. Autopsies are permitted; cremation is preferred.

Food Practices and Intolerances: White rice and vegetables are staples.

Infant Feeding Practices: Most infants are breastfed; however, breastfeeding may be delayed because the people believe that colostrum is not good for infants.

National Childhood Immunizations: BCG at birth and 6 weeks; DPT at 6, 10, and 14 weeks; OPV at 6, 10, and 14 weeks; measles at 9 months.

BIBLIOGRAPHY

Boyle JS, Andrews MM: *Transcultural concepts in nursing care,* Glenview, Ill, 1989, Scott, Foresman/Little, Brown College Division.
Falla J: Rebels with a cause, *Nurs Times* 84(26):36, 1988.
Fawcett B: Midwifery training in Burma, *Nurs Times* 86(30):30, 1990.
Forbes C: Burma: the royal and golden country, *Health Visit* 62(4):119, 1989.
Kington M: *Great journeys,* Oct 27, 1991, PBS-TV.
Lally MM: Last rites and funeral customs of minority groups, *Midwife Health Visit Comm Nurse* 14(7):224, 1978.
Parker T: Born in Burma, *Nurs Times* 14:44, 1987.
Samovar LA, Porter RE: *Intercultural communication: a reader,* Belmont, Calif, 1985, Wadsworth.

◆ NAMIBIA

MAP PAGE (317)

Location: Namibia (formerly South-West Africa) is bounded in part by South Africa. It is a sparsely populated part of the high plateau of southern Africa. The country is currently experiencing severe drought.

Major Languages	Ethnic Groups		Major Religions	
Afrikaans	Ovanbi	50%	Lutheran	50%
English	Kavangos	9%	Other Christian	30%
German	Herero	7%	Indigenous	20%
African	Damara	7%	Beliefs	
Languages	White	6%		
	Other Black	21%		

Ethnic/Race Specific or Endemic Diseases: ENDEMIC: Poliovirus. RISK: Chloroquine-resistant malaria; schistosomiasis. The AIDS rate per 100,000 is 119.14.

National Childhood Immunizations: BCG at birth; DPT at 6, 10, and 14 weeks; OPV at 6, 10, and 14 weeks; measles at 9 months.

BIBLIOGRAPHY

Pauley J: *NBC News,* June 22, 1992.

van Niekerk ABW et al.: Outbreak of paralytic poliomyelitis in Namibia, *Lancet* 344(8923):661, 1994.

◆ NAURU

MAP PAGE (311)

Location: A remote island nation of only 18.2 square miles (21 square km) and 8000 people, Nauru lies just south of the equator in the western Pacific Ocean. It is ringed by dying, ashen-gray coral reefs. The water is so deep that ships cannot anchor. The nearly exhausted phosphate reserves (the island's only natural resource) have provided one of the world's highest per-capita incomes. Strip mining has left all but one fifth of the land useless.

Major Languages	Ethnic Groups		Major Religions	
Nauruan	Nauruan	58%	Christian	95%
English	Pacific Islander	26%	Other	5%
	Chinese	8%		
	European	8%		

Ethnic/Race Specific or Endemic Diseases: ENDEMIC: Highest rate of diabetes in the world. RISK: High blood pressure; heart disease; obesity. The life expectancy rate is low. Because immigrant laborers are available to do the mining, most Nauruans follow a sedentary lifestyle. The AIDS rate per 100,000 is reported by the country as zero.

Health Team Relationships: Nauruans do not respond well to aggressive, argumentative people. A friendly, nonassertive approach will most likely achieve a successful interaction.

Families' Role in Hospital Care: Most services are free. On weekdays free consultations are available at the general hospital.

Food Practices and Intolerances: Nearly all food is imported from Australia. Water is also shipped into the island. Local fish (tainted by cadmium) are usually eaten raw, especially by children. Eating processed foods is considered a sign of affluence that contributes to obesity.

National Childhood Immunizations: No data located.

Other Characteristics: Native Nauruans are large physically. Few males survive beyond age 50. Traffic accidents cause many deaths.

BIBLIOGRAPHY

Cousteau JM: *Nauru—the island planet,* July 19, 1992, CBS News.
Mellor B: Paradise or hell? *Time,* Aug 24, 1992, p 30.
Stanley D: *Micronesia handbook: guide to an American lake,* Chico, Calif, 1985, Moon.

◆ NEPAL

MAP PAGE (320)

Location: Nepal is a landlocked country in southern Asia that has many mountain peaks over 20,000 feet (6096 m), including Mt. Everest, which is the earth's tallest mountain. The literacy and life expectancy rates are low. Geography and altitude influence the types of health problems and also the availability of health care. People in rural areas make up 92% of the population.

Major Languages	Ethnic Groups		Major Religions	
Nepali	Indigenous	80%	Hindu	90%
Newari	Groups		Buddhist	5%
Tibetan	East Indian	5%	Muslim	3%
Other	Tibetan and	15%	Other	2%
	Other			

High-altitude groups include Sherpas, Tamang, and Kirantis. Midmountain groups include Tamang, Magyars, Tharus, Danuars, and Chepang. The lowland group is mostly Indian immigrants.

Predominant Sick Care Practices: Biomedical; magico-religious; traditional. Health care treatments include indigenous and Western, as well as Ayurvedic medicine, which is based on identifying and maintaining a balance that is identified for a particular individual. Belief in the "evil eye" exists.

Ethnic/Race Specific or Endemic Diseases: ENDEMIC: Chloroquine-resistant malaria, with no risk in urban areas. RISK: Cholera; Japanese encephalitis; leprosy; diarrhea; nutritional deficiencies; pneumonia; communicable diseases. Accidents are common causes of death in children. The AIDS rate per 100,000 is 0.07.

Health Team Relationships: People are considered strangers if they are outside the patient's caste system or ethnic background. People are reluctant to call on strangers for help. Most health service positions are held by men. Nurses implement doctors' orders, and most people do not find it culturally acceptable for nurses to give physical care to men. Who one knows or how one is connected is important.

Dominance Patterns: The family unit is important. Gender inequities exist within the society. The status of women is determined by marriage.

Death Rites: Some Sherpa people express grief through singing sad songs.

Infant Feeding Practices: Breastfeeding mothers do not eat vegetables because vegetables are believed to cause diarrhea and colds. Solids and salt are begun at 6 months. Fluids may not be given to infants with diarrhea in the belief that they will cause more diarrhea.

Child Rearing Practices: Sons are preferred. Contraceptive techniques are not well known. Infants up to 6 months old are massaged in oil, particularly mustard oil, and placed in the sun several times a day. The oil, which is absorbed by the body, adds fatty tissue. The head and face are shaped to produce high noses and wide foreheads, which are highly valued. This is achieved by having the infants sleep on pillows that are shaped with seeds. Personal feelings and opinions are rarely expressed. Discipline and obedience are encouraged.

National Childhood Immunizations: BCG at birth; DPT at 6, 10, and 14 weeks; OPV at 6, 10, and 14 weeks; measles at 9 months.

BIBLIOGRAPHY

Desjarlais RR: Poetic transformations of Yolmo "sadness," *Cult Med Psychiatry* 15(4):387, 1991.

Jones CM: The meaning of being an elder in Nepal, *Nurs Sci Q* 5(4):171, 1992.

Justice J: Can socio-cultural information improve health planning? A case study of Nepal's assistant nurse-midwife, *Soc Sci Med* 19(3):193, 1984.

Mahat G, Phiri M: Promoting assertive behaviours in traditional societies, *Int Nurs Rev* 38(5):153, 1991.

Ogilvie L: Nursing in Nepal, *Can Nurse* 91(6):25, 1995.

Sharma A, Ross J: Nepal: integrating traditional and modern health services in the remote area of Bashkharka, *Int J Nurs Stud* 27(4):343, 1990.

Storti C: *The art of crossing cultures,* Yarmouth, Me, 1990, Intercultural Press.

Subedi J: Modern health services and health care behavior: a survey in Kathmandu, Nepal, *J Health Soc Behav* 30(4):412, 1989.

◆ NETHERLANDS

MAP PAGE (314)

Location: The Netherlands, also known as Holland, is located on the North Sea in northwestern Europe. Most of the land is low, flat farmland. Approximately 50% is below sea level. The land is protected by dikes. The islands of the Netherlands Antilles lie in the Caribbean north of Venezuela; the largest islands are Curaçao and Bonaire. The islands have complete autonomy in domestic affairs.

Major Language	Ethnic Groups		Major Religions	
Dutch	Dutch	96%	Catholic	34%
	Indonesian	1%	Protestant	25%
	and Other		Unaffiliated	41%
	Other	3%	and Other	

Ethnic/Race Specific or Endemic Diseases: The AIDS rate per 100,000 is 3.08.

Pain Reactions: During birthing, analgesia is neither expected nor required.

Birth Rites: There are many home births that are assisted by midwives. Home births are increasing. Overall fertility rates are decreasing.

Death Rites: Euthanasia and assisted suicide are against the law, but more people are choosing to end their own life. Active euthanasia is permitted under special circumstances.

Child Rearing Practices: Breastfeeding is very popular. Children begin school when they are 4 years old. Children can request and receive inoculations without parental consent.

National Childhood Immunizations: BCG at 6 months; DPT at 3, 5, 7, and 11 months and 4 and 9 years; IPV at 3, 5, 7, and 11 months and 4 and 9 years; MMR at 14 months and 9 years.

BIBLIOGRAPHY

Arrindell WA et al.: Cross-national generalizability of dimensions of perceived parental rearing practices: Hungary and The Netherlands: a correction and repetition with healthy adolescents, *Psychol Rep* 65(3-2):1079, 1989.

Branegan J: I want to draw the line myself, *Time* 149(11):30, 1997.

Bull MJ: Health care reform and community health nursing in the Netherlands, *Minn Nurs Accent* 65(8):3, 1993.

Davis AJ, Slater PV: U.S. and Australian nurses' attitudes and beliefs about the good death, *IMAGE: J Nurs Sch* 21(1):34, 1989.

Gamel C et al.: Factors that influence the provision of sexual health care by Dutch cancer nurses, *Int J Nurs Stud* 32(3):301, 1995.

Glover E: Going Dutch, *Nurs Standard* 42:47, 1994.

Mander R: The relevance of the Dutch system of maternity care to the United Kingdom, *J Adv Nurs* 22(6):1023, 1995.

Melchior M et al.: The tasks of psychiatric nurses in long-term residential settings in the Netherlands, *Int J Nurs Stud* 32(4):398, 1995.

Tijhuis MA, Peters L, Foets M: An orientation toward help-seeking for emotional problems, *Soc Sci Med* 31(9):989, 1990.

◆ NEW ZEALAND

MAP PAGE (311)

Location: Located below the equator, New Zealand lies about 1200 miles (2012 km) east of Australia. It consists primarily of two islands: North Island and South Island, which are separated by Cook Strait. Though both islands are hilly and mountainous, South Island has the Southern Alps, which have glaciers and many high mountain peaks.

Major Languages	Ethnic Groups		Major Religions	
English	European	88%	Christian	81%
Maori	Maori	9%	Hindu and	1%
	Pacific Islander	2%	Confucian	
	Other	1%	Other	18%

Predominant Sick Care Practices: Biomedical.

Ethnic/Race Specific or Endemic Diseases: RISK: Mortality from asthma, which is higher than expected; tuberculosis. The AIDS rate per 100,000 is 1.40.

Health Team Relationships: Equality is valued.

Food Practices and Intolerances: A yeast spread called Vegemite is popular.

National Childhood Immunizations: DPT at 5 weeks and 3 and 5 months; OPV at 3, 5, and 18 months and 5 years; measles at 15 months and 11 years; hep B at birth, 3 months, and between 12 and 15 months.

BIBLIOGRAPHY

Clarke A, Higgins C: Tuberculosis: a risk to nurses, *Kai Tiaki: Nurs NZ* 1(8):16, 1995.

Clements CJ, Patel AC, Pearce NE: 1988 New Zealand national immunisation survey: methodology, *NZ Med J* 102(870):320, 1989.

Davidson GP: Grief, death and bereavement among New Zealand's Polynesian people: a community affair, *NZ Nurs J* 76(7):12, 1983.

Golden P: Thinking of working in New Zealand?, *Midwives* 109(1299):90, 1996.

Sears MR et al.: Asthma mortality comparison between New Zealand and England, *BMJ* 293(6558):1342, 1986.

Sears MR et al.: Deaths from asthma in New Zealand, *Arch Dis Child* 61(1):6, 1986.

Sherrard I: Cross-cultural studies, *NZ Nurs J* 77(11):22, 1984.

◆ NICARAGUA

MAP PAGE (312)

Location: Nicaragua is the largest yet most sparsely populated Central American country. Its Pacific coast is volcanic and fertile. The Caribbean "Mosquito Coast" is swampy.

Major Languages	Ethnic Groups		Major Religions	
Spanish	Mestizo	69%	Catholic	95%
English	White	17%	Other	5%
Indian Languages	Black	9%		
	Native American	5%		

Health Care Beliefs: Active involvement, often with self-medication. In rural areas more than 80% of all illnesses are treated with traditional medicine; the remainder are treated with a combination of traditional and Western medicine. Most medicines can be obtained over the counter. Private physicians may prescribe unnecessary medicine for demanding clients.

Ethnic/Race Specific or Endemic Diseases: RISK: Chloroquine-sensitive malaria (minimal risk in urban areas); dengue fever; diarrhea. The AIDS rate per 100,000 is 0.20.

Health Team Relationships: The Nicaraguans may be reluctant to go to a hospital.

National Childhood Immunizations: BCG at birth; DPT at 1 month, between 2 and 3 months, between 3 and 4 months, and at 15 months and 6 years; OPV at 1 month, between 2 and 3 months, between 3 and 4 months, at 15 months, and at 6 years; measles at 9 months.

BIBLIOGRAPHY

Fitzgerald K: UConn researcher documents use of plants to treat maladies in the wilds of Nicaragua, *Univ CT Traditions* 2(3):8, 1996.

Hudelson PM: ORS and the treatment of childhood diarrhea in Managua, Nicaragua, *Soc Sci Med* 37(1):97, 1993.

Radcliffe M: Nicaragua: a good example in health, *Nurs Standard* 5(38):22, 1991.

◆ NIGER

MAP PAGE (316)

Location: Located in the interior of northern Africa, Niger is mostly arid desert that is part of the southern Sahara. The country experiences periods of famine and drought. Four fifths of the land is uninhabitable desert. Larger cities may not always have electricity and running water.

Major Languages	Ethnic Groups		Major Religions	
French	Hausa	56%	Muslim	80%
Hausa	Djerma	22%	Other	20%
Djerma	Fula	9%		
	Tuareg	8%		
	Beri-Beri and Other	5%		

Predominant Sick Care Practices: Holistic; traditional. Primary health care and medical practice are based on an ancient and complex, traditional set of practices, including herbs, Islamic treatments of religious prayers, verses, and appeals to different spirits.

Health Care Beliefs: There are linguistic taboos against speaking words related to sexuality, even by midwives.

Ethnic/Race Specific or Endemic Diseases: ACTIVE: Cholera. ENDEMIC: Yellow fever; chloroquine-resistant malaria. The AIDS rate per 100,000 is 6.79.

Health Team Relationships: Because of a belief that the mention of an illness can cause it to occur, patients may describe illness in broad and general terms, especially when children are involved.

Dominance Patterns: Polygamy is practiced. The wife is responsible for all activities related to raising children and maintaining the household.

Birth Rites: The maternal mortality rate is very high. Women refuse to push during labor because they fear that it will result in after-pains. Shouting or crying are not condoned. The placenta is buried in or near the house with the maternal side facing the sky. In traditional groups the first-time mother delivers in her parents' house, where she is isolated in a room with her mother or a traditional birth attendant and delivers in the squatting position. A 40-day period of rest is observed.

Death Rites: Muslim belief forbids organ donations or transplants. Muslim physicians may recommend transfusions to save lives. Autopsy is uncommon because the deceased must be buried intact. Cremation is not permitted. For Muslim burial the body is wrapped in special pieces of cloth and buried without a coffin in the ground.

Infant Feeding Practices: Based on the belief that breast-feeding weakens the mother, infants are quickly weaned if the mother discovers she is pregnant again.

Child Rearing Practices: Children are sent to live with grandparents or an older female for an unspecified period of time if the mother must work in the fields, if she becomes pregnant again, or if the children become ill. The surrogate parent assumes all responsibility (except financial) for the child. Female circumcision and excision is widespread within some groups.

National Childhood Immunizations: BCG at birth; DPT at 6, 10, and 14 weeks; OPV at 6, 10, and 14 weeks; measles at 9 months, hep B at 9 months.

BIBLIOGRAPHY

Amadou M: The sun rose more than twice on Amina, *Safe Motherhood* 18(2):11, 1995.

Chmielarczyk V: Transcultural nursing: providing culturally congruent care to the Hausa of northwest Africa, *J Transcultural Nurs* 3(1):15, 1991.

Jaffre Y, Prual A: Midwives in Niger: an uncomfortable position between social behaviours and health care constraints, *Soc Sci Med* 38(8):1069, 1994.

Khassis U, Windsor RA: Building an infrastructure for health: a conceptual framework and application, *Hygie* 2(3):27, 1983.

Ross HM: Societal/cultural views regarding death and dying, *Top Clin Nurs* 1(1):1, 1981.

Wright J: Female genital mutilation: an overview, *J Adv Nurs* 24:251, 1996.

◆ NIGERIA

MAP PAGE (316)

Location: Black Africa's most populous nation is located in western Africa on the Gulf of Guinea. The southern coast has swamps, mangrove forests, tropical rain forests, and a plateau of open woodland. A semidesert region is found in the north.

Major Languages	Ethnic Groups		Major Religions	
English	Hausa	21%	Muslim	50%
Hausa	Yoruba	21%	Christian	40%
Yoruba	Ibo	18%	Other	10%
Ibo	Fulani	11%		
Fulani and Other	Other	29%		

Predominant Sick Care Practices: Biomedical; magico-religious; traditional. Illnesses from religious or magical causes are thought not to be best treated by Western medicine. Hausa traditional healers called "surgeons" treat sprains, swellings, and other selected problems. There are surgeons who specialize in circumcision and making traditional facial markings, which may have medicinal herbs rubbed into them. Pharmacists and patent medicine shop operators routinely prescribe antibiotics for childhood diarrhea, but rarely do they prescribe oral rehydration therapy.

Ethnic/Race Specific or Endemic Diseases: ENDEMIC: Chloroquine-resistant malaria (in urban and rural areas). RISK: Cholera; yellow fever; schistosomiasis; tetanus among infants, especially in rural areas.

Dominance Patterns: Men are considered superior to women, and lineage is primarily patrilineal. Males are polygamous.

Pain Reactions: Many Muslim Nigerians are stoic, and they may offer their pain to Allah.

Birth Rites: Traditional birth attendants are often used for deliveries outside the hospital.

Death Rites: Muslim belief forbids organ donations or transplants. Muslim physicians may recommend transfusions to save lives. Autopsy is uncommon because the deceased must be buried intact. Cremation is not permitted. For Muslim burial the body is wrapped in special pieces of cloth and buried without a coffin in the ground.

Food Practices and Intolerances: Women who are overweight by Western standards are admired.

Child Rearing Practices: Children are taught to honor their parents and elders to the point where they have no right to question, just to obey. All the children of one wife may be calculated as one child. Large families are common. Female circumcision and excision is widespread within some groups.

National Childhood Immunizations: BCG at birth; DPT at 6, 10, and 14 weeks; OPV at 6, 10, and 14 weeks; measles at 9 months; hep B at birth and 4 weeks.

Other Characteristics: Nigeria has the highest incidence of twins in the world. The thumbs-up gesture is rude.

BIBLIOGRAPHY

A planet for the taking, March 15, 1989, Discovery Channel.

Adetunji JA: Infant mortality and mother's education in Ondo State, Nigeria, *Soc Sci Med* 40(2):253, 1995.

Ajuwon AJ et al.: Indigenous surgical practices in rural southwestern Nigeria, *Health Educ Res* 10(3):379, 1995.

Etkin NL, Ross PJ, Muazzamu I: The indigenization of pharmaceuticals: therapeutic transitions in rural Hausaland, *Soc Sci Med* 30(8):919, 1990.

Fajemilehin RB: Factors influencing high rate of 'born-before-arrival' babies in Nigeria—a case control study in Ogbomosho, *Int J Nurs Stud* 28(1):13, 1991.

Fajemilehin RB: Neonatal tetanus among rural-born Nigerian infants, *Matern Child Nurs J* 23(2):39, 1995.

Fakeye O: Contraception with subdermal levonorgestrel implants as an alternative to surgical contraception at Llorin, Nigeria, *Int J Gynaecol Obstet* 35(4):331, 1991.

Galanti GA: *Caring for patients from different cultures,* ed 2, Philadelphia, 1997, University of Pennsylvania Press.

Igun UA: Reported and actual prescription of oral rehydration therapy for childhood diarrhoeas by retail pharmacists in Nigeria, *Soc Sci Med* 39(6):797, 1994.

Iiechukwu STC: Food dreams and illness among Nigerians: a pilot study, *Psychiatr J Univ Ottawa* 10(2):89, 1985.

Laoye JA: Selling health in the market place: the Araromi approach, *Int J Health Educ* 23(2):87, 1980.

Odebiyi AI: The sociocultural factors affecting health care delivery in Nigeria, *J Trop Med Hyg* 80(11):249, 1977.

Omorodion FI: Child sexual abuse in Benin City, Edo State, Nigeria: a sociological analysis, *Issues Compr Pediatr Nurs* 17(1):29, 1994.

Onyejiaku EE et al.: Evaluation of a primary health care project in Nigeria, *Int Nurs Rev* 37(3):265, 1990.

Ross HM: Societal/cultural views regarding death and dying, *Top Clin Nurs* 1(1):1, 1981.

Stewart EC, Bennett MJ: *American cultural patterns: a cross-cultural perspective,* rev ed, Yarmouth, Me, 1991, Intercultural Press.

Westbrook MT, Nordholm LA, McGee JE: Cultural differences in reactions to patient behaviour: a comparison of Swedish and Australian health professionals, *Soc Sci Med* 19(9):939, 1984.

Wright J: Female genital mutilation: an overview, *J Adv Nurs* 24:251, 1996.

◆ NORWAY

MAP PAGE (314)

Location: Norway occupies the western part of the Scandinavian peninsula in northwestern Europe and extends approximately 300 miles (483 km) above the Arctic Circle. More than two thirds of the country is uninhabitable because of glaciers, mountains, moors, and rivers.

Major Languages	Ethnic Groups		Major Religions	
Norwegian	Norwegian	99%	Lutheran	88%
Lapp	Lappish	1%	Other Christian	8%
Finnish			Other	4%

Predominant Sick Care Practices: Biomedical; holistic.

Health Care Beliefs: Active involvement; health promotion important. Cleanliness, rest, and taking cod liver oil are believed to promote health.

Ethnic/Race Specific or Endemic Diseases: RISK: Cholestasis-lymphedema; Krabbe's disease; phenylketonuria. Suicide takes more lives than traffic accidents. The AIDS rate per 100,000 is 1.48.

Health Team Relationships: The people want to be given options and to be helped in making decisions. Politeness is practiced; however, it is subject to reciprocity. The word for "sir" does not exist in the Norwegian language, and some may feel uncomfortable if "sir" is used to address them. In communication the understatement is preferred.

Families' Role in Hospital Care: Staff provides all care in the hospital. Visiting hours are fairly liberal, and young children can visit.

Dominance Patterns: Decisions are usually not made quickly; matters are debated at length. Those in the home share decision making, caring for children, and duties.

Eye Contact Practices: Direct eye contact occurs during conversations, but the eyes may shift back and forth at times.

Touch Practices: This culture has little or no touching contact. Younger people are beginning to touch more often when greeting or when saying farewell. In familiar situations, touching may be increased.

Perceptions of Time: The people are present and future oriented. A general attitude persists that if things are going okay, why worry? The people are rather punctual and may give themselves a 5- to 10-minute leeway.

Birth Rites: The perinatal mortality rate is among the lowest in the world. Prenatal care and natural childbirth are common. Skin-to-skin care (Kangaroo Care) is practiced. Deliveries at home are becoming more common. The father is often in the delivery room to support the mother. Nonmedical analgesia such as acupuncture, bathing, sterile water packs, or massage may be preferred. Circumcision is not practiced.

Death Rites: The closest family members are usually with the dying person because they believe that no one should die alone. A ceremony accompanies cremation and burial in the ground.

Food Practices and Intolerances: The main meal is at midday in rural areas. For people who work in the cities, the main meal is in the early evening. City people have a sandwich for lunch, and breakfast is a heavy meal. Potatoes with meat or meatballs and boiled fish are the food staples. Great quantities of milk are consumed. Another light meal is eaten between 8 and 10 PM.

Infant Feeding Practices: Breastfeeding is encouraged and common. Milk substitute advertisements are banned.

Child Rearing Practices: Because child rearing practices are permissive, children are allowed to participate in decision making and generally have a great deal of autonomy. Children begin school at 7 years old.

National Childhood Immunizations: BCG at 13 years; DPT at 3, 5, and 10 months and 11 years; OPV at 6, 7, and 16 months and 7 years; IPV at 6, 7, and 16 months and 7 years; MMR at 15 months and 12 years.

Other Characteristics: Homeopathic medicine and holistic approaches with acupuncture are on the increase.

BIBLIOGRAPHY

Aarnes T: Norway: where legislation recognises the importance of midwives, *Midwives* 109(1296):8, 1996.

Andrews MM, Boyle JS: *Transcultural concepts in nursing care,* ed 2, Philadelphia, 1995, Lippincott.

Dahl O: Contributor.

Geissler EM: Personal observations, Aug 15-21, 1992.

Gloppestad K: Initial separation time between fathers and their premature infants: comparison between two periods of time, *Vard-I-Norden* 15(2):10, 1995.

Grimsmo A, Siem H: Factors affecting primary health care utilization, *Fam Pract* 1(3):155, 1984.

Habert K, Lillebo A: *Made in Norway: Norwegians as others see them,* 1988, The Sons of Norway Viking, n.p.

Hopp Z: *Norwegian folklore simplified,* 1991, John Grieg Produksjon A/S (translated by Toni Ramholt), n.p.

Ro OC et al.: Intervention studies among elderly people, *Scand J Prim Health Care* 5(3):163, 1987.

Sogaard AJ, Fonnebo V: The Norwegian mental health campaign in 1992: Part II: Changes in knowledge and attitudes, *Health Educ Res* 10(3):267, 1995.

Spector RE: *Cultural diversity in health & illness,* ed 4, Stamford, Conn, 1996, Appleton & Lange.

◆ OMAN

MAP PAGE (318)

Location: Oman is located on the tip of the Arabian Peninsula. It has a narrow coastal plain, a wide, mostly waterless plateau, and a range of barren mountains. Oil has become the major source of income.

Major Languages	Ethnic Groups		Major Religions	
Arabic	Arab	74%	Ibadhi Muslim	75%
English	Pakistani	21%	Other Muslim	20%
Baluchi	Other	5%	Other	5%
Urdu				
Indian Languages				

Predominant Sick Care Practices: Health preservation and well-being.

Ethnic/Race Specific or Endemic Diseases: ENDEMIC: Chloroquine-sensitive malaria. The AIDS rate per 100,000 is 0.32.

Health Team Relationships: There is about a 2:1 ratio of female nurses to male nurses.

Death Rites: Muslim belief forbids organ donations or transplants. Muslim physicians may recommend transfusions to save lives. Autopsy is uncommon because the deceased must be buried intact. Cremation is not permitted. For Muslim burial the body is wrapped in special pieces of cloth and buried without a coffin in the ground.

Food Practices and Intolerances: Pork, carrion, and blood are forbidden. Food tends to be spicy. Ramadan fasting is practiced, with exemptions for the sick and children.

National Childhood Immunizations: OPV at birth; DPT at 3, 5, 7 and 15 months; DT at 6 and 12 years; OPV at birth and 1½, 3, 5, 7, and 15 months; measles at 9 and 15 months; hep B at birth and 1½ and 7 months.

BIBLIOGRAPHY

Jeetun AR: Nurse education in the Sultanate of Oman, *Nurs Standard* 6(49):37, 1992.

Jeetun AR: Using continuous assessment in Oman, *Nurs Standard* 8(4):37, 1993.

Ross HM: Societal/cultural views regarding death and dying, *Top Clin Nurs* 1(1):1, 1981.

◆ PAKISTAN

MAP PAGE (320)

Location: Pakistan's Hindu Kush and Himalayan mountains contain the second highest peak in the world. There are desert lands in the east and areas of alluvial plains along the Indus River.

Major Languages	Ethnic Groups		Major Religions	
Urdu	Punjabi	66%	Sunni Muslim	77%
English	Sindhi	13%	Shi'a Muslim	20%
Punjabi	Pashtun	9%	Other	3%
Sindhi	Balochi and	12%		
Pashtu and	Other			
Other				

Predominant Sick Care Practices: Allopathic and indigenous medical practitioners are used concurrently by some.

Health Care Beliefs: Acute sick care. Approximately one third of the population has access to safe drinking water, and approximately one sixth has access to sanitation facilities.

Ethnic/Race Specific or Endemic Diseases: ENDEMIC: Chloroquine-resistant malaria (including urban areas); tuberculosis; acute respiratory infections; bacillary dysentery; amoebiasis; rabies. Diarrhea is the chief cause of death among children. Almost two thirds of children under age 5 have mild to moderate protein-energy malnutrition. The AIDS rate per 100,000 is 0.01.

Health Team Relationships: Women may object to being examined by a male physician. Criticizing someone of higher status or rank is viewed as unacceptable. Traditionally men fill positions of authority; therefore female health care workers are under the authority of male physicians and hospital administrators. Nursing is perceived as a menial occupation, and nurses are not trained to make decisions or as change agents. Nurses may expect to be tipped. Traditional practitioners are called "hakims."

Families' Role in Hospital Care: Hospitals do not supply meals, so family does. The patient lacking needed medicines must buy them from an outside pharmacy or do without. A male member of the family must stay with a woman at the hospital 24 hours a day.

Dominance Patterns: Women are governed by different laws than men are. Women are expected to be obedient to male authority; women are not encouraged to make decisions. Decent women, as defined by the culture, remain in their homes and go out only if they are completely covered, unrecognizable, and with the protection of a male relative.

Eye Contact Practices: The peripheral gaze or no eye contact may be preferred during interactions.

Touch Practices: Both male and female health care professionals are reluctant to expose the patient, even for an examination.

Birth Rites: The maternal and infant mortality rates are high. Approximately one fourth of births are attended by trained health personnel. Traditional birth attendants are called "dai."

Death Rites: Muslim belief forbids organ donations or transplants. Muslim physicians may recommend transfusions to save lives. A Holy Iman does not have to be present at death; however, a Muslim should recite the Declaration of the Faith or help the patient recite it; it is as follows: "There is no God but God, and Muhammed is his Messenger." According to Islamic tradition the family members must wash the body before the funeral. Autopsy is uncommon because the deceased must be buried intact. Cremation is not permitted. For Muslim burial the body is wrapped in special pieces of cloth and buried without a coffin in the ground.

Food Practices and Intolerances: During hot weather the foods that are considered hot (beef, pork, potatoes, and whiskey) are avoided. Cold foods (chicken, fish, fruit, and beer) are avoided in the winter. Pork, carrion, and blood are forbidden to Muslims. Food tends to be spicy. Ramadan fasting is practiced, with exemptions for the sick. Diet is high in saturated fat (ghee).

Child Rearing Practices: Some associate dehydration and malnutrition, even marasmus, and inevitable death with spirits and close contact with unclean women, meaning women who are menstruating or who had not taken a ritual bath after sexual intercourse. The most traditional may wrap their infants in cow dung to give them the strength and warmth needed for growth. Some mothers do not connect lack of growth with lack of food. A sick child reflects the mother's carelessness and social disgrace; this can cause the family to be ostracized. The duration of breastfeeding is declining. The high fat content in buffalo milk fed to some babies makes it hard to digest.

National Childhood Immunizations: BCG at birth; DPT at 6, 10, and 14 weeks; OPV at birth and 6, 10, and 14 weeks; measles at 9 months.

Other Characteristics: Mortality statistics are higher for women than men, possibly because men receive preferential treatment. Most women are not literate. Elimination is done from a squatting position, as the toilet is flush to the floor, and water is used for cleaning oneself.

BIBLIOGRAPHY

Ahmad WI: Patients' choice of general practitioner: intolerance of patients' fluency in English and the ethnicity and sex of the doctor, *J R Coll Gen Pract* 39(321):153, 1989.

David S, Lobo ML: Childhood diarrhea and malnutrition in Pakistan: Part I: Incidence and prevalence, *J Pediatr Nurs* 10(2):131, 1995.

David S, Lobo ML: Childhood diarrhea and malnutrition in Pakistan: Part II: Treatment and managements, *J Pediatr Nurs* 10(3):204, 1995.

David S, Lobo ML: Childhood diarrhea and malnutrition in Pakistan: Part III: Social policy issues, *J Pediatr Nurs* 10(4):273, 1995.

Edwards N: McMaster's link with Pakistan, *Can Nurse,* March 1989, p 30.

Galanti GA: *Caring for patients from different cultures,* ed 2, Philadelphia, 1997, University of Pennsylvania Press.

Haq MB: Lady health visitors: public health nursing education in Pakistan, *J Cult Diversity Health* 1(2):36, 1994.

Harnar R et al.: Health and nursing services in Pakistan: problems and challenges for nurse leaders, *Nurs Adm Q* 16(2):52, 1992.

Hezekiah J: The pioneers of rural Pakistan: the lady health visitors, *Health Care Women Int* 14(6):493, 1993.

Irujo S: An introduction to intercultural differences and similarities in nonverbal communication. In Wurzel JS, editor: *Toward multiculturalism,* Yarmouth, Me, 1988, Intercultural Press.

Kamal IT: The traditional birth attendant, *World Health,* Sept-Oct 1992, p 6.

Lally MM: Last rites and funeral customs of minority groups, *Midwife Health Visit Comm Nurse* 14(7):224, 1978.

Raftery KA: Emergency medicine in southern Pakistan, *Ann Emerg Med* 27(1):79, 1996.

Ross HM: Societal/cultural views regarding death and dying, *Top Clin Nurs* 1(1):1, 1981.

Sbaih LC: Women in the 'developing world' and their perceptions of health: an area for examination by the nurse from the 'developed world,' *J Adv Nurs* 18:1524, 1993.

Schmidt RL: Women and health care in rural Pakistan, *Soc Sci Med* 17(7):419, 1983.

Weisfeld GE: Sociobiological patterns of Arab culture, *Ethnol Sociobiol* 11:23, 1990.

Zindani N: Pakistani nurses vision for change, *Int Nurs Rev* 43(3):85, 1996.

◆ PALAU

MAP PAGE (311)

Location: Palau is an archipelago of 26 islands located in the western Pacific Ocean southeast of the Philippines.

Major Languages	Ethnic Groups	Major Religions
English	Polynesian	Catholic
Palauan	Malayan	Protestant
Sonsorolese	Melanesian	Modeknegi
Anguar	Japanese	Tobian

Ethnic/Race Specific or Endemic Diseases: The AIDS rate per 100,000 is reported by the country as zero.

National Childhood Immunizations: DPT at 6 weeks, 4, 6, and 15 months, and between 4 and 6 years; OPV at 6 weeks, 4, 6, and 15 months, 3 years, and between 4 and 6 years; measles at 15 months and between 5 and 13 years; hep B at birth and 2 and 6 months.

BIBLIOGRAPHY

No data located.

◆ PANAMA

MAP PAGE (312)

Location: Panama is the southernmost of the Central American nations. Eastern Panama is tropical rain forest; the country has moderate-sized hills in the interior and volcanic mountains in the west.

Major Languages	Ethnic Groups		Major Religions	
Spanish	Mestizo	70%	Catholic	85%
English	Native American	14%	Protestant	15%
	White and Other	16%		

Ethnic/Race Specific or Endemic Diseases: ENDEMIC: Yellow fever. RISK: Chloroquine-sensitive and chloroquine-resistant malaria. The AIDS rate per 100,000 is 7.72.

National Childhood Immunizations: BCG at birth and 6 years; DPT at 2, 4, 6, and 15 months and between 4 and 5 years; Td at 12 years; OPV at birth, 2, 4, 6, and 15 months, and between 4 and 5 years; measles at 9 months; MMR at 15 months.

Other Characteristics: Having body fat is considered healthy in women and a sign of fertility.

BIBLIOGRAPHY

Contreras S: Support workers in Panama, *Int Nurs Rev* 38(6):178, 1991.

Galanti GA: *Caring for patients from different cultures,* ed 2, Philadelphia, 1997, University of Pennsylvania Press.

◆ PAPUA NEW GUINEA

MAP PAGE (311)

Location: Papua is located 1° below the equator on the eastern half of the island of New Guinea. The island supports one of the largest unspoiled rain forests in the world. Papua New Guinea's center is thickly forested, with dense jungle and relatively unexplored mountains. The climate is temperate in places, whereas the coastal lowlands are tropical. Over time the inhabitants were isolated by the topography, and an extremely large number of diverse tribes evolved. Over 700 different languages and dialects are spoken. Because of the vast number of languages and dialects, pidgin English, or Melanesian pidgin, is the universal language used.

Major Languages	Ethnic Groups		Major Religions	
Pidgin English	Papuan/	95%	Protestant	44%
Motu	Melanesian		Indigenous	34%
English	Other	5%	Beliefs	
Other			Catholic	22%

Predominant Sick Care Practices: Biomedical; magico-religious; traditional. It is believed that evil spirits inhabit some jungle and forest areas.

Health Care Beliefs: Acute sick care; health promotion important.

Ethnic/Race Specific or Endemic Diseases: ENDEMIC: Chloroquine-resistant malaria in the lowlands and coastal areas. Chloroquine drug resistance problems are beginning. RISK: Burkitt's lymphoma in children; pigbel (enteritis necroticans) in the highlands; anemia in all age groups; tuberculosis in children. The AIDS rate per 100,000 is 1.00.

Health Team Relationships: Government aid posts are staffed by people trained in first aid and basic hygiene and are scattered throughout the country.

Families' Role in Hospital Care: Almost all parents actively participate in giving care to their children in the hospital. Families consider it both duty and obligation to remain with and care for the sick family member; this includes provision of food.

Dominance Patterns: Obtaining the husband's approval for initiation of contraceptives is important. Male dominance and individuality are important to some. Polygamy is practiced. In rural areas women are responsible for food, children, and tending animals. Girls may be married by age 14.

Touch Practices: Strong value, particularly among same sex and with children.

Birth Rites: Approximately two thirds of women receive some antenatal care. The majority of births are unsupervised. Almost all mothers breastfeed.

Death Rites: Women in some cultural groups are expected to express grief; however, men are not. A woman left widowed hacks off her fingers as a sign of her sorrow in traditional bush country.

Food Practices and Intolerances: Sweet potatoes are eaten in the highlands, and sago palm (almost pure starch) is eaten in the lowlands. Taro, bananas, and greens are common.

Infant Feeding Practices: To encourage breastfeeding, prescriptions are required to obtain infant feeding bottles.

Child Rearing Practices: Parents are firm, and punishment is given for breaking cultural rules. In traditional bush country, infants with physical anomalies may be left to die.

National Childhood Immunizations: BCG at birth and 7 and 13 years; DPT at 1, 2, and 3 months; OPV at birth and 1, 2, and 3 months; measles at 6 months; hep B at birth and 1 and 2 months.

BIBLIOGRAPHY

Alto WA, Albu RE, Irabo G: An alternative to unattended delivery: a training programme for village midwives in Papua New Guinea, *Soc Sci Med* 32(5):613, 1991.

Avue B, Freeman P: Some factors affecting acceptance of family planning in Manus, *P N G Med J* 34(4):270, 1991.

Biddulph J: Child health in Papua New Guinea: a 30 year personal perspective, *Med J Aust* 154(7):439, 1991.

Discovery Channel: *Jungle Trek,* Sept 9, 1992.

Frankel S, Smith D: Conjugal bereavement amongst the Huli people of Papua New Guinea, *Br J Psychiatry* 141:302, 1982.

Hetzel BS: From Papua New Guinea to the United Nations: the prevention of mental defect due to iodine deficiency, *Aust J Public Health* 19(3):231, 1995.

Leininger MM: Transcultural care diversity and universality: a theory of nursing, *Nurs Health Care* 6(4):209, 1985.

Leininger MM: Gadsup of Papua New Guinea revisited: a three decade view, *J Transcultural Nurs* 5(1):21, 1993.

Marshall LB, Lakin JA: Antenatal health care policy, services and clients in urban Papua New Guinea, *Int J Nurs Stud* 21(1):19, 1984.

Reuben R: Women and malaria: special risks and appropriate control strategy, *Soc Sci Med* 37(4):473, 1993.

Ruffolo DC: Trauma nursing in the bush country of Papua New Guinea, *Int J Trauma Nurs* 1(3):61, 1995.

Sharaz J: Motherhood in Papua New Guinea, *Midwives* 107(1299):102, 1996.

Spear SF et al.: Nurses as a key PHC link in Papua New Guinea, *Int Nurs Rev* 37(1):207, 1990.

◆ PARAGUAY

MAP PAGE (314)

Location: Paraguay is a landlocked country located in south central South America. Eastern Paraguay has grassy lands and fertile plains, whereas western Paraguay is covered with marshes, lagoons, dense forests, and jungles. Because Paraguay is below the equator, the seasons are reversed from those in North America and Europe.

Major Languages	Ethnic Groups		Major Religions	
Spanish	Mestizo	95%	Catholic	90%
Guarani	Other	5%	Other	10%

Ethnic/Race Specific or Endemic Diseases: Chloroquine-sensitive malaria. The AIDS rate per 100,000 is 0.46.

Touch Practices: The conversation space for talking with friends is close. Men may embrace when greeting after long absences. Close friends of both sexes may walk arm-in-arm.

National Childhood Immunizations: BCG at birth; DPT at 2, 4, 6, and 18 months and 4 years; OPV at 2, 4, 6, and 18 months; measles at 9 and 15 months and between 6 and 7 years.

BIBLIOGRAPHY

Grossman S: Thoughts from a Peace Corps PT, *Clin Manage* 5(3):26, 1985.

Taylor VL, editor: *Culturgrams: the nations around us,* Provo, Utah, 1987, Brigham Young University, David M Kennedy Center for International Studies.

◆ PERU

MAP PAGE (314)

Location: This South American country along the Pacific Ocean is divided by the Andes mountains into three zones: the arid coastline, the mountains—with peaks over 20,000 feet (6096 m) and deep valleys—and the heavily forested eastern mountain slopes.

Major Languages	Ethnic Groups		Major Religions	
Spanish	Native American	45%	Catholic	95%
Quechua	Mestizo	37%	Other	5%
Aymara	White	15%		
	Other	3%		

Ethnic/Race Specific or Endemic Diseases: ACTIVE: Yellow fever. RISK: Chloroquine-sensitive and chloroquine-resistant malaria (not in urban areas); cholera; measles; whooping cough; gastrointestinal and bronchial-pulmonary problems. The AIDS rate per 100,000 is 3.82.

Dominance Patterns: Males dominate.

National Childhood Immunizations: BCG at birth and 6 years; DPT at 2, 3, and 4 months; OPV at birth and 2, 3, and 4 months; measles at 9 months.

BIBLIOGRAPHY

Bonner R: A reporter at large: Peru's war, New Yorker, Jan 1988, p 31.

Penny M, Paredes P: A competition to promote weaning foods, *World Health Forum* 10(1):99, 1989.

Soucy G: Primary health care in the Amazon jungle of Peru, *Info Nurs* 26(2):11, 1995.

World Monitor TV: April 11, 1991.

◆ PHILIPPINES

MAP PAGE (321)

Location: An archipelago off the southeast coast of Asia, the Philippines consists of about 7000 volcanic islands. The larger islands are crossed with mountain ranges. More than half of the 60 million people live in extreme poverty.

Major Languages	Ethnic Groups		Major Religions	
Pilipino (Tagalog)	Christian	92%	Catholic	83%
English	Malay		Protestant	9%
Other	Muslim	4%	Muslim	5%
	Malay		Buddhist and	3%
	Chinese	2%	Other	
	Other	2%		

Predominant Sick Care Practices: Biomedical; magico-religious. A combination of home remedies, professional providers, and traditional healers is consulted. Fatalism accompanies beliefs that ghosts and spirits control life and death. Usurping the powers of the gods is believed to have a cause-and-effect relationship to subsequent bad happenings.

Health Care Beliefs: Acute sick care; health promotion important. Mental illness is highly stigmatized in the Filipino culture. It is believed that the "evil eye" can be cast upon someone through the eyes or the mouth.

Ethnic/Race Specific or Endemic Diseases: ENDEMIC: Chloroquine-sensitive and chloroquine-resistant malaria (not in urban areas). RISK: Japanese encephalitis; schistosomiasis. Vitamin A deficiency is a common cause of childhood blindness. The AIDS rate per 100,000 is 0.07.

Health Team Relationships: Authority is respected, and it is believed that the professional's time is valuable; therefore the problem must be serious, or it is left unmentioned. Nurses may carry out a physician's order rather than question it. Rather than give a "no" answer, the patient may remain silent or respond with a hesitant "yes." Group decisions are often made by an influential group member. An intermediary may be used for confrontational situations.

Families' Role in Hospital Care: A child may feel an obligation to the parent who is ill and spend hours giving care. The family may desire to give physical care.

Dominance Patterns: The self is perceived in the context of the family. Protection against outsiders, dependency, harmony, and reciprocity of obligation are group values. Dependence strengthens relationships among people.

Eye Contact Practices: Some may fear eye contact; however, if it is established, it is important to return and to maintain eye contact.

Touch Practices: In some parts of the country it is believed that the evil eye may be neutralized on a child by putting a bit of saliva on the finger and making the sign of the cross on a child's forehead when giving a compliment. Touch is stressed.

Perceptions of Time: Time generally moves ahead slowly. Life is lived from day to day.

Pain Reactions: People may appear stoic if they believe that pain is the will of God and that God will give them the strength to bear it.

Birth Rites: It is believed that daily bathing and shampooing during pregnancy will produce a clean baby and that sexual intercourse may cause harm to the woman and the infant. Some type of symbolic unlocking or opening act during labor using keys or flowers may be practiced. A traditional postpartum lying-in period of 10 days prohibits bathing or showering. A special bath after 2 weeks removes the debris of pregnancy that is believed to be found in perspiration. Regardless of room temperature the new mother may wear warm clothing and keep covered with blankets.

Death Rites: Patients should be protected from knowing about a poor prognosis because it will only add to their suffering. After death, emotional grief responses may occur.

Food Practices and Intolerances: Rice is preferred with every meal.

Infant Feeding Practices: The percentage of the population involved in breastfeeding and its duration have declined in the past 2 decades.

National Childhood Immunizations: BCG at birth and 7 years; DPT at 6, 10, and 14 weeks; OPV at 6, 10, and 14 weeks; measles at 9 months; hep B at 6, 10, and 14 weeks.

Other Characteristics: The Filipino gesture that invites others to approach uses the whole hand, with palm in and fingers up. A Quackdoctor is a completely acceptable folk health practitioner. Premature birth weight is suggested at 2200 g. An invitation must be extended more than once and must be reluctantly accepted. The value of shared rather than private possessions or property is practiced.

BIBLIOGRAPHY

Aguilar DD: The social construction of the Filipino woman, *Int J Intercult Relations* 13:527, 1989.

Althen GL, Jaime J: Assumptions and values in Philippine, American and other cultures, class materials, Summer Institute of Intercultural Communication, Portland, Ore, 1991.

Andrews MM, Boyle JS: *Transcultural concepts in nursing care*, ed 2, Philadelphia, 1995, Lippincott.

Bates B, Turner AN: Imagery and symbolism in the birth practices of traditional cultures, *Birth* 12(1):29, 1985.

Chernack C: Speak up . . . Dula Pacquaio, *NJ Nurse* 25(6):3, 1995.

Condon JC, Yousef F: *An introduction to intercultural communication,* New York, 1975, Macmillan.

Davis CF: Culturally responsive nursing management in an international health care setting. In Brown BJ, editor: On the scene, *Nurs Adm Q* 16(2):36, 1992.

Galanti GA: *Caring for patients from different cultures,* ed 2, Philadelphia, 1997, University of Pennsylvania Press.

Giger JN, Davidhizar RE: *Transcultural nursing: assessment and intervention,* ed 2, St. Louis, 1995, Mosby.

Horn BM: Cultural concepts and postpartal care, *Nurs Health Care* 2(9):516, 1981.

Lieban RW: Urban Philippine healers and their contrasting clienteles, *Cult Med Psychiatry* 5(3):217, 1981.

Luyas G: How Filipino mothers care for their young children, *UT Nurse* 5(1):7, 1991.

Marcos I: *The Today Show,* Oct 9, 1991, NBC.

Overfield T: *Biologic variation in health and illness,* Menlo Park, Calif, 1985, Addison-Wesley.

Prosser MH: *The cultural dialogue,* Washington, DC, 1985, SIETAR.

Ross HM: Societal/cultural views regarding death and dying, *Top Clin Nurs* 1(1):1, 1981.

Rowell M: Eradication of vitamin A deficiency with 5 cents and a vegetable garden, *J Ophthalmic Nurs Tech* 12(5):217, 1993.

Samovar LA, Porter RE: *Intercultural communication: a reader,* Belmont, Calif, 1985, Wadsworth.

Spector RE: *Cultural diversity in health & illness,* ed 4, Stamford, Conn, 1996, Appleton & Lange.

Utley G, anchor: *NBC News,* Nov 3, 1991.

Williamson NE: Breastfeeding trends and the breastfeeding promotion program in the Philippines, *Int J Gynaecol Obstet Suppl 1,* 30(1):35, 1990.

Wilson S: The Filipino elder: implications for nursing practice, *J Gerontol Nurs* 20(8):31, 1994.

◆ POLAND

MAP PAGE (314)

Location: Other than the Carpathian Mountains in the south, this north central European country is primarily rich, agricultural, lowland plains.

Major Language	Ethnic Groups		Major Religions	
Polish	Polish	98%	Catholic	95%
	Ukrainian and Other	2%	Uniate and Other	5%

Predominant Sick Care Practices: Biomedical; magico-religious; folk. Older generations believe in the "evil eye" (Szatan) and in praying and wearing religious medals and scapulars to help protect them against illness. Folk healers and miracle workers are also sought. Feldshers are similar to physician assistants or nurse practitioners. Elective procedures or surgeries are done on a space-available schedule.

Health Care Beliefs: Passive role; acute sick care.

Ethnic/Race Specific or Endemic Diseases: RISK: Phenylketonuria. The AIDS rate per 100,000 is 0.28.

Health Team Relationships: Many physicians accept gifts from patients who can pay for additional services or for hospital admission. For adults, dental care is almost exclusively in the private sector. Patients have a bit of choice among several doctors or regarding which polyclinic to use. Despite a law that gives patients the right to know their diagnosis, many doctors do not inform them.

Families' Role in Hospital Care: Parents may wish to be involved in caring for their hospitalized child.

Dominance Patterns: Traditionally the man of the family is the chief disciplinarian and decision maker; however, Poland's legal Family Code stresses equality between husband and wife. Sons are preferred over daughters.

Eye Contact Practices: Direct eye contact is made.

Touch Practices: Hugging and kissing on the cheek are acceptable between sexes.

Pain Reactions: Tolerance of pain is valued. Pain may be expressed, however, by facial grimaces or by crying out.

Birth Rites: Among the more traditional people, preparations for birth may be made in secret to avoid evil spells. Circumcision is not universal. Recent political and economic events have influenced an increase in premature deliveries and low-birth weight newborns. To deliver, women report to their assigned hospital, which is close to home. No family is present during labor because delivery rooms are too small. In general, midwives practice under the direction of physicians. After a normal delivery, the length of stay is 5 to 7 days.

Death Rites: The body is not embalmed; it is placed in the home for the wake. Church services and burial in the ground follow. Feelings of grief may be verbally expressed.

Food Practices and Intolerances: The diet tends to be high in starch and fat. Potatoes and rye and wheat products are staples.

Child Rearing Practices: A wide variety of family planning methods are used, and abortion is an option. Strict discipline, respect for elders, and development of strength, individualism, and self-sufficiency are important. The grandmother has a valued position in child rearing.

National Childhood Immunizations: BCG at birth, between 11 and 12 months, and at 7, 12, and 18 years; OPV at 3 months, between 4 and 5 months, at 6 months, between 19 and 24 months, and at 6 and 11 years; measles at between 13 and 15 months and at 9 years.

BIBLIOGRAPHY

Andrews MM, Boyle JS: *Transcultural concepts in nursing care*, ed 2, Philadelphia, 1995, Lippincott.

Blunt E: Emergency nursing in Poland, *J Emerg Nurs* 19(6):22A, 1993.

Chilicki CR: Contributor.

Cook LJ: Notes from work in Poland with a perinatal education program, *Neonatal Net* 5:61, 1992.

Frackiewicz L: The importance of social policy in the protection of people's health in Poland, *Acta Med Leg Soc (Liege)* 36(2):35, 1986.

Lagowska U: System of nursing care in Poland, *Int Nurs Rev* 34(5):131, 1987.

Lenartowicz H: Polish nursing in action, *Nurs Adm Q* 16(2):64, 1992.

Nelson F: Citizen Ambassador Program of People to People International's hospice delegation to Russia and Poland, *Am J Hospice Palliat Care* 12(4):6, 1995.

Ostrowska A: Elements of the health culture of Polish society, *Soc Sci Med* 17(10):631, 1983.

Reid J: A trip to Poland examines their midwifery, *KY Nurse* 42(4):15, 1994.

Roemer MI: Recent health system development in Poland and Hungary, *J Community Health* 19(3):153, 1994.

Spector RE: *Cultural diversity in health & illness,* ed 4, Stamford, Conn, 1996, Appleton & Lange.

Wronska I, Lidbrink M: Letter from Poland, *Nurs Times* 92(3):221, 1996.

◆ PORTUGAL

MAP PAGE (314)

Location: Portugal is located at the extreme southwestern edge of Europe on the Iberian Peninsula. It is crossed by many small rivers; the three largest arise in Spain and flow into the Atlantic. North of the Tajus River it is mountainous, cool, and rainy, whereas in the south dry plains and warm climate prevail. The nine islands of the Azores provide an important link in the air route across the Atlantic Ocean.

Major Language	Ethnic Groups		Major Religions	
Portuguese	Portuguese	99%	Catholic	97%
	African and	1%	Protestant	1%
	Other		Other	2%

Ethnic/Race Specific or Endemic Diseases: Joseph disease. The AIDS rate per 100,000 is 6.61.

Birth Rites: Childbirth is not highly ritualized. Rural villagers rely on lay midwives to assist at birth. At home women may wish to deliver while kneeling on a clean sheet on the floor. Chicken soup or melted butter that is consumed after delivery may help the uterus to go back in place.

Death Rites: The traditional widow is expected to remain unmarried and to wear black clothing for the rest of her life. She visits the grave frequently and has a picture of the deceased spouse evident in the home.

National Childhood Immunizations: BCG at birth and 5 and 11 years; DPT at 2, 4, 6, and 18 months and 5 years; OPV at 2, 4, and 6 months and 5 years; MMR at 15 months.

BIBLIOGRAPHY

Andrews MM, Boyle JS: *Transcultural concepts in nursing care*, ed 2, Philadelphia, 1995, Lippincott.

Boavida J, Borges L: Community involvement in early intervention: a Portuguese perspective, *Infants Young Child* 7(1):42, 1994.

Cobb AK: The role of the lay midwife in childbirth in rural Portugal, *West J Nurs Res* 17(4):353, 1995.

Eisenbruch M: Cross-cultural aspects of bereavement. II. Ethnic and cultural variations in the development of bereavement practices, *Cult Med Psychiatry* 8(4):315, 1984.

Patient education in selected countries, *J Hum Hypertens,* Feb 1990, p 107.

◆ QATAR

MAP PAGE (318)

Location: This Islamic republic occupies a small peninsula in the Persian Gulf. The barren, stony land is low lying; the highest point is 344 feet (105 m) above sea level. The climate is hot and humid. Most of the people live in the urban capital area, and the nomadic bedouins are being encouraged to live there also.

Major Languages	Ethnic Groups		Major Religions	
Arabic	Arab	40%	Muslim	95%
English	Pakistani	18%	Other	5%
	East Indian	18%		
	Iranian	10%		
	Other	14%		

Predominant Sick Care Practices: Modern health and dental care, including primary, secondary, and tertiary services, are readily available and free.

Ethnic/Race Specific or Endemic Diseases: RISK: The fumes from Bokhour, an Arabian Gulf incense, are a common precipitator of asthma attacks in children. The AIDS rate per 100,000 is 0.91.

Death Rites: Muslim belief forbids organ donations or transplants. Muslim physicians may recommend transfusions to save lives. Autopsy is uncommon because the deceased must be buried intact. Cremation is not permitted. For Muslim burial the body is wrapped in special pieces of cloth and buried without a coffin in the ground.

Food Practices and Intolerances: Pork, carrion, and blood are forbidden. Food tends to be spicy. Ramadan fasting is practiced, with exemptions for the sick and children.

National Childhood Immunizations: BCG at birth; DPT at 2, 4, and 6 months, between 18 and 24 months, and at 4 years; OPV at 2, 4, and 6 months, between 18 and 24 months, and at 4 years; measles at 9 and 15 months; hep B at birth and 1 and 9 months.

BIBLIOGRAPHY

Dawod S, Hussain AAW: Childhood asthma in Qatar, *Ann Allergy Asthma Immunol* 75(4):360, 1995.

Green J: Death with dignity: Islam, *Nurs Times* 85(5):56, 1989.

Nagelkerk J: Nursing in the State of Qatar, *J Nurs Adm* 24(11):15, 1994.

Ross HM: Societal/cultural views regarding death and dying, *Top Clin Nurs* 1(1):1, 1981.

◆ ROMANIA

MAP PAGE (314)

Location: This eastern European republic opens onto the Black Sea. The highest peak of the Carpathian Mountains and Transylvanian Alps is 8346 feet (2544 m); the two mountain ranges have a plateau and plains between them. Warm summers and cold, snowy winters are characteristic.

Major Languages	Ethnic Groups		Major Religions	
Romanian	Romanian	89%	Romanian	70%
Hungarian	Hungarian	9%	Orthodox	
German	German	2%	Catholic	6%
			Protestant	6%
			Other	18%

Predominant Sick Care Practices: Biomedical; magico-religious. Superstitions and rituals are incorporated into daily life.

Health Care Beliefs: Acute sick care only.

Ethnic/Race Specific or Endemic Diseases: RISK: Industrial pollution influences health. Cardiovascular diseases, hypertension, viral hepatitis, and cancer are major adult problems, whereas malnutrition among AIDS victims and respiratory illnesses are more common among children than adults. The AIDS rate per 100,000 is 2.85. Approximately 80% of the water supply is not potable.

Health Team Relationships: Physicians were the only health care professionals when nursing schools were closed in 1978. Midwives are now available, and redevelopment of the health care system and professionals is the goal.

Families' Role in Hospital Care: Patient care is at a minimum. The majority of hospitals accommodate two patients per bed. Medical equipment is not readily available, or it is kept for personal use or sold on the black market.

Dominance Patterns: The traditional pattern is patriarchal and is based on male decision making in the public domain. Although men agree that physical abuse is unacceptable, female abuse is a societal male coping mechanism. Females have authority over domestic affairs. Couples often live with the husband's parents, and the mother-in-law manages domestic affairs.

Perceptions of Time: Time schedules are followed more precisely in urban areas than they are in rural areas.

Pain Reactions: Without any analgesia, women do not make any sounds during labor in hospitals.

Birth Rites: Most deliveries are assisted by midwives in hospitals. The maternal mortality rate has dropped since the legalization of abortion.

Death Rites: Romanians believe in an afterlife.

Child Rearing Practices: Milk may be unavailable, so parents may try to obtain calcium tablets on the black market. Approximately 700 orphanages or dystrophic centers exist for children. Dystrophia includes AIDS, metabolic disorders, congenital anomalies, malnutrition, and failure to thrive.

National Childhood Immunizations: BCG at birth and 7 and 14 years; DPT at 3, 4, 5, 18, and 36 months; DT/Td at 7 and 14 years; OPV at between 2 and 7 months, between 4 and 9 months, between 10 and 15 months, and at 9 years; measles at between 9 and 15 months and at 7 years.

Other Characteristics: Abortion and contraceptives are legal. Only since the 1989 revolution has the government acknowledged the existence of AIDS. Children are often left at orphanages.

BIBLIOGRAPHY

Awlasewicz A: Contributor.

Betrothal and marriage, Life 14(2):54, 1991.

Buchanan J: Ceausescu's legacy, *Nurs Times* 86(7):16, 1990.

Campbell NN, Harbonne DJ, Norwich R: Medicine in Romania, *Br Med J* 300(6726):699, 1990.

Cassidy MD: Romania: haemodialysis, handicap and a sense of humor, *Lancet* 337(8737):353, 1991.

Cole JW, Nydon JA: Class, gender and fertility, *East Eur Q* 23(4):469, 1989.

Death and remembrance, Life 14(2):72, 1991.

Dickman S: AIDS in children adds to Romania's troubles, *Nature* 343:579, 1990.

Ember L: Pollution chokes East-bloc nations, *Chem Engin News* 68(16):7, 1990.

Freedman DC: Gender identity and dance style, *East Eur Q* 23(4):419, 1990.

Hale J: Customs and folklore. In *The land and people of Romania,* New York, 1972, Lippincott.

Houston S: Birth, abortion, family planning and child care in Romania, *Prof Care Mother Child* 3(2):41, 1993.

Lakey CK: Romania: a nursing journey, *Nurs Health Care* 16(3):144, 1995.

Lakey CK et al.: Health care and nursing in Romania, *J Adv Nurs* 23(5):1045, 1996.

Lass A: The wedding of the dead, *Am Anthropol* 92(3):784, 1990.

Life after Ceausescu, *Economist* 314(7636):43, 1990.

Lutz S: Nurses begin Romanian mission, *Mod Healthcare* 21(34):13, 1990.

Lutz S: U.S. execs find Romanian health system "depraved," *Mod Healthcare* 20(37):2, 1990.

Nolan P, Nolan M: Child of hardship, *Nurs Times* 87(12):16, 1991.

Rawlinson JW: Developing mental health nursing education in Romania, *Nurse Ed Today* 13(3):225, 1993.

Rudin C et al.: HIV-1, hepatitis (A, B, and C) and measles in Romanian children, *Lancet* 336(8730):1592, 1990.

◆ RUSSIA

MAP PAGE (315)

Location: Massive disintegration of the former Soviet Union's Communist Party and territory occurred in 1992. Declarations of independence by the republics of Latvia, Estonia, and Lithuania were followed rapidly by declarations of other republics. Russia extends from the western Black and Baltic Seas to the Pacific Ocean. Its vast areas of plains and plateaus are relieved by some low mountain ranges. The climate varies from arctic severity in winters to subtropical heat in summers.

Major Languages	**Ethnic Groups**		**Major Religions**
Russian	Russian	82%	Russian Orthodox
Ukrainian	Tatar	4%	Muslim
Belarussian	Other	14%	
Uzbek			
Armenian			

The practice of religion became legal in 1989.

Predominant Sick Care Practices: Biomedical. Holistic, folk, and Western medical practices coexist. Health promotion and illness prevention do not predominate. Mortality and morbidity statistics have increased since the change to a free market economy.

Health Care Beliefs: Passive role; acute sick care; health promotion important. Health promotion practices encourage maternal and child care. Health care addresses acute problems and tertiary care; however, rehabilitation is not emphasized.

Ethnic/Race Specific or Endemic Diseases (in former Soviet Union): ENDEMIC: Chloroquine-sensitive malaria in scattered areas bordering Iran and Afghanistan; diphtheria nearing epidemic proportions; whooping cough; measles. RISK: Japanese encephalitis. The AIDS rate per 100,000 is 0.02.

Health Team Relationships: Health care paraprofessionals (nurses in particular) are under the control of physicians and have no independent roles. Questioning a physician's order is unacceptable. The rigid and highly specialized health care system provides separate hospitals for children and adults. The dividing age is 15. Rural hospitals, however, serve all ages.

Families' Role in Hospital Care: Patients in general hospital units wear street clothes and take on a passive role. Family members usually bathe, feed, and comfort the patient and change the bed linen; when hospitals lack a nursing staff, family members clean bedpans and bring food from home.

Dominance Patterns: The father usually assumes the dominant role, and the mother and grandmother share domestic and child health decisions.

Eye Contact Practices: Direct, sustained eye contact is the norm.

Touch Practices: Three kisses on the cheek for greetings and farewells are common. Touch is an important part of nonverbal communication.

Perceptions of Time: Punctual or even early for appointments.

Pain Reactions: Some are communicative about pain, and others are stoic. Some prefer injections for pain relief.

Birth Rites: Most infants are born in hospitals. A wide range of care may not be available in all areas. Hospitalization lasts approximately 5 to 10 days, and no visitors, including the father, are allowed for the first 2 days or at all. The mother and child can be viewed through a glass window to protect them against infection. At time of hospital discharge all mothers are breastfeeding and desire to continue as long as there is milk. Breastfeeding in dim light to protect the infant's eyesight may be preferred. Male circumcision is not usually done by Russian Christians.

Death Rites: First the family is told of a serious prognosis, and they decide if the patient should be informed.

Food Practices and Intolerances: The heaviest of the three meals is at noon. The diet is high in starch, fat, and salt. No ice is desired in drinks. Vodka made from potatoes is sold without age restrictions or government regulations. It is served free with meals at restaurants unless water or soda is specifically requested.

Child Rearing Practices: The child is encouraged to focus on the mother and may continue to do so throughout life. Children are taught to depend heavily on their parents. Because of the economic burden, children with defects as simple as a lazy eye are placed in orphanages for adoption.

National Childhood Immunizations (former Soviet Union): BCG at between 4 and 7 days, at 7 years, between 14 and 15 years, and between 27 and 30 years; DPT at 3 months, between 4 and 5 months, and at 6 and 18 months; DT/Td at between 6 and 7 years, between 11 and 12 years, and every 10 years thereafter; OPV at 3 months, between 4 and 5 months, and at 6 months, between 1 and 2 years, at 3 years, between 7 and 8 years, and between 15 and 16 years; measles at 12 months and between 6 and 7 years.

Other Characteristics: Attempting to control or suppress emotions is considered unfriendly, insincere, and dishonest. Hands clasped above the head is a traditional gesture of friendship. Many establish an area of personal space by displaying an impassive facial expression; however, such demeanor should not automatically be interpreted as unfriendly.

BIBLIOGRAPHY

Allen A: Old enemies practice teamwork, *J Post Anesth Nurs* 9(4):247, 1994.

Braaten KM, Meyers J, Anderson J: Visit inside Russian health care, *Prairie Rose* 62(2):8, 1993.

Bridges LB, Clacy BJ: An American perception of Soviet health care, *Kansas Nurse,* March 1988, p 1.

Condon JC, Yousef F: *An introduction to intercultural communication,* New York, 1975, Macmillan.

Dennis LI: Nursing within the Soviet health care system, *Int Nurs Rev* 32(5):149, 1985.

Edwards DJ: Transcultural nursing: a view of the Russian health care system, *Orthop Nurs* 13(2):47, 1994.

Elliott RL: Life experiences of Russian nurses with health care systems, *J Multicult Nurs & Health* 1(1):13, 1994.

Evanikoff LJ: Russians. In Lipson JG, Dibble SL, Minarik PA: *Culture and nursing care: a pocket guide,* San Francisco, 1996, UCSF Nursing Press.

Galanti GA: *Caring for patients from different cultures,* ed 2, Philadelphia, 1997, University of Pennsylvania Press.

Galkin VV et al.: Health system development and infection control in Russia, *Asepsis* 18(2):4, 1996.

Harper B: The new Russia: a hope for maternity care, *Int J Childbirth Educ* 9(3):3032, 1994.

Harris-Offutt R: Inside Russia: a look at alcohol and other drug use, treatment methodologies, and effectiveness of treatment, *Addictions Nurs* 7(3):71, 1995.

Kinsey D: The moral and professional role of the Russian nurse, *Nurs Health Care* 13(8):426, 1992.

Kluny R: From Russia with love, *News Am Holistic Nurses Assoc* 15(6):1, 1995.

Korb MM: Expectations in giving and receiving help among nurses and Russian refugees, *Int J Nurs Stud* 33(5):479, 1996.

MacAvoy S: A cross-cultural learning opportunity: USSR, *J Cont Educ Nurs* 19(5):196, 1988.

Miner J, Witte DJ, Nordstrom DL: Infant feeding practices in a Russian and a United States City: patterns and comparisons, *J Hum Lact* 10(2):95, 1994.

Monks P: Go private or die, *Nurs Times* 90(25):44, 1994.

Picard C, Perfiljeva G: Nursing education in Russia: visions and realities, *Nurs Health Care* 16(3):126, 1995.

Prosser MH: *The cultural dialogue,* Washington, DC, 1985, SIETAR.

Rahlin M: Mother and child in Russian healthcare, *Pediatr Phys Ther* 7(4):187, 1995.

Samovar LA, Porter RE: *Intercultural communication: a reader,* Belmont, Calif, 1985, Wadsworth.

Schecter J et al.: *Back in the U.S.S.R.,* New York, 1988, Macmillan.

Smith H: *The new Russians,* New York, 1990, Random House.

Storey PB: Emergency medical services in the U.S.S.R. In Schwartz GR, editor: *Principles and practice of emergency medicine,* vol 2, Philadelphia, 1978, Saunders.

Storti C: *The art of crossing cultures,* Yarmouth, Me, 1990, Intercultural Press.

Szwez D: Contributor.

Wenge R, anchor: *CNN News,* March 20, 1994.

◆ RWANDA

MAP PAGE (317)

Location: This landlocked nation in eastern Africa has grassy hills and deep valleys that support subsistence farming. It is one of Africa's most densely populated countries, and all arable land is being used.

Major Languages	Ethnic Groups		Major Religions	
Kinyarwanda	Hutu	90%	Catholic	65%
French	Tutsi	9%	Indigenous	25%
Kiswahili	Twa (Pygmoid)	1%	Beliefs	
			Protestant	9%
			Muslim	1%

Ethnic/Race Specific or Endemic Diseases: ENDEMIC: Yellow fever; cholera; shigellosis; malaria that is currently chloroquine resistant. Diarrheal diseases and malnutrition are major problems resulting from the displacement and genocide of about one eighth of the population in 1994. AIDS case rate is 30.5/100,000 people. HIV was estimated at 30% of the population before the start of the 1994 war. **RISK:** Tuberculosis. The AIDS rate per 100,000 is reported by the country as zero.

Dominance Patterns: Fathers eat first and get the better food.

National Childhood Immunizations: BCG at birth; DPT at 6, 10, and 14 weeks and 15 months; OPV at 6, 10, and 14 weeks; measles at 9 months.

Other Characteristics: Menarche may occur later than age 15. The Tutsi are extremely tall people.

BIBLIOGRAPHY

Adler MW, editor: Statistics from the World Health Organization and the Centers for Disease Control, *AIDS* 6(10):1229, 1992.

Dodd R: Rwanda, one year on, *Nurs Times* 11(19):42, 1995.

Jones AG: Relief organization provides valuable service—AmeriCares, *Minn Nurs Accent* 67(1):1, 1995.

Lambert MI: Rebuilding in Rwanda: about nurses and nursing, *Home Health Focus* 2(11):84, 1996.

Lyons T: A nurse's experience in a world gone temporarily mad, *Alaska Nurse* 46(3):1, 1996.

Ninger LJ: New hope for Rwanda: NP leads the way, *NPnews* 3(4):3, 1995.

Overfield T: *Biologic variation in health and illness,* Menlo Park, Calif, 1985, Addison-Wesley.

◆ ST. KITTS-NEVIS

MAP PAGE (313)

Location: Also known as St. Christopher-Nevis, St. Kitts-Nevis is located in the eastern Caribbean among the northern Leeward Islands. The population is primarily rural and concentrated along the coast.

Major Language	Ethnic Groups		Major Religions	
English	Black	95%	Protestant	76%
	Other	5%	Catholic	11%
			Other	13%

Ethnic/Race Specific or Endemic Diseases: The AIDS rate per 100,000 is 12.20.

National Childhood Immunizations: BCG at 5 years; DPT at 3 months, between 4 and 5 months, between 5 and 6 months, and at 18 months; DT at 5 years; OPV at 3 months, between 4 and 5 months, between 5 and 6 months, at 18 months, and at 4 years; MMR at between 12 and 15 months.

BIBLIOGRAPHY

Adler MW, editor: Statistics from the World Health Organization and the Centers for Disease Control, *AIDS* 6(10):1229, 1992.

◆ ST. LUCIA

MAP PAGE (313)

Location: St. Lucia is one of the Windward Islands of the eastern Caribbean. It is a volcanic island, and mountains run from north to south. St. Lucians are primarily descendants of black African slaves. The island has a tropical climate.

Major Languages	Ethnic Groups		Major Religions	
English	Black	90%	Catholic	90%
French Patois	Mixed	6%	Protestant	7%
	East Indian	3%	Anglican and	3%
	White and	1%	Other	
	Other			

Ethnic/Race Specific or Endemic Diseases: RISK: Schistosomiasis. The AIDS rate per 100,000 is 7.04.

National Childhood Immunizations: BCG at 3 months; DPT at 3, 4½, 6, and 15 months; DT at 5 years; Td at 18 years; OPV at 3, 4½, 6, and 15 months and 5 years; MMR at 12 months.

BIBLIOGRAPHY

Adler MW, editor: Statistics from the World Health Organization and the Centers for Disease Control, *AIDS* 6(10):1229, 1992.

◆ ST. VINCENT AND THE GRENADINES

MAP PAGE (313)

Location: These islands are among the Windward Islands of the eastern Caribbean. St. Vincent has forested mountains and a volcano that became active in 1979, and The Grenadines are a chain of hundreds of little islets. The people are primarily descendants of black African slaves. The climate is hot and humid.

Major Languages	**Ethnic Groups**		**Major Religions**	
English	African	95%	Anglican	70%
French Patois	Other	5%	Methodist	15%
			Catholic	10%
			Other	5%

Predominant Sick Care Practices: Biomedical.

Ethnic/Race Specific or Endemic Diseases: The AIDS rate per 100,000 is 5.36.

Health Team Relationships: Nurses are authoritarian and dominate the patients. Slapping patients is acceptable behavior.

Dominance Patterns: Women are often dominant, especially in the home.

Food Practices and Intolerances: Great quantities of fruits and vegetables are eaten, and meat is rarely in the diet. Food is cooked outside.

Child Rearing Practices: The pregnancy rate is high because the child mortality rate is high. The percentage of children who die before age 5 is high; 50% die before adulthood. School is voluntary.

National Childhood Immunizations: BCG at birth; DPT at 3, 4½, and 6 months; DT at 4½ years; OPV at 3, 4½, and 6 months and 5 years; MMR at 12 months.

Other Characteristics: No records of births, deaths, or diseases are kept.

BIBLIOGRAPHY

Steel J: Lecture notes, Nursing 309, Storrs, Conn, University of Connecticut, Nov 13, 1991.

◆ SAN MARINO

MAP PAGE (314)

Location: Tiny San Marino is the oldest republic in the world. It has a strong, independent history, even though it is completely surrounded by Italy. Its landlocked location in the

Apennine mountains affords a rugged terrain. People remain citizens and have voting privileges no matter where they live.

Major Language	Ethnic Groups		Major Religions	
Italian	Italo-Sanmarinese	99%	Catholic	99%
	Other	1%	Other	1%

Ethnic/Race Specific or Endemic Diseases: RISK: Lipid metabolism disorders; anxiety; depression; irritable bowel syndrome; stomach-gastritis problems. The AIDS rate per 100,000 is reported by the country as zero.

National Childhood Immunizations: No data located.

BIBLIOGRAPHY

Mamon J, Paccagnella B: Patient counseling by general practitioners: Republic of San Marino's experience, *Health Educ Q* 18(1):135, 1991.

◆ SÃO TOMÉ AND PRÍNCIPE

MAP PAGE (317)

Location: These small volcanic islands are located 150 miles (240 km) off the west coast of Africa in the Gulf of Guinea. São Tomé has dense mountainous jungle, and Príncipe has jagged mountains.

Major Language	Ethnic Groups		Major Religions	
Portuguese	Portuguese-African	98%	Catholic	80%
			Protestant	10%
	African	2%	Other	10%

Ethnic/Race Specific or Endemic Diseases: ACTIVE: Cholera. **ENDEMIC:** Yellow fever; chloroquine-sensitive malaria. **RISK:** The AIDS rate per 100,000 is 3.01.

National Childhood Immunizations: BCG at birth; DPT-1 at 3 months; DPT-2 at 4 months; DPT-3 at 5 months; measles at 9 months; OPV-1 at 3 months; OPV-2 at 4 months; OPV-3 at 5 months.

BIBLIOGRAPHY

No data located, including no updated WHO immunization schedule.

◆ SAUDI ARABIA

MAP PAGE (318)

Location: Most of the Arabian Peninsula of the Middle East is occupied by Saudi Arabia. The Red Sea and the Gulf of Aqaba lie to the west; the Arabian (Persian) Gulf lies to the east. A mountain range spans the length of the western coastline; east of the mountains is a massive plateau, the Rub Al-Khali (Empty Quarter), which contains the world's largest sand desert.

Major Language	Ethnic Groups		Major Religions	
Arabic	Arab	90%	Muslim	99%
	Afro-Asian	10%	Other	1%

Predominant Sick Care Practices: Biomedical; holistic; magico-religious; traditional. Islamic beliefs and culture pervade all aspects of health care. Although advanced technologic medical care is available, many among the nomadic tribes in remote villages favor traditional practices. For example, it is believed that healing by cauterization, which results in many scars on the body, burns out evil spirits.

Health Care Beliefs: Active involvement; health promotion important. The practice of healthy ways, performance of roles, and harmony in life are valued. Nomadic tribes and people in remote areas seek treatment only when they are extremely ill and are possibly beyond curative treatment. Many believe that intrusive procedures such as injections and intravenous fluids are more effective than are those procedures that are not intrusive. Women hold an inferior social position, and their somatic complaints are often signs of emotional distress.

Ethnic/Race Specific or Endemic Diseases: Dental caries caused by the high consumption of dates and poor oral hygiene are a major problem. ENDEMIC: Chloroquine-sensitive malaria; schistosomiasis. RISK: High prevalence of diabetes mellitus. Trachoma; syphilis; leprosy; filariasis in western Saudi Arabia; cutaneous leishmaniasis in Bisha; cholera in the Jizan district; rickets and malnutrition diseases in rural areas. The AIDS rate per 100,000 is 0.21.

Health Team Relationships: Health care professionals and support personnel who are the same sex as the patient are important to male and female patients and may be essential for females. Male nurses may not give direct care or enter the room of an adult female patient who is alone. Some male patients may accept female nurses. Elaborate and prolonged greeting rituals are practiced with polite expressions and inquiries. To avoid conflict or to avoid admitting ignorance, people may say "yes" when they mean "no."

Families' Role in Hospital Care: Most patients have one or more family members or sitters staying with them, and most hospitals provide couches in each room. Family and friends may be demanding of health care personnel to ensure that care and attention are given to the patient. The sitter also expects services from nursing staff.

Dominance Patterns: The husband is the family leader and decision maker. A woman cannot sign an operative consent form; two male family members sign for her. The man may answer questions directed to his spouse. He may decide when the family member should eat and bathe, or the female may decide basic care patterns such as when to bathe, eat, and breastfeed. Extended families live together in the same compound. The Saudi mother is revered, and most sons will seek their mothers' opinion on family issues.

Eye Contact Practices: For a woman, direct eye contact is limited to other women or family members. Educated Saudis generally respect direct eye contact as a sign of honesty and integrity. An approximate 2-foot separation permits conversationalists to evaluate each other's pupil responses. Pupils dilate with interest and contract with dislike.

Touch Practices: Males may touch only those women who are in the family. It is common for males to hold hands in public. Handshakes are continued for a lengthy period.

Perceptions of Time: Time has little meaning except in business. Enshalla (as Allah wills), or whenever it happens, is the norm. Social rituals continue while appointments go by unattended.

Pain Reactions: Pain is expressed verbally and nonverbally and with emotion, especially to the family. Immediate pain relief is desired. A great deal of analgesia may be needed for pain relief. Some patients may wish to remain sufficiently alert to be able to pray. Some Arabic cultures make use of analogies and metaphors to describe their pain.

Birth Rites: The father, grandfather, and many female family members are present for birthing. The father may move into the hospital room after delivery; he will be a constant visitor.

Death Rites: Confronting the patient with a grave diagnosis shatters hope and creates mistrust. It is believed that only God knows the true prognosis, and death is discussed with extreme reluctance. After death the body must be washed by a family member before removal from the hospital or the home. No menstruating female can touch the body because she is unclean and will affect the afterlife of the deceased. Embalming and autopsies are rarely permitted. Females express grief by wailing. Muslim belief forbids organ donations or transplants. Muslim physicians may recommend transfusions to save lives. Cremation is not permitted. For Muslim burial the body is wrapped in special pieces of cloth and buried without a coffin in the ground.

Food Practices and Intolerances: Ramadan fasting is practiced from sunup to sundown. The sick person must receive permission not to fast from the Iman during this month. Lamb and rice are common foods. Fresh fruits and vegetables are included among the more up-to-date people. Pork and alcoholic beverages are forbidden. Food deprivation is considered a precursor to illness. It is customary to have food or beverages offered several times before accepting.

Infant Feeding Practices: Breastfeeding is the predominant practice, and it continues for an average of 1 year. Nomadic people give infants ghee, a semifluid and clarified form of butter, for the first 3 days of life to lubricate and clean the intestines and to give nourishment. A wet nurse may breastfeed until the mother begins lactating. Older children may be fed powdered goat's or camel's milk.

Child Rearing Practices: If a wife does not produce a son and heir, her husband divorces her. Contraceptive methods are not used, and women may have 15 or more children. Because of the high infant mortality rate, a welcoming party for an infant is delayed for 3 months. Boys are raised in the female section of the household until they are 10 years old; then the boys are segregated. Boys and girls are educated separately. A traditional practice that is on the decline is to remove the female clitoris at puberty; the vagina may also be partially sewn up to prevent premarital sex and to curtail the sex drive. Females begin wearing the veil by age 12. Premarital and extramarital sex are strongly forbidden by Islamic law and may be punishable by death.

National Childhood Immunizations: BCG at birth; DPT at 1½, 3, 5, and 18 months and at between 4 and 6 years; OPV at 1½, 3, 5, and 18 months and between 4 and 6 years; measles at 6 and 12 months; hep B at birth and 1½ and 6 months.

Other Characteristics: Religious police (Matowa) enforce the cultural laws governing segregation of the sexes, dress codes, and the use of alcohol and illegal drugs. Covering the hair is required for women. Polygamy is more common among the older generations and is practiced with the condition that the wives will be treated equally. Hope, optimism, and the positive advantages of treatment should be stressed.

BIBLIOGRAPHY

Adelman MB, Lustig MW: Intercultural communication problems as perceived by Saudi Arabian and American managers. Paper presented to the Intercultural Communication Division of the Western Speech Communication Association, San Jose, Calif, 1981.

al-Nasser AN, Bamgboye EA, Alburno MK: A retrospective study of factors affecting breast feeding practices in a rural community of Saudi Arabia, *East Afr Med J* 68(3):174, 1991.

al-Shammari SA: Help-seeking behavior of adults with health problems in Saudi Arabia, *Fam Pract Res J* 12(1):75, 1992.

Anderson R: Saudi Arabian culture. In On the scene, *Nurs Adm Q* 16(2):20, 1992.

Ballas E: Health meanings of Saudi women, *J Adv Nurs* 21(5):853, 1995.

Boyles C, Nordhaugen N: An employee health service in Saudi Arabia, *AAOHN J* 37(11):459, 1989.

Brown BJ: Contributor.

Dahlberg N: Innovative management of acute pain: a collaborative approach. Paper presented at the Second International Middle East Nursing Conference, Irbid, Jordan, April 27, 1992.

Daly E: Personal communication, April 26, 1992.

Davis CF: Culturally responsive nursing management in an international health care setting. In On the scene, *Nurs Adm Q* 16(2):36, 1992.

El Hazmi et al.: Diabetes mellitus and impaired glucose tolerance in Saudi Arabia, *Ann Saudi Med* 16(4):381, 1996.

Galanti GA: *Caring for patients from different cultures,* ed 2, Philadelphia, 1997, University of Pennsylvania Press.

Green J: Death with dignity: Islam, *Nurs Times* 85(5):56, 1989.

Hall ET: Learning the Arabs' silent language, *Psychol Today,* Aug 1979, p 45.

Hathout MM: Comment on ethical crises and cultural differences, *West J Med* 139(3):380, 1983.

Meleis AI, Jonsen AR: Medicine in perspective: ethical crises and cultural differences, *West J Med* 138(6):889, 1980.

Racy J: Somatization in Saudi women: a therapeutic challenge, *Br J Psychiatry* 137:212, 1980.

Reece D: Covering and communication: the symbolism of dress among Muslim women, *Howard J Commun* 7(1):35, 1996.

Reizian A, Meleis AI: Arab-Americans' perceptions of and responses to pain, *Crit Care Nurse* 6(6):30, 1986.

Ross HM: Societal/cultural views regarding death and dying, *Top Clin Nurs* 1(1):1, 1981.

Sebai ZA, Bella H: Laying the foundations of good health care, *World Health Forum* 11(4):385, 1990.

Storti C: *The art of crossing cultures,* Yarmouth, Me, 1990, Intercultural Press.

◆ SENEGAL

MAP PAGE (316)

Location: Senegal is the westernmost nation in Africa and is located on the Atlantic coast. It consists primarily of a rural population that lives by subsistence farming. The country has one of the best transportation systems in Africa. Much of Senegal is low lying and flat, with differentiated dry and wet seasons.

Major Languages	Ethnic Groups		Major Religions	
French	Wolof	36%	Muslim	92%
Wolof	Fulani	17%	Indigenous	6%
Pulaar	Serer	17%	Beliefs	
Diola	Toucouleur	9%	Christian	2%
Mandingo and Other	Diola and Other	21%		

Ethnic/Race Specific or Endemic Diseases: ENDEMIC: Yellow fever; chloroquine-resistant malaria. RISK: Schistosomiasis. Vitamin A deficiency is a major cause of childhood blindness. The AIDS rate per 100,000 is 4.76.

Death Rites: Muslim belief forbids organ donations or transplants. Muslim physicians may recommend transfusions to save lives. Autopsy is uncommon because the deceased must be buried intact. For Muslim burial the body is wrapped in special pieces of cloth and buried without a coffin in the ground. Cremation is not permitted.

Food Practices and Intolerances: Pork, carrion, and blood are forbidden. Food tends to be spicy. Ramadan fasting is practiced, with exemptions for the sick.

Child Rearing Practices: Female circumcision and excision is widespread in some groups.

National Childhood Immunizations: BCG at birth; DPT at 6, 10, and 14 weeks; OPV at birth and 6, 10, and 14 weeks; measles at 9 months; hep B at 9 months.

Other Characteristics: Children under age 5 who migrate from rural to urban areas continue to have a much higher mortality rate.

BIBLIOGRAPHY

Brockerhoff M: Rural-to-urban migration and child survival in Senegal, *Demography 1990* 27(4):601, 1990.

Fassin D et al.: Who consults and where? Sociocultural differentiation in access to health care in urban Africa, *Int J Epidemiol* 17(4):858, 1988.

McEvers NC: Health and the assault on poverty in low income countries, *Soc Sci Med* 14(1):41, 1980.

Ross HM: Societal/cultural views regarding death and dying, *Top Clin Nurs* 1(1):1, 1981.

Rowell M: Eradication of vitamin A deficiency with 5 cents and a vegetable garden, *J Ophthalmic Nurs Tech* 12(5):217, 1993.
Wright J: Female genital mutilation: an overview, *J Adv Nurs* 24:251, 1996.

◆ SERBIA AND MONTENEGRO (Yugoslavia)

MAP PAGE (314)

Location: The "new" Yugoslavia is located in southeastern Europe on the Balkan Peninsula along the Adriatic Sea. Present-day Yugoslavia consists of its former republics of Serbia and Montenegro. Serbia contains the fertile Danube River plain, whereas Montenegro is very mountainous.

Major Languages	Ethnic Groups		Major Religions	
Serbo-Croatian	Serb	63%	Greek	65%
Albanian	Albanian	14%	Orthodox	
	Montenegrin	6%	Muslim	19%
	Other	17%	Catholic	4%
			Other	12%

Ethnic/Race Specific or Endemic Diseases: RISK: Coronary heart disease; colon cancer; adult-onset insulin-dependent diabetes. The AIDS rate per 100,000 is 0.89.

National Childhood Immunizations: No data located.

BIBLIOGRAPHY

Aspell T: *NBC News,* June 15, 1992.
Benson ER: The legend of the Maiden of Kosovo and nursing in Serbia, *IMAGE: J Nurs Sch* 23(1):57, 1991.
Brokaw T, anchor: *NBC News,* June 25, 1991.
Reeser DS: An international experience, *Imprint* 32(1):46, 1985.
Solomon J: Critical care nursing, *Focus Crit Care* 13(3):10, 1986.
Sutton J: Why Bosnia lies bleeding, *World Vision Childlife* IX(2):6, 1996.

◆ SEYCHELLES

MAP PAGE (317)

Location: Approximately 100 islands in the Indian Ocean east of Africa and northeast of Madagascar form the Seychelles. Many of the islands are uninhabited atolls. The country's culture contains French and African influences.

Major Languages	Ethnic Groups		Major Religions	
English	Black/Mulatto	99%	Catholic	90%
French	Other	1%	Anglican	8%
Creole			Other	2%

Ethnic/Race Specific or Endemic Diseases: The AIDS rate per 100,000 is 8.22.

National Childhood Immunizations: BCG at birth; DPT at 3, 4, 5, and 18 months; OPV at 3, 4, and 5 months; measles at 15 months.

BIBLIOGRAPHY

No data located.

◆ SIERRA LEONE

MAP PAGE (316)

Location: This western African coastal nation on the Atlantic has a heavily indented coastline with mangrove swamps, wooded hills, and a plateau inland.

Major Languages	Ethnic Groups		Major Religions	
English	Temne	30%	Muslim	60%
Krio	Mende	30%	Indigenous	30%
Mende	Creole and	40%	Beliefs	
Temne	Other		Christian	10%

Predominant Sick Care Practices: Fatalistic attitude and attributing illness to God's will. Traditional health care workers include bone setters, snake bite healers, herbalists, and birth attendants.

Ethnic/Race Specific or Endemic Diseases: ENDEMIC: Yellow fever; chloroquine-resistant malaria. RISK: Schistosomiasis; contaminated fresh and tap water. The AIDS rate per 100,000 is 0.64.

Health Team Relationships: Singing used for teaching method in neonatal clinic.

Families' Role in Hospital Care: In rural hospitals families provide meals.

Perceptions of Time: Afternoon naps are common. People tend to be oriented to the present. Because of lack of infrastructure for communication and transportation, being on time is impractical. Things happen when they happen.

Birth Rites: Highest neonatal deaths are caused by tetanus and gastroenteritis.

Child Rearing Practices: Female circumcision and excision is widespread in some groups. Age may not be known in a significant number of children.

National Childhood Immunizations: BCG at birth; DPT at 6, 10, and 14 weeks; OPV at birth and 6, 10, and 14 weeks; measles at 9 months.

Other Characteristics: Women rarely wear slacks.

BIBLIOGRAPHY

Cunningham ME, Beal CS, Nerderman RM: Nursing institute in Sierra Leone, Africa: a continuing education experience, *J Cult Diversity* 1(2):44, 1994.

Edwards NC: Traditional birth attendants in Sierra Leone: key providers of maternal and child health in West Africa, *West J Nurs Res* 9(3):335, 1987.

Seely DR et al.: Hearing loss prevalence and risk factors among Sierra Leonean children, *Arch Otolaryngol Head Neck Surg* 121(8):853, 1995.

Williams B, Yumbella F: An evaluation of the training of traditional birth attendants in Sierra Leone and their performance after training, *World Health Organ Offset Publ* (95):35, 1986.

Wright J: Female genital mutilation: an overview, *J Adv Nurs* 24:251, 1996.

◆ SINGAPORE

MAP PAGE (321)

Location: An island nation off the southeast coast of Malaysia, Singapore is one of the most densely populated areas in the world and is a leading economic power with one of the world's largest ports. Its economic power has contributed to its high standards of health, education, and housing. Most people live in the city of Singapore on the main island.

Major Languages	Ethnic Groups		Major Religions	
Malay	Chinese	76%	Buddhist	70%
Chinese	Malay	15%	Taoist	14%
Tamil	East Indian	6%	Muslim	9%
English	Other	3%	Hindu	7%

Health Care Beliefs: Fatalistic belief that life and death are beyond one's control.

Ethnic/Race Specific or Endemic Diseases: RISK: Japanese encephalitis. The AIDS rate per 100,000 is 1.96.

Touch Practices: The head is considered sacred. It is an offense to pat a child on the head. Reaching over the patient's head to pass something to another person may be impolite.

Food Practices and Intolerances: Female adolescent obesity risk is related to parents who were food vendors and male adolescent obesity with eating supper out.

National Childhood Immunizations: BCG at birth; DPT at 3, 4, 5, and 18 months; OPV at 3, 4, 5, and 18 months; measles at 12 months; hep B at birth and 1 and 6 months.

BIBLIOGRAPHY

Boon WH: Child health in Singapore: past, present and future, *J Sing Paediatr Soc Suppl*:4, 1979.

Fong NP, Basir H, Seow A: Awareness and acceptance of hepatitis B vaccination in Clementi, Singapore, *Ann Acad Med Singapore* 19(6):788, 1990.

Kong SG et al.: Some aspects of child-rearing practices and their relationship to behavioural deviance, *J Sing Paediatr Soc* 28(1-2):94, 1986.

Soo KS: My child is ill, what shall I do? *J Sing Paediatr Soc* 24(1-2):93, 1982.

Straughan PT, Seow A: Barriers to mammography among Chinese women in Singapore: a focus group approach, *Health Educ Res* 10(4):431, 1995.

Wong ML et al.: Influence of lifestyle behaviours on obesity among Chinese adolescents in Singapore, *Health Educ J* 54(2):198, 1995.

◆ SLOVAKIA

MAP PAGE (314)

Location: A part of the former Czechoslovakia with the Czech Republic, Slovakia is a rugged, mountainous area located in east central Europe. It has vast forests and pastureland.

Major Languages	Ethnic Groups		Major Religions	
Slavak	Slovak	86%	Catholic	60%
Hungarian	Hungarian	11%	Protestant	8%
	Other	3%	Orthodox	4%
			Other	28%

Predominant Sick Care Practices: Primarily biomedical state system. Some hope to introduce elements of natural healing into the system.

Ethnic/Race Specific or Endemic Diseases: The AIDS rate per 100,000 is 0.04.

National Childhood Immunizations: BCG at 4 days, 6 months, and 6, 13, and 18 years; DPT at 3, 5, and 12 months and 3 and 6 years; OPV 4 times between birth and 2 years and at 13 years; MMR at 2 and 14 years; hep B at birth and 1 and 6 months.

BIBLIOGRAPHY

Michalkova DM et al.: Incidence and prevalence of childhood diabetes in Slovakia, *Diabetes Care* 18(3):315, 1995.

Rubens D, Gyurkovics B, Hornacek K: The cultural production of bioterapia: psychic healing and the natural medicine movement in Slovakia, *Soc Sci Med* 41(9):1261, 1995.

◆ SLOVENIA

MAP PAGE (314)

Location: Slovenia, formerly a part of Yugoslavia, is located in southeastern Europe. The terrain is hilly, and almost one half of the land is forested.

Major Languages	Ethnic Groups		Major Religions	
Slovenian	Slovene	91%	Catholic	96%
Serbo-Croatian	Croat	3%	Other	4%
	Other	6%		

Ethnic/Race Specific or Endemic Diseases: The AIDS rate per 100,000 is 0.82.

National Childhood Immunizations: BCG at birth and 14 years; DPT at 3 months, between 4 and 5 months, and at 18 months; DT/Td at 6 and 14 years; TT at 18 years; OPV at 3, 4, 5, and 18 months and 6 and 14 years; MMR at 16 months.

BIBLIOGRAPHY

Malin M et al.: Careprovider and obstetrical interventions: a comparative study of four European countries, *Scand J Caring Sci* 7(3):161, 1993.

◆ SOLOMON ISLANDS

MAP PAGE (311)

Location: The islands are located in the Pacific Ocean east of Papua New Guinea. Approximately 90% of the people are Melanesian, and many different local languages are spoken. The population is primarily rural. The land consists of forested mountains and low atolls, with 10 large and rugged volcanic islands and four groups of smaller islands.

Major Languages	Ethnic Groups		Major Religions	
English	Melanesian	93%	Anglican	34%
Melanesian	Polynesian	4%	Catholic	19%
Papuan	Micronesian	1%	Baptist	17%
	European and Other	2%	Other Christian	26%
			Other	4%

Ethnic/Race Specific or Endemic Diseases: ENDEMIC: Chloroquine-resistant malaria. The AIDS rate per 100,000 is reported by the country as zero.

National Childhood Immunizations: BCG at birth; DPT at 6 weeks and 3 and 5 months; OPV at 6 weeks, 3, 5, and 9 months, and 6 years; measles at 9 months; hep B at birth and 3 and 5 months.

BIBLIOGRAPHY

Lysack CL: Community participation and community-based rehabilitation: an Indonesian case study, *Occup Ther Int* 2(3):149, 1995.

Mullard T: An experience of a lifetime: VSA volunteer to the Solomon Islands, *NZ Nurs J* 78(2):29, 1985.

◆ SOMALIA

MAP PAGE (316)

Location: Situated in eastern Africa along the Gulf of Aden and the Indian Ocean, Somalia is unique for its homogenous language and culture. The majority of people are nomads. The arid, barren land is subject to severe droughts and famine and is currently experiencing a drought that is especially severe. The literacy and life expectancy rates are low.

Major Languages	Ethnic Groups		Major Religions	
Somali	Somali	85%	Sunni	97%
Arabic	Bantu Groups	5%	Muslim	
English	Arab and Other	10%	Other	3%
Italian				

Predominant Sick Care Practices: Traditional. The use of traditional healers, including respected and skilled bone setters, is widespread throughout the rural and urban parts of the country. Self-medication, herbal medicines, religious acts, and traditional dances are part of traditional treatment procedures.

Ethnic/Race Specific or Endemic Diseases: ENDEMIC: Yellow fever; chloroquine-resistant malaria. RISK: Schistosomiasis; vector-borne diseases. The AIDS rate per 100,000 is reported by the country as zero.

Health Team Relationships: Women prefer female health care workers who are knowledgeable about female circumcision.

Dominance Patterns: Rigid sex differentiation dictates the female role within domestic and maternal functions. Women may walk behind men.

Birth Rites: Use of traditional midwives (daya) is common in rural areas. At delivery, opening of the mother's genital infibulation is necessary, and reinfibulation often follows delivery.

Death Rites: Muslim belief forbids organ donations or transplants. Muslim physicians may recommend transfusions to save lives. Autopsy is uncommon because the deceased must be buried intact. Cremation is not permitted. For Muslim burial the body is wrapped in special pieces of cloth and buried without a coffin in the ground.

Food Practices and Intolerances: Pork, carrion, and blood are forbidden. Food tends to be spicy. Ramadan fasting is practiced, with exemptions for the sick and children. A shrub with stimulant properties, khat, is chewed at celebrations.

Child Rearing Practices: The practice of the most extreme form of female infibulation and excision remains almost universal (99.5%). Circumcision is valued by women as a source of full womanhood and an instrument to control female sexuality.

National Childhood Immunizations: BCG at birth; DPT at 6, 10, and 14 weeks; OPV at birth and 6, 10, and 14 weeks; measles at 9 months.

BIBLIOGRAPHY

Arbesman M, Kahler L, Buck GM: Assessment of the impact of female circumcision on the gynecological, genitourinary and obstetrical health problems of women from Somalia: literature review and case series, *Women Health* 20(3):27, 1993.

Beine K et al.: Conceptions of prenatal care among Somali women in San Diego, *J Nurse Midwife* 40(4):376, 1995.

Brown Y: Female circumcision, *Can Nurse,* April 1989, p 19.

Carlisle D: Chewing it over, *Nurs Times* 90(30):14, 1994.

Hartman WJ, Dufresne GW: Development of a trauma center in Somalia, *J Emerg Nurs* 20(1):30A, 1994.

McCleary PH: Female genital mutilation and childbirth: a case report, *Birth* 21(4):221, 1994.

Ntiri DW: Circumcision and health among rural women of southern Somalia as part of a family life survey, *Health Care Women Int* 14:215, 1993.

Ross HM: Societal/cultural views regarding death and dying, *Top Clin Nurs* 1(1):1, 1981.

Spaulding HS: Can I make a difference? *J Christ Nurs* 11(2):28, 1994.

Walker LR, Morgan MC: Female circumcision: a report of four adolescents, *J Adolesc Health* 17(2):128, 1995.

Wright J: Female genital mutilation: an overview, *J Adv Nurs* 24:251, 1996.

Yusuf HI et al.: Traditional medical practices in some Somali communities, *J Trop Pediatr* 30(2):87, 1984.

◆ SOUTH AFRICA

MAP PAGE (317)

Location: South Africa is situated on the southern tip of Africa. It has the Atlantic on its west and the Indian Ocean on its south and east. The former apartheid rule by the minority white race ended in steps during the 1990s. The new constitution, which guarantees equal rights, was adopted in 1996 and is to be implemented over 3 years. For the first time, in this edition, the dominant culture is the black culture.

Major Languages	Ethnic Groups		Major Religions	
Afrikaans	African	75%	Christian	60%
English	White	14%	Hindu	2%
Ndebele	Mixed	9%	Muslim	38%
Sotho	East Indian	3%	and Other	

Predominant Sick Care Practices: Biomedical; magico-religious. As many as 50% of the people may consult a traditional healer before practitioners of Western medicine or concurrently with them, which results in a mixture of both forms of treatments. Treatments used by traditional healers may include ashes, amulets, and holy water. The two separate and unequal health care delivery systems that formerly existed for white and black races are no longer legal; however, segregation continues.

Ethnic/Race Specific or Endemic Diseases: ENDEMIC: Chloroquine-resistant malaria. Tuberculosis has reached nearly epidemic proportions and is estimated at 40% of the population. **RISK:** Chest infections; diarrhea; tuberculosis; schistosomiasis; trachoma. The AIDS rate per 100,000 is 6.76.

Health Team Relationships: Many white South African health care professionals and white patients have difficulty accepting care from—and especially supervision by—black health care professionals.

Food Practices and Intolerances: Unrefined maize in rural areas and sifted maize, white bread, and few vegetables in urban areas.

Infant Feeding Practices: Breastfeeding is widespread.

National Childhood Immunizations: BCG at birth; DPT at 6, 10, and 14 weeks and 18 months; Td at 5 years; OPV at birth and 6, 10, and 14 weeks; measles at 9 and 18 months; hep B at 6, 10, and 14 weeks.

Other Characteristics: The U.S.'s finger gestures for thumbs up and the V held palm are insulting gestures.

BIBLIOGRAPHY

Findlay J: Democratic health care, *Nurs Times* 12(91):40, 1995.

Galanti GA: *Caring for patients from different cultures,* ed 2, Philadelphia, 1997, University of Pennsylvania Press.

Hildebrandt E: Building community participation in health care: a model and example from South Africa, *IMAGE: J Nurs Sch* 28(2):155, 1996.

Hildebrandt E, Robertson B: Self-care of older black adults in a South African community, *Nurs Health Care* 16(3):136, 1995.

Kuhn L et al.: *S Afr Med J* 77(9):471, 1990.

Lubanga N: The legacy of apartheid in a changing South Africa, *Nurs Health Care* 14(10):512, 1993.

Masipa A: Transcultural nursing in South Africa: prospects for the 1990's, *J Transcultural Nurs* 3(1):3, 1991.

Miller K: *NBC Nightly News,* March 23, 1997.

Nightingale EO et al.: Apartheid medicine: health and human rights in South Africa, *JAMA* 264(16):2097, 1990.

Nzimakwe D: Primary health care in South Africa: private practice nurse practitioners and traditional healers form partnerships, *J Am Acad Nurse Pract* 8(7):311, 1996.

Oldshue R, Shange E, Vost DA: Maternal and child care services in rural Kwazulu, *S Afr Med J* 55(9):344, 1979.

Sutter EE, Ballard RC: A community approach to trachoma control in the Northern Transvaal, *S Afr Med J* 53(16):622, 1978.

Van Der Walt AM: Patient classification in the Groote Schuur Hospital region, Republic of South Africa, *Nurs Adm Q* 16(2):43, 1992.

Westaway MS: Health complaints, remedies and medical assistance in a peri-urban area, *S Afr Med J* 77(1):34, 1990.

◆ SPAIN

MAP PAGE (314)

Location: Spain occupies most of the Iberian Peninsula in southwestern Europe. Spain is bordered by the Atlantic on the west and the Mediterranean on the south; Africa is only 10 miles (16 km) away. The Pyrenees Mountains in the northeast separate Spain from France. The Spanish people include groups that are originally from other parts of Europe and from the Mediterranean.

Major Languages	Ethnic Groups		Major Religions	
Castilian Spanish	Spanish	73%	Catholic	99%
Catalan	Catalan	16%	Other	1%
Galician	Galician	8%		
Basque	Basque and Other	3%		

Health Care Beliefs: Health promotion is important. It is believed that disease is caused by an upset in body balance.

Ethnic/Race Specific or Endemic Diseases: The AIDS rate per 100,000 is 15.72.

Health Team Relationships: People of higher socioeconomic groups ask about and expect to be fully informed about their problems and treatments. Children do not remain in bed in the hospital unless it is indicated. The nurse is moving from a dependent to a more collaborative role, but both nurse and physician still have specific tasks separating their respective roles. In selected areas nurse practitioners practice without physician supervision. Friendliness, patience, efficacy, and professionalism are the qualities in the nurse that are most highly valued by patients. Communication between nurse and patient is usually better than that between patient and physician.

Families' Role in Hospital Care: Hospitals encourage the collaboration of patient and family in care. The family, as an integral part of the patient's life, is involved in planning care. School for children is continued in some hospitals.

Dominance Patterns: The father is the undisputed head of the family; however, this tradition is changing in younger families. Family ties are strong, and the extended family pattern is prevalent.

Eye Contact Practices: Direct eye contact prevails among the younger generations.

Touch Practices: The tendency is toward touching frequently.

Perceptions of Time: People take a casual attitude toward punctuality. An exception is the 1 PM to 4 PM afternoon siesta, which is always observed promptly. Bedtime can be very late.

Pain Reactions: In general, pain is not well tolerated and pain relief medication will be requested.

Birth Rites: The birth rate is decreasing while the age at which women become pregnant is increasing. Deliveries usually occur in the hospital. Fathers may attend an uncomplicated delivery. Contraceptive methods used are (in their order of frequency) the condom, pill, IUD, diaphragm, and biologic rhythm, which is used by religious couples who do not approve of other contraceptive methods.

Death Rites: The deceased is waked for 24 hours, and some prefer a Mass before burial. The deceased is either buried or cremated according to his or her wishes.

Food Practices and Intolerances: Spanish food is not spiced liberally, although olive oil is an important ingredient. Breakfast is light, and the main meal is eaten during the afternoon siesta period. An early evening snack is taken, and a several-course dinner is eaten late in the evening.

Child Rearing Practices: Formerly infant care was primarily the job of the women, but today infant care is beginning to be shared by the father. Learning the sex role differences begins early. The opportunity to enter a desired field of education is based on passing the competitive qualifying examinations.

National Childhood Immunizations: DPT at 3, 5, and 7 months; DT/Td at 18 months; TT at 6 and 14 years; OPV at 3, 5, 7, and 18 months; MMR at 15 months and 11 years; hep B at birth, 2 and 6 months, and 12 years.

Other Characteristics: Women are expected to be loyal to their husbands, yet they are to tolerate extramarital relationships. The influence of the woman extends beyond the home into business, education, and government. The woman's traditional submissive role is currently being modified. The traditional "OK" sign has a vulgar connotation in Spain. Prescriptions are not required for many medications.

BIBLIOGRAPHY

Beunza I et al.: Diversity and commonality in international nursing, *Int Nurs Rev* 41(2):47, 1994.

Brigham Young University Language and Intercultural Research Center: *España,* Provo, Utah, 1977.

Calvet IC et al.: The role of the nurse from a user's point of view, *Enfermeria Clin* 5(2):61, 1995.

Cubel PML et al.: A study of the demand for self care in the Medical Department of the Son Dureta Hospital in Palma de Mallorca, Spain, *Enfermeria Clin* 4(6):260, 1994.

Elsden C, Yarritu C: Development of nursing services in the Basque Autonomous Region, Spain, *Nurs Adm Q* 16(2):68, 1992.

Galanti GA: *Caring for patients from different cultures,* ed 2, Philadelphia, 1997, University of Pennsylvania Press.

Geissler EM, Dick MJ: Spanish hospitals: personal observations and impressions, *Sigma Theta Tau Reflect* 9:2, 1983.

Giger JN, Davidhizar RE: *Transcultural nursing: assessment and intervention,* ed 2, St. Louis, 1995, Mosby.

Mondragón D: Health status and nursing's contribution in Catalonia, *Nurs Health Care* 14(10):520, 1993.

Moroan PL et al.: The qualities of the nurse from the point of view of the patient, *Enfermeria Clin* 4(2):68, 1994.

Plata CB: Personal communication, July to Aug 1990, June and Sept 1997.

Rendon DC et al.: The living experience of aging in community-dwelling elders in Valencia, Spain: a phenomenological study, *Nurs Sci Q* 8(4):152, 1995.

Sims J: Nursing in Spain: times of change, *Nurs Times* 21(86):30, 1990.

◆ SRI LANKA

MAP PAGE (320)

Location: Sri Lanka, formerly Ceylon, is an island located just off the southeastern tip of India. It has a tropical climate with flat, rolling land and mountains in the south central area.

Major Languages	Ethnic Groups		Major Religions	
Sinhala	Sinhalese	74%	Buddhist	69%
Tamil	Tamil	18%	Hindu	15%
English	Moor	7%	Christian	8%
	Other	1%	Muslim	8%

Predominant Sick Care Practices: Biomedical; magico-religious; traditional. Choice of health systems may be based on availability of practitioners. Traditional healers may refer patients to the physician or hospital when it is believed that modern medicine can save the client's life. Mental health problems are believed to be within the realm of indigenous practitioners.

Ethnic/Race Specific or Endemic Diseases: ENDEMIC: Chloroquine-resistant malaria. RISK: Japanese encephalitis. The AIDS rate per 100,000 is 0.09.

Health Team Relationships: Nurses do not enjoy a position of status. Patients may consider titles more important than names and use the health professional's title.

Families' Role in Hospital Care: Traditionally older parents are cared for by their children. Changes are being seen, however, now that young people are often emigrating for work or to escape violence.

Dominance Patterns: The male is dominant. Women may be restricted from evening activities. In traditional homes, guests are separated into male and female groups for social interactions.

Touch Practices: Greeting is done by placing the palms together in a praying motion.

Birth Rites: Most deliveries occur in hospitals.

Death Rites: Preference is for quality of life over quantity because of the Buddhist belief in reincarnation and the expectation of less suffering in the next life. The dying are helped to remember their past good deeds and to achieve a fitting mental state. Autopsies are permitted and cremation is preferred.

Food Practices and Intolerances: The right hand is used for eating, and the left hand is reserved for cleaning oneself after elimination.

Infant Feeding Practices: Early breastfeeding of colostrum is common. Formula is introduced at around 6 months.

National Childhood Immunizations: BCG at birth and 5 years; DPT at 3, 5, 7, and 18 months; DT at 5 years; OPV at 3, 5, 7, and 18 months and 5 years; measles at 9 months.

Other Characteristics: Mortality statistics are higher for women than men, apparently because males receive preferential treatment. Elimination is accomplished by squatting over a receptacle on the floor. Toilets with seats may be a safety hazard for people who are unfamiliar with them. It may be preferred that bedpans be placed on the floor because elimination is considered unclean and is not done in bed.

BIBLIOGRAPHY

Caldwell J et al.: Sensitization to illness and the risk of death: an explanation for Sri Lanka's approach to good health for all, *Soc Sci Med* 28(4):365, 1989.

Factors that influence patients in Sri Lanka in their choice between Ayurvedic and Western medicine (letter), *Br Med J* 291(6499):899, 1985.

Galanti GA: *Caring for patients from different cultures,* ed 2, Philadelphia, 1997, University of Pennsylvania Press.

Geissler EM: Personal observations, 1968-1969.

Jeyarajah R: Factors that influence patients in Sri Lanka in their choice between Ayurvedic and Western medicine. Response to article in *Br Med J* 291(6499):899, 1985.

Lally MM: Last rites and funeral customs of minority groups, *Midwife Health Visit Comm Nurse* 14(7):224, 1978.

Malini A: Women in Sri Lanka: patience and progress, *World Vision Childlife,* Autumn 1996, p 5.

Nichter M, Nordstrom C: A question of medicine answering health commodification and the social relations of health in Sri Lanka, *Cult Med Psychiatry* 13(4):367, 1989.

Reid T: Age-old problem, *Nurs Times* 27(91):18, 1995.

Soysa PE, Fernando DN, Abbeywickrama K: Role of health personnel in the promotion of breast feeding practices, *J Trop Pediatr* 34(2):75, 1988.

Thapa S, deSilva V, Farr MG: Potential acceptors of Norplant implants in comparison with recently sterilized women in Sri Lanka, *Fam Health Internal Adv Contraception* 5(3):147, 1989.

Waxler NE: Behavioral convergence and institutional separation: an analysis of plural medicine in Sri Lanka, *Cult Med Psychiatry* 8(2):187, 1984.

Weisfeld GE: Sociobiological patterns of Arab culture, *Ethnol Sociobiol* 11:23, 1990.

Wolfers I: Factors that influence patients in Sri Lanka in their choice between Ayurvedic and Western medicine. Response to article in *Br Med J* 291:970, 1985.

◆ SUDAN

MAP PAGE (316)

Location: This northeastern African country (formerly Anglo-Egyptian Sudan) is the largest country on the continent. Parts of the Libyan Desert are in the north. The Nile river runs through Sudan, and the southern region and its tropical climate support fertile land and forests. African blacks are concentrated in the south, and Arabs are in the central and northern regions. The two cultures are quite distinct. The country is experiencing drought, famine, and civil war.

Major Languages	Ethnic Groups		Major Religions	
Arabic	Black	52%	Sunni Muslim	70%
English	Arab	39%	Indigenous Beliefs	25%
Nubian	Beja	6%	Christian and	5%
Ta Bedawie	Other	3%	Other	
Other				

Predominant Sick Care Practices: Biomedical; magico-religious. Money for biomedical health care is currently being used for the civil war.

Ethnic/Race Specific or Endemic Diseases: ACTIVE: Yellow fever. ENDEMIC: Chloroquine-resistant malaria. RISK: Schistosomiasis. The AIDS rate per 100,000 is 0.91.

Birth Rites: Spacing of children is preferred over limiting the number.

Death Rites: Muslim belief forbids organ donations or transplants. Muslim physicians may recommend transfusions to save lives. Autopsy is uncommon because the deceased must be buried intact. Cremation is not permitted. For Muslim burial the body is wrapped in special pieces of cloth and buried without a coffin in the ground.

Food Practices and Intolerances: Pork, carrion, and blood are forbidden. Food tends to be spicy. Ramadan fasting is practiced, with exemptions for the sick and children.

Infant Feeding Practices: Many mothers breastfeed for 1 year; however, a trend toward a shorter duration is occurring among educated women. The belief that children's fluid intake should be reduced and that breastfeeding should be stopped or reduced during episodes of diarrhea is popular.

Child Rearing Practices: Family planning may be perceived as being against the wishes of the husband or against religious teachings. Though it is illegal, female circumcision and excision is widespread in some groups.

National Childhood Immunizations: BCG at birth; DPT at 6, 10, and 14 weeks; OPV at birth and 6, 10, and 14 weeks; measles at 9 months.

BIBLIOGRAPHY

Ali BH, Roese PM: Children and youth in a population of the Shendi area, Sudan, *Arztl Jugendkd* 80(3):135, 1989.

Beasley A: Breastfeeding studies: culture, biomedicine, and methodology, *J Hum Lact* 7(1):7, 1991.

El Tom AR et al.: Family planning in the Sudan: a pilot project success story, *World Health Forum* 10:333, 1989.

Grotberg EH: Research in Sudan on child and family concerns, *Child Today* 12(5):18, 1983.

Ross HM: Societal/cultural views regarding death and dying, *Top Clin Nurs* 1(1):1, 1981.

Rushwan HE, Ferguson JG, Bernard RP: Hospital counseling in Khartoum: a study of factors affecting contraceptive acceptance after abortion, *Int J Gynaecol Obstet* 15(5):440, 1978.

Taha TET: Family planning practice in Central Sudan, *Soc Sci Med* 37(5):685, 1993.

Wright J: Female genital mutilation: an overview, *J Adv Nurs* 24:251, 1996.

Zaki V: Personal communication, Sept 28, 1992.

◆ SURINAME

MAP PAGE (314)

Location: Suriname (formerly Dutch Guiana) is situated on the northeast coast of South America. The interior has tropical rain forests, and the narrow coastal area is swampland.

Major Languages	Ethnic Groups		Major Religions	
Dutch	Hindustani	37%	Christian	48%
English	Creole	31%	Hindu	27%
Sranan Tongo	Javanese	15%	Muslim	20%
Hindustani	Bush Black	10%	Other	5%
Javanese	Native American and Other	7%		

Ethnic/Race Specific or Endemic Diseases: ENDEMIC: Yellow fever; chloroquine-resistant malaria (in the interior, with no risk in urban areas). RISK: Schistosomiasis. The AIDS rate per 100,000 is 4.72.

National Childhood Immunizations: DPT at 3, 4, 5, and 18 months and 5 years; OPV at 3, 4, 5, and 18 months and 5 years; measles at 9 months.

BIBLIOGRAPHY

Rozendaal JA: Epidemiology and control of malaria in Suriname, *Bull Pan Am Health Organ* 25(4):336, 1991.

◆ SWAZILAND

MAP PAGE (317)

Location: Swaziland is landlocked and located near the Indian Ocean in southern Africa. The climate is temperate.

Major Languages	Ethnic Groups		Major Religions	
English	Swazi	90%	Christian	60%
Siswati	Zulu	2%	Indigenous Beliefs	40%
	European	3%		
	Other	5%		

Predominant Sick Care Practices: There is a high proportion of indigenous healers, including sangomas, inyangas, faith healers, throat scratchers, and traditional birth attendants, who attribute illness primarily to the supernatural, to a violation of indigenous beliefs, to the environment, or to the influence of their ancestors.

Health Care Beliefs: Patients are actively involved in determining their illness and its source within the indigenous health care system.

Ethnic/Race Specific or Endemic Diseases: RISK: Tuberculosis; schistosomiasis; kwashiorkor; infantile diarrhea; dysentery; enteric fever; advanced periodontal disease. Malaria and leprosy are decreasing. The AIDS rate per 100,000 is 18.01.

Birth Rites: Approximately one half of deliveries are assisted by untrained, traditional birth attendants. Free family planning and birth control opportunities are available but relatively unused.

Infant Feeding Practices: Mothers often return to work soon after delivery to supplement families' incomes; therefore soft table foods are usually introduced to infants at 6 to 8 weeks. This early introduction may slow the infants' growth.

Child Rearing Practices: Working mothers require alternate caregivers. National policy supports an intensive program that monitors and promotes growth in children and works to eliminate stunted growth.

National Childhood Immunizations: BCG at birth; DPT at 3, 4, and 5 months; OPV at 3, 4, and 5 months; measles at 9 months.

Other Characteristics: There are no rural villages. Families who do not live in towns live in beehive-shaped huts in the fields.

BIBLIOGRAPHY

Chaudhuri SN: National policy on growth monitoring and promotion: Swaziland leads the way, *Indian J Pediatr Suppl* 55:S106, 1988.

Douglas P: Rehabilitation work in Swaziland, *Physiother Frontline* 2(6):17, 1996.

Moran R: Swazi safari, *Nurs Times* 88(40):54, 1992.

Upvall MJ: A Swazi nursing perspective on the role of indigenous healers, *J Cult Diversity* 2(1):16, 1995.

Yoder RA: Are people willing and able to pay for health services? *Soc Sci Med* 29(1):35, 1989.

◆ SWEDEN

MAP PAGE (314)

Location: This northern European country is located in eastern Scandinavia along the Baltic Sea. It is a land of many lakes. Half of Sweden is covered by forests. Its northern boundary extends into the Arctic Circle. Sweden has one of the world's highest standards of living.

Major Languages	Ethnic Groups		Major Religions	
Swedish	Swedish	90%	Lutheran	94%
Lapp	Lappish	4%	Catholic	1%
Finnish	Finnish	2%	Other	5%
	Other	4%		

Predominant Sick Care Practices: Biomedical.

Health Care Beliefs: Active involvement; health promotion important. Health promotion is emphasized primarily in maternal and child care. Free universal health care is provided. People are expected to be responsible for self-care and health; however, many social services are available. The focus of care is on health care facilities and not on the community-family setting.

Ethnic/Race Specific or Endemic Diseases: RISK: Sjögren-Larsson syndrome; Krabbe's disease; Rett syndrome; phenylketonuria. Alcoholism is widespread and results in severe fetal alcohol syndrome in some infants. The AIDS rate per 100,000 is 2.12.

Health Team Relationships: Receptionist nurses who are contacted by telephone are the first point of contact in the health care system. The physician holds an authoritarian role and is not questioned. Although patients are expected to say what they feel, the expression of feelings is not encouraged by health care professionals. Patients expect to have influence in planning medical treatment and nursing care.

Families' Role in Hospital Care: Staff provides for all the patient's needs; however, the family may assist if they like. Flexible visiting hours are observed. Stipends are paid to individuals who provide care for a sick family member at home.

Dominance Patterns: This is an egalitarian society; however, the woman is usually responsible for household chores and food purchases and preparation.

Eye Contact Practices: Direct eye contact is observed when speaking.

Touch Practices: This is a society that touches infrequently.

Perceptions of Time: Northern Swedes are not as time conscious as those from large cities in southern Sweden. A 15- to 30-minute delay is tolerated. Swedes are present and future oriented and plan for that which may be important in the future.

Pain Reactions: Nonexpressive or expressive reactions to pain are acceptable. To express pain, muscles may be contracted in the body or the face with accompanying verbal expression. Immediate pain relief is expected.

Birth Rites: Sweden has one of the lowest infant mortality rates. Women may choose any position in which to deliver, even underwater. ABC Clinics provide many choices for delivery, including father-sibling participation. Under some options the father cuts the umbilical cord, the baby is placed on the mother's abdomen, and the family is left alone for several hours. Rooming in during the day is common. The infant is returned to the nursery at night.

Death Rites: Quiet and open grief are both acceptable. The dying person is not to be left alone or without family present. After death a closed coffin is used. The body is not viewed after death.

Food Practices and Intolerances: Breakfast often consists of coffee or tea and a sandwich of meat and cheese or porridge. A large meal is eaten at lunch and dinner. Meatballs with potatoes and gravy are popular. Coffee breaks may include a sandwich at mid-morning and mid-afternoon. Fish, meat, and bananas are foods that are eaten often.

Infant Feeding Practices: Breastfeeding is preferred and encouraged and continues for about 1 year. Other foods are introduced at 4 or 5 months. Bottle-feeding is discouraged.

Child Rearing Practices: Children are raised in a permissive environment but with safety limits. School starts at age 7. Nurses from government-sponsored day care centers care for the preschool child. Most mothers work.

National Childhood Immunizations: BCG after 6 months; DT/Td at 3, 5, and 12 months and 10 years; IPV at 3, 5, and 12 months and between 5 and 6 years; MMR at 18 months and 12 years.

BIBLIOGRAPHY

Andrews MM, Boyle JS: *Transcultural concepts in nursing care,* ed 2, Philadelphia, 1995, Lippincott.

Bergh I: Contributor.

Carr C: A four-week observation of maternity care in Finland, *J Obstet Gynecol Neonatal Nurs* 18(2):100, 1989.

Dahlen T: Contributor.

Ekblad S: Influence of child-rearing on aggressive behavior in a transcultural perspective, *Acta Psychiatr Scand Suppl* 344:133, 1988.

Engquist A: Personal communication, Aug 14, 1992.

Forni PR: Health care delivery in Sweden and Finland: a challenge to the American system, *J Prof Nurs* 2(4):234, 1986.

Geissler EM: Personal observations, Aug 11-15, 1992.

Götherström C, Hamrin E, Gullberg M: Development of a tool for measuring the concept of good care among patients and staff in relation to Swedish legislation, *Int J Nurs Stud* 32(3):277, 1995.

Granger R: Effects of maternal alcohol/drug use on the infant/child: issues and interventions. Lecture presented at the Hole in the Wall Gang Camp, Ashford, Conn, May 14, 1992.

Marklund B et al.: Evaluation of the telephone advisory activity at Swedish primary health care centres, *Fam Pract* 7(3):184, 1990.

Morgensen E: Personal communication, Aug 13, 1992.

Morris J: Rett's syndrome: a case study, *J Neurosci Nurs* 22(5):285, 1990.

Nettelbladt P, Uddenberg N, Englesson I: Sex-role patterns, paternal rearing attitudes and child development in different social classes, *Acta Psychiatr Scand* 64(1):12, 1981.

Sheehy B: Ideological exchange, *Nurs Times* 86(3):36, 1990.

Solheim JS: A cross-cultural examination of use of corporal punishment on children: a focus on Sweden and the United States, *Child Abuse Negl* 6(2):147, 1982.

Timpka T, Arborelius E: The primary-care nurse's dilemmas: a study of knowledge use and need during telephone conversations, *J Adv Nurs* 15:1457, 1990.

Waldenstrom U, Swenson A: Rooming-in at night in the postpartum ward, *Midwifery* 7(2):82, 1991.

Westbrook MT, Nordholm LA, McGee JE: Cultural differences in reactions to patient behaviour: a comparison of Swedish and Australian health professionals, *Soc Sci Med* 19(9):939, 1984.

Whetstone WR, Hansson AO: Perceptions of self-care in Sweden: a cross-cultural replication, *J Adv Nurs* 14:962, 1989.

◆ SWITZERLAND

MAP PAGE (314)

Location: Switzerland is a landlocked nation of central Europe, and the topography consists of the Alps, glaciers, lakes, and a large plateau where most people reside. Four official languages are used. The rugged landscape does not support much agriculture. Banking and tourism are important industries.

Major Languages	Ethnic Groups		Major Religions	
German	German	65%	Catholic	48%
French	French	18%	Protestant	44%
Italian	Italian	10%	Other	8%
Romansch	Romansch	1%		
	Other	6%		

Predominant Sick Care Practices: Biomedical.

Ethnic/Race Specific or Endemic Diseases: The AIDS rate per 100,000 is 6.24.

Health Team Relationships: Each of the 26 cantons (states) has its own government; therefore there are 26 ministries of health with different laws regulating health care. Nurses fulfill a primarily technical role under the direction of the physician.

Perceptions of Time: The Swiss are punctual.

Food Practices and Intolerances: Plain, hearty food, heavy, filling soups, and cheese dishes are common.

National Childhood Immunizations: BCG at birth and 5 and 12 years; DPT at 2, 4, 6, and 15 months and between 5 and 7 years; DT/Td at 15 months and 5 and 12 years; OPV at 2, 4, 6, and 15 months; MMR at 15 months.

BIBLIOGRAPHY

Abelin T: Getting health promotion off the ground in Switzerland, *J Public Health Policy* 9(2):284, 1988.

Clift JM: Nursing education in Austria, Germany, and Switzerland, *IMAGE: J Nurs Sch* 29(1):89, 1997.

Condon JC, Yousef F: *An introduction to intercultural communication,* New York, 1975, Macmillan.

Language Research Center: *German-speaking people of Europe,* Provo, Utah, 1976, Brigham Young University.

Panchaud C: Enhancing ethical thinking: the role of a national nurses' association, *Nurs Ethics* 2(3):243, 1995.

◆ SYRIA

MAP PAGE (318)

Location: One of the world's oldest civilizations, Syria is located at the eastern end of the Mediterranean Sea. The east is desert, and coastal plains, fertile lowlands, and mountains can be found in the remainder of the country.

Major Languages	Ethnic Groups		Major Religions	
Arabic	Arab	90%	Sunni Muslim	74%
Kurdish	Kurdish and	10%	Other Muslim	16%
Armenian	Other		Christian	10%
French				
English				

Ethnic/Race Specific or Endemic Diseases: ENDEMIC: Chloroquine-sensitive malaria (no risk in urban areas). RISK: Schistosomiasis. The AIDS rate per 100,000 is 0.04.

Families' Role in Hospital Care: Family members or close friends accompany the patient and expect to participate in care or take a vigilant supervisory role.

Perceptions of Time: Planning ahead has the potential of defying God's will. Lack of planning is not an indication of lack of interest.

Pain Reactions: Immediate pain relief is expected and may be persistently requested. The belief in conserving energy for recovery is in conflict with therapies that require exertion. Pain is expressed only privately or with close relatives and friends. The exception occurs during labor and delivery, when pain is expressed vehemently.

Death Rites: Families may insist that loved ones are not to be told about a terminal diagnosis. Muslim belief forbids organ donations or transplants. Muslim physicians may recommend transfusions to save lives. Autopsy is uncommon because the deceased must be buried intact. Cremation is not permitted. For Muslim burial the body is wrapped in special pieces of cloth and buried without a coffin in the ground.

Food Practices and Intolerances: Pork, carrion, and blood are forbidden. Food tends to be spicy. Ramadan fasting is practiced, with exemptions for the sick and children.

National Childhood Immunizations: BCG at birth; DPT at 2, 3, 4, and 18 months; DT at 6 years; OPV at birth and 2, 3, 4, and 18 months; measles at 9 and 15 months; hep B at birth and 2 and 9 months.

Other Characteristics: Hope, optimism, and the positive advantages of treatment should be stressed.

BIBLIOGRAPHY

Green J: Death with dignity: Islam, *Nurs Times* 85(5):56, 1989.

Meleis AI, Sorrell L: Arab American women and their birth experiences, *MCN Am J Matern Child Nurs* 6:171, 1981.

Racy J: Death in an Arab culture: discussion of the paper, *Ann NY Acad Sci* 871:1969.

Reizian A, Meleis AI: Arab-Americans' perceptions of and responses to pain, *Crit Care Nurse* 6(6):30, 1986.

Ross HM: Societal/cultural views regarding death and dying, *Top Clin Nurs* 1(1):1, 1981.

◆ TAJIKISTAN

MAP PAGE (315)

Location: This central Asian country is more than 90% mountainous; glaciers are the source of its rivers. The land is earthquake prone. The country became an independent state with the dissolution of the USSR.

Major Languages	Ethnic Groups		Major Religions	
Tajik	Tajik	65%	Sunni Muslim	80%
Russian	Uzbek	25%	Other	20%
	Russian	4%		
	Other	6%		

Ethnic/Race Specific or Endemic Diseases: The AIDS rate per 100,000 is reported by the country as zero.

National Childhood Immunizations: BCG at between 3 and 6 days, at 6 years, and between 16 and 17 years; OPV at between 3 and 6 days, at 2, 4, 6, and 16 months, between 5 and 7 years, and between 12 and 15 years; measles at 9 months and 3 years.

BIBLIOGRAPHY

No data located.

◆ TANZANIA

MAP PAGE (317)

Location: Tanzania is located in eastern Africa on the Indian Ocean. Africa's highest point, Mt. Kilimanjaro at 19,340 feet (5895 m), and lowest point, the floor of Lake Tanganyika at −1174 feet (−358 m), are found here. The climate, which is influenced by altitude, is hot and humid on the coast, arid in the central area, and temperate in the highlands. Tanzania is one of the less-developed countries of the world.

Major Languages	Ethnic Groups		Major Religions	
Swahili	African	99%	Christian	45%
English	Other	1%	Muslim	35%
			Indigenous	20%
			Beliefs	

Most of the tribes are Bantus.

Predominant Sick Care Practices: Traditional. The goal of the Bantus is to acquire vital force to make life stronger. Illnesses, wounds, disappointments, suffering, and death deplete this vital force. In varying degrees the sources of vital force are strongest in God, Spirit, or Creator, next in ancestors, then living people, and weakest in animals, plants, minerals, sand, and clay. Traditional healers use evil spirits as part of care. Witch doctors, who have been given legitimate status by the government, use local herbs.

Health Care Beliefs: Acute sick care. The trend is toward health promotion among infants and children.

Ethnic/Race Specific or Endemic Diseases: ENDEMIC: Chloroquine-resistant malaria (including urban areas); tsetse fly infestation. RISK: Cholera; schistosomiasis. The common causes of morbidity and mortality among infants are communicable diseases and parasitic infections. There are as many as 29 words used by the population to describe diarrhea. The AIDS rate per 100,000 is 95.47.

Health Team Relationships: Professional nursing status is symbolized by wearing a uniform. Greetings are very important before anything else is said; they show the patients that the health care provider is in their service.

Families' Role in Hospital Care: Assistance with hygiene, elimination, nutrition, and surveillance is provided by family members who remain near the bedside. Families may force sick relatives to take local herbs prescribed by witch doctors.

Dominance Patterns: Because the family, rather than the individual, is valued, language that reflects group ownership, rather than individual ownership, is used. Traditionally the status of women is inferior to that of men. The mother-in-law plays a key role during the wife's pregnancy in some tribes.

Eye Contact Practices: Looking straight in the eye is acceptable.

Touch Practices: Touch is used.

Perceptions of Time: Time is not a major concern.

Birth Rites: Traditional birth attendants are often used, although nurse midwives assist most births in health care facilities. Many women prefer home births. Abstinence from sexual intercourse during pregnancy is relatively common. A tendency to prefer boys over girls exists. Various tribes may not touch the umbilical cord until it falls off; some may put cow dung on the cord.

Death Rites: Among the dominant Bantus death is only a normal part of life when it occurs in old age. In younger age groups death may have been caused on purpose, possibly by enemies.

Food Practices and Intolerances: Children may drink alcohol freely in a few tribes.

Infant Feeding Practices: Breastfeeding begins with colostrum the first or second day after birth and may continue for 2 to 3 years. Weaning onto a soft maize soup begins at 3 to 4 months.

Child Rearing Practices: A woman's most important role is to bear as many children as possible and to take full responsibility for their care. During the preschool years child care may be shared by female relatives or baby-sitters. Female circumcision and excision is widespread in some groups. Traditional females remain indoors for a year during puberty to learn proper behavior; they have limited contact with males. Traditional practices for family planning include breastfeeding, abstinence, and polygamy.

National Childhood Immunizations: BCG at birth; DPT at 6, 10, and 14 weeks; OPV at birth and 6, 10, and 14 weeks; measles at 9 months.

Other Characteristics: An interaction may begin by first establishing a "laughing relationship": one person laughs gently and another echoes the laugh.

BIBLIOGRAPHY

Adler MW, editor: Statistics from the World Health Organization and the Centers for Disease Control, *AIDS* 6(10):1229, 1992.

Carlisle D: The real Makoye, *Nurs Times* 89(43):42, 1993.

Condon JC, Yousef F: *An introduction to intercultural communication,* New York, 1975, Macmillan.

Heggenhougen HK: Will primary health care efforts be allowed to succeed? *Soc Sci Med* 19(3):217, 1984.

Hounsa AM et al.: An application of Ajzen's theory of planned behaviour to predict mothers' intention to use oral rehydration therapy in a rural area of Benin, *Soc Sci Med* 37(2):253, 1993.

Juntunen A, Nikkonen M: Professional nursing care in Tanzania: a descriptive study of nursing care in Ilembula Lutheran Hospital in Tanzania, *J Adv Nurs* 24:536, 1996.

Karungula J: Measures to reduce the infant mortality rate in Tanzania, *Int J Nurs Stud* 29(2):113, 1992.

Mella PP: Effects of educated professionals on the health and care of women in Tanzania, *Health Care Women Int* 8(4):239, 1987.

Pedersen B: A pilot project for training traditional birth attendants, *J Nurse Midwifery* 30(1):43, 1985.

Wright J: Female genital mutilation: an overview, *J Adv Nurs* 24:251, 1996.

◆ THAILAND

MAP PAGE (321)

Location: Thailand (formerly Siam) is located in the western Indochinese and the northern Malay peninsulas. It enjoys a variety of forested mountains, plateaus, and alluvial valleys, with rain forests in its southern peninsula.

Major Languages	Ethnic Groups		Major Religions	
Thai	Thai	75%	Buddhist	95%
English	Chinese	14%	Muslim	4%
Lao	Other	11%	Christian	1%
Chinese				
Malay				

Predominant Sick Care Practices: Biomedical; magico-religious.

Health Care Beliefs: Conditions known as "thinking too much" or "thinking a lot" may be associated with stress, poverty, and life cycle stages. Folk beliefs include menstrual restrictions, some based on ideas of symbolic pollution.

Ethnic/Race Specific or Endemic Diseases: ENDEMIC: There is an explosive epidemic of AIDS. Chloroquine- and Fansidar-resistant malaria (no risk in urban areas). RISK: Japanese encephalitis; schistosomiasis; adult lactase deficiency; hemoglobin E disease; opium addiction in northern areas. The AIDS rate per 100,000 is 30.53.

Health Team Relationships: If the Thai suggests a course of action cautiously and hesitantly, he or she wants that course of action to be followed. More nurses hold doctoral degrees than other females do in other occupational fields.

Dominance Patterns: Men are dominant, yet women have considerable authority in domestic and commercial aspects of family life. Thai society is structured more on social hierarchy than it is on equality; however, self is perceived as an autonomous individual rather than as part of a family or of an extended group.

Touch Practices: Because the head is considered sacred, it is inappropriate to pat a child on the head. Also, reaching over the patient's head to pass something to another person may be considered impolite.

Pain Reactions: Childbirth pain may be expressed quietly and nonverbally by some.

Birth Rites: The new mother keeps warm regardless of the ambient temperature because of the belief that this will help lactation. In the north it is believed that the wrists of the child must be bound with string to prevent loss of the soul. A common position for birth at home has the husband sitting on the mattress with his knees supporting his wife's shoulders and her head between his thighs. He may stroke her face and hair for emotional support. After delivery the husband buries the placenta. A ritual postpartum month may be observed, and some mothers eat only rice gruel during the first postpartum week.

Death Rites: For those who adhere to Buddhist beliefs of reincarnation, preference is for quality of life over quantity because it is believed that there will be less suffering in the next life. Therefore the dying should be helped to recall their past good deeds and to achieve a fitting mental state. Autopsies are permitted, and cremation is preferred.

Food Practices and Intolerances: Rice is a staple.

Infant Feeding Practices: Breastfeeding is common; however, some indications of decline are apparent. Children are bottle-fed supplemental foods and liquids at early ages.

Child Rearing Practices: Grandmothers play an important role in child rearing. Children are taught to be polite, modest, self-controlled, and deferential—values that are espoused in Buddhism. There are thousands of street children. At 6 or 7 years of age, rural children are in charge of younger siblings while mothers are away for several days working in rice fields.

National Childhood Immunizations: BCG at birth and 1 year; DPT at 2, 4, 6, and 18 months and between 4 and 6 years; Td and rubella at primary school entry and leaving; OPV at 6, 10, and 14 weeks; measles at 9 months; hep B at birth and 2 and 6 months.

Other Characteristics: The higher the hands are held (the norm being chest level), the more respect is shown during greeting; however, if the hands are held above eye level, it is an insult. Because the head is sacred, placing a piece of clothing worn on a lower part of the body on a pillow where the head is to be placed is unacceptable behavior. Pointing your feet at a person is unacceptable. Some prefer injections rather than pills.

BIBLIOGRAPHY

Andrews MM, Boyle JS: *Transcultural concepts in nursing care,* ed 2, Philadelphia, 1995, Lippincott.

Bazell R: *NBC News,* Jan 25, 1997.

Beardslee C et al.: Nursing care of children in developing countries: issues in Thailand, Botswana and Jordan, *Recent Adv Nurs* 16:31, 1987.

Blease DA: The Asian mother and her expectations, *Midwives Chron Nurs Notes* 98(1171):xiii, 1985.

Cassidy J: The unseen menace: Thailand, child health, HIV/AIDS, *Nurs Times* 92(8):50, 1996.

Chayovan N, Knodel J, Wongboonsin K: Infant feeding practices in Thailand: an update from the 1987 demographic and health survey, *Stud Fam Plann* 21(1):40, 1990.

Chow DC: AIDS in Thailand: a medical student's perspective, *J Community Health* 19(6):417, 1994.

Fox PG, Komchum S: Primary health care in an unsettled area of northern Thailand, *Int Nurs Rev* 39(2):49, 1992.

Fungladda W, Sornmani S: Health behavior, treatment-seeking patterns, and cost of treatment for patients visiting malaria clinics in western Thailand, *Southeast Asian J Trop Med Public Health* 17(3):379, 1986.

Gualtieri V: Preventing is better than fixing, *Am J Nurs* 91(2):110, 1991.

Horn BM: Cultural concepts and postpartal care, *Nurs Health Care* 2(9):516, 1981. Reprint in *J Transcultural Nurs* 2(1):48, 1990.

Lally MM: Last rites and funeral customs of minority groups, *Midwife Health Visit Comm Nurse* 14(7):224, 1978.

Muecke MA: Health care systems as socializing agents: childbearing the north Thai and western ways, *Soc Sci Med* 10:177, 1976.

Muecke MA: Worries and worriers in Thailand, *Health Care Women Int* 15(6):503, 1994.

Muecke MA, Srisuphan W: From women in white to scholarship: the new nurse leaders in Thailand, *J Transcultural Nurs* 1(2):21, 1990.

Pathanapong P: Childbirth pain communicative behaviors among selected laboring Thai women, doctoral dissertation, 1990, Tucson, Ariz, University of Arizona.

Rittenhouse CA: Commentary on gender and health: some Asian evidence, *Awhonns Womens Health Nurs Scan* 8(2):16, 1994.

Sikkema M, Niyekawa A: *Design for cross-cultural learning,* Yarmouth, Me, 1987, Intercultural Press.

Stewart EC, Bennett MJ: *American cultural patterns: a cross-cultural perspective,* rev ed, Yarmouth, Me, 1991, Intercultural Press.

Storti C: *The art of crossing cultures,* Yarmouth, Me, 1990, Intercultural Press.

Weisberg DH: Northern Thai health care alternatives: patient control and the structure of medical pluralism, *Soc Sci Med* 16(16):1507, 1982.

Weisz JR et al.: Over- and undercontrolled referral problems among children and adolescents from Thailand and the United States: the Wat and Wai of cultural differences, *J Consult Clin Psychol* 55(5):719, 1987.

◆ TOGO

MAP PAGE (316)

Location: Togo (formerly Togoland) is located in western Africa with a small coastline on the Gulf of Guinea. Most of Togo's people are black Africans. Togo consists of mountains and a small coastal plain. The climate is primarily hot and humid.

Major Languages	Ethnic Groups		Major Religions	
French	Ewe	35%	Indigenous	70%
Ewe	Kabye	22%	Beliefs	
Mina	Mina	6%	Christian	20%
Dagomba	Other	37%	Muslim	10%
Kabye and Other				

Ethnic/Race Specific or Endemic Diseases: ENDEMIC: Yellow fever; chloroquine-resistant malaria (including urban areas). **RISK:** Schistosomiasis. The AIDS rate per 100,000 is 41.33.

Child Rearing Practices: Female circumcision and excision is widespread in some groups.

National Childhood Immunizations: BCG at birth; DPT at 6, 10, and 14 weeks, 16 months, and 7 years; OPV at birth and 6, 10, and 14 weeks; measles at 9 months; yellow fever at 10 months.

BIBLIOGRAPHY

Adler MW, editor: Statistics from the World Health Organization and the Centers for Disease Control, *AIDS* 6(10):1229, 1992.

Wright J: Female genital mutilation: an overview, *J Adv Nurs* 24:251, 1996.

◆ TONGA

MAP PAGE (311)

Location: Tonga (also called the Friendly Islands) is a series of volcanic and coral islands. Less than one third of the islands are inhabited. The country is located in the western South Pacific northeast of New Zealand. The majority of the population lives on the largest island, Tongatapu. Tonga has the highest percentage of arable land of any country in the world. School enrollment is high, and most people are literate. The climate is subtropical.

Major Languages	Ethnic Groups		Major Religions	
Tongan	Polynesian	99%	Christian	88%
English	Other	1%	Other	12%

Health Care Beliefs: Acute sick care only.

Ethnic/Race Specific or Endemic Diseases: Obesity with related diabetes, heart attacks, and strokes as the greatest causes of mortality. The AIDS rate per 100,000 is reported by the country as zero.

Dominance Patterns: Two clearly defined social classes, the nobles and the commoners.

Death Rites: Funerals are important social events.

Food Practices and Intolerances: Feasting is a national pastime because for centuries big was considered beautiful. Today exercise and dieting are being encouraged.

National Childhood Immunizations: BCG at birth and 5 years; DPT at 6, 12, and 18 weeks and 2 and 5 years; OPV at 6, 12, and 18 weeks; measles at 9 months; hep B at birth and 6 and 12 weeks.

Other Characteristics: Raising the eyebrows is a "yes" answer to a question. It is forbidden to do anything outdoors on Sundays.

BIBLIOGRAPHY

Finau SA, Taummoepeau B, To'a L: Review of the village health worker pilot scheme in Tonga, *NZ Med J* 99(807):592, 1986.

Storti C: *The art of crossing cultures,* Yarmouth, Me, 1990, Intercultural Press.

Tenn L et al.: Getting the community involved in developing a PHC curriculum in Tonga, *Int Nurs Rev* 41(5):141, 1994.

Theroux P: *NBC Today Show,* June 22, 1992.

Tibbles K: *NBC Today,* Jan 24, 1996.

◆ TRINIDAD AND TOBAGO

MAP PAGE (313)

Location: Trinidad and Tobago are located in the Caribbean just off the Venezuelan coast. Trinidad is the larger of the two and has the majority of the predominantly black African or East Indian people.

Major Languages	Ethnic Groups		Major Religions	
English	Black	43%	Catholic	32%
Hindi	East Indian	40%	Protestant	25%
French	Mixed	14%	Hindu	24%
Spanish	White	1%	Muslim	6%
	Chinese and Other	2%	Other	13%

Health Care Beliefs: Health promotion is important.

Ethnic/Race Specific or Endemic Diseases: ENDEMIC: Yellow fever. RISK: Dengue fever. The AIDS rate per 100,000 is 25.99.

Health Team Relationships: Health care administration is often hierarchical, authoritarian, and based on seniority.

Families' Role in Hospital Care: Materials for physical care (food and clean clothing) are expected from male relatives, whereas emotional support comes from female relatives, especially sisters.

Dominance Patterns: The male is dominant and the female is more yielding.

Perceptions of Time: Rewards for current activity are preferred over delayed gratification.

National Childhood Immunizations: DPT at 3 months, between 4 and 5 months, between 5 and 6 months, and at 18 and 36 months; OPV at 3 months, between 4 and 5 months, between 5 and 6 months, and at 18 and 36 months; MMR at between 12 and 15 months.

BIBLIOGRAPHY

Adler MW, editor: Statistics from the World Health Organization and the Centers for Disease Control, *AIDS* 6(10):1229, 1992.

Andrews MM, Boyle JS: *Transcultural concepts in nursing care,* ed 2, Philadelphia, 1995, Lippincott.

Green HB: Temporal attitudes in four Negro subcultures, *Studium Generale* 23(6):571, 1970.

Hezekiah J: Colonial heritage and nursing leadership in Trinidad and Tobago, *IMAGE: J Nurs Sch* 20(3):155, 1988.

Hezekiah J: Postcolonial nursing education in Trinidad and Tobago, *Adv Nurs Sci* 12(2):28, 1990.

McKee PL: A cultural exchange of values, *Act Adapt Aging* 19(2):17, 1994.

◆ TUNISIA

MAP PAGE (316)

Location: Tunisia is located in northern Africa near the dividing point between the eastern and western Mediterranean Sea. Its people are descendants of several Berber and Arab groups. It is an agricultural country in the wooded fertile north and the central coastal plains. The south becomes more arid toward the part of the Sahara where it reaches −56 feet (−17 m) sea level. Among Arab nations, Tunisia is a leader in advocating women's rights.

Major Languages	Ethnic Groups		Major Religions	
Arabic	Arab	98%	Muslim	98%
French	European	2%	Christian	1%
			Jewish	1%

Predominant Sick Care Practices: Traditional healers include scribes, herbalists, bone setters, and healers of specific afflictions.

Ethnic/Race Specific or Endemic Diseases: RISK: Schistosomiasis. The AIDS rate per 100,000 is 0.69.

Health Team Relationships: A "yes" followed by "N'sha'llah" (God willing) reflects a supernatural control over the future and therefore may mean "no."

Families' Role in Hospital Care: Family members or close friends accompany the patient and expect to participate in care or to take a vigilant, supervisory role.

Pain Reactions: Immediate pain relief is expected and may be persistently requested. The belief in conserving energy for recovery is in conflict with therapies that require exertion. Pain is expressed only privately or with close relatives and friends; however, during labor and delivery, pain may be expressed vehemently.

Birth Rites: The choices for assistance with childbirth include staying at home with a lay midwife (qabla) or trained midwife (sage femme) or going to the hospital. Traditionally henna is applied as decoration to the hands and feet before going into labor; the purpose is to attract beneficial forces.

Death Rites: Muslim belief forbids organ donations or transplants. Muslim physicians may recommend transfusions to save lives. Autopsy is uncommon because the deceased must be buried intact. Cremation is not permitted. For Muslim burial the body is wrapped in special pieces of cloth and buried without a coffin in the ground.

Food Practices and Intolerances: Ramadan fasting is practiced.

National Childhood Immunizations: BCG at birth and 6 years; DPT at 3, 4, 5, and 18 months; OPV at 3, 4, 5, and 18 months; measles at 9 and 15 months; hep B at 2, 4, and 9 months.

Other Characteristics: Crowding up to be served is a common and accepted behavior. Hope, optimism, and the positive advantages of treatment should be stressed.

BIBLIOGRAPHY

Auerbach LS: Childbirth in Tunisia: implications of a decision-making model, *Soc Sci Med* 16(16):1499, 1982.

Green J: Death with dignity: Islam, *Nurs Times* 85(5):56, 1989.

Reizian A, Meleis AI: Arab-Americans' perceptions of and responses to pain, *Crit Care Nurse* 6(6):30, 1986.

Ross HM: Societal/cultural views regarding death and dying, *Top Clin Nurs* 1(1):1, 1981.

Storti C: *The art of crossing cultures,* Yarmouth, Me, 1990, Intercultural Press.

◆ TURKEY

MAP PAGE (318)

Location: Turkey is a southeastern European and southwestern Asian (Anatolia) country at the northeastern end of the Mediterranean Sea. The Black Sea is to the north, and the Aegean Sea is to the west. The European area is hilly, and the central Asian region is a treeless plateau that is rimmed with high mountains. The climate is hot and dry in summer and cold in winter.

Major Languages	Ethnic Groups		Major Religions	
Turkish	Turkish	80%	Muslim	99%
Kurdish	Kurdish	20%	Other	1%
Arabic				

Predominant Sick Care Practices: Biomedical; holistic. A strong preventive health care system is currently being established. Bone setters are important alternative health care practitioners. The patient may choose a health care system and change if the desired results are not realized.

Health Care Beliefs: Passive role; acute sick care only. People accept treatment passively. Some Muslims may wish to postpone elective medical treatment until the end of the month of Ramadan.

Ethnic/Race Specific or Endemic Diseases: ENDEMIC: Chloroquine-sensitive malaria (including urban areas); leishmaniasis; trachoma (along the Mediterranean and in the southeast); regional typhoid fever; viral hepatitis. RISK: Goiter in northern Black Sea area; dental problems. The AIDS rate per 100,000 is 0.04.

Health Team Relationships: Most physicians are male and have absolute authority. Patients do not question physicians. They do not want to bother them or take their time. Patients usually comply with physician orders if the physician's good will is apparent. Professional dialogue rarely occurs between doctors and nurses. Most nurses are female. Women prefer a nurse or midwife for discussions about family planning.

Families' Role in Hospital Care: A family member usually stays with the patient day and night.

Dominance Patterns: Decisions are generally made by males. Women are perceived as having lower status in society, with variations between urban and rural areas. Rural women pass through four stages: young bride (ages 15 to 30), with low status; middle age (ages 30 to 45), with medium status; mature (ages 45 to 65), with highest status; and finally old (age 65 and above), when women are respected but not powerful. Women are the quietly dominant decision makers in their homes, especially when health care decisions are necessary. Husbands are responsible for the paperwork, such as insurance forms that need to be filled out before a hospital visit.

Eye Contact Practices: Sustained eye contact with authority figures is considered impolite and disrespectful by traditional groups.

Touch Practices: Unlike that of a social setting, no physical contact occurs during greetings among health care professionals and patients, in part due to overloaded working conditions of health care personnel. The abdomen and part of the legs are covered for gynecologic examinations. Outside the health care environment, kissing the cheek and handshaking are customary for greetings.

Perceptions of Time: A relaxed attitude is taken toward time.

Pain Reactions: Tolerating pain and keeping quiet about it is a common trend. Pain is regarded as a part of life.

Birth Rites: In rural areas approximately 47% of the babies are born in health care institutions; however, in urban areas approximately 72% of the babies are born in them. The majority of deliveries are assisted by official or traditional midwives or experienced women in rural areas and by physicians or midwives in urban areas. A kneeling position and a prone position on a flat surface are the most common delivery positions. Fathers are not present during deliveries nor are relatives in hospital deliveries. Relatives and neighbors help with housework and baby care for 40 days postpartum.

Death Rites: The deceased is buried as soon as possible—the same day or the next day. Time of burial depends on the amount of paperwork involved or the arrival time of close relatives. For Muslim burial the body is wrapped in special pieces of cloth and buried without a coffin in the ground. The imam offers a short prayer during the burial ceremony, with additional prayers at home or at the local mosque on the seventh, fortieth, and fifty-second days. These days are dictated by beliefs regarding the time for decaying of certain parts of the body. Live organ donations are done, but cadaver donations are uncommon because the preference is for the body to be buried intact. The same reason makes autopsies uncommon. Cremation is not permitted.

Food Practices and Intolerances: People along the Black Sea consume a great deal of cabbage. Pork is a forbidden food. Legumes, vegetables, and bread are food staples. Fish is consumed throughout the country, and seafood is eaten in the big cities. Three meals per day is routine. Breakfast is the main meal in rural areas, and dinner is the main meal in urban areas. Ramadan fasting is practiced, with exemptions for the sick and children.

Infant Feeding Practices: Approximately 95% of babies are breastfed until they are 10 to 12 months old. Boys are breastfed longer because of a belief that breastfeeding will make them stronger. Working mothers may breastfeed for only 4 to 6 months. Plain, fresh yogurt, fresh fruit juices, fruit puree, vegetable soup, and soups with grains are advocated for babies who are 4 to 5 months old.

Child Rearing Practices: The mother is the primary child care giver; however, the paternal grandmother is also an important influence. Strict discipline is practiced. Permissive attitudes exist toward boys, and girls are taught to become productive, hard workers. Girls start helping with household chores when they enter school. Mothers are very protective of their sons.

National Childhood Immunizations: (A more recent immunization schedule is not on file with WHO.) BCG at birth and repeated every 5 years with PPD test; measles at 8 (rural) to 12 (urban) months; measles booster at 15 months; OPV-1 at 2 months; OPV-2 at 4 months; OPV-3 at 6 months; OPV booster at 18 to 24 months; DPT-1 at 2 months; DPT-2 at 4 months; DPT-3 at 6 months; DPT booster at 18 to 24 months; DT at 6 years or at entry into school; tetanus toxoid at 10 years.

Other Characteristics: Families commonly believe in the "evil eye." Mothers may fasten an evil eye pin on the child's shoulder or may say short prayers for protection.

BIBLIOGRAPHY

Akaslan S, Akasian I: Cutaneous leishmaniasis in Sanli Urfa, Turkiye Parazi-
toioji Dergisi, *Acta Parasitol Turcica* 13(304):43, 1989.

Aksit B: *Rural health seeking, culture and the economy: changes in Turkish
villages,* Cambridgeshire, 1993, Eothen Press (edited by Stirling P).

Bedük T, Özhan N: Inservice education in Turkey, *J Cont Educ Nurs*
25(2):86, 1994.

Dardick KR, Neumann HH: *Foreign travel and immunization guide,* ed 13,
Oradell, NJ, 1990, Medical Economics Books.

Erefe I: Turkey faces the challenge of Alma-Ata, *Int Nurs Rev* 31(6):169,
1984.

Hatipoglu S, Tatar K: The strengths and weaknesses of Turkish bone-setters,
World Health Forum 16(2):203, 1995.

Institute of Population Studies: Turkish population and health survey, Ankara, Turkey, 1989, Hacettepe University.

Maternal and Child Situation Analysis of Turkey: National Program 1991-
95, Serial No. 2, Ankara, Turkey, 1991, Yenicag Press.

1988 Turkish Population and Health Survey, Hacettepe University Institute
of Population Studies, Ankara, Turkey, 1989.

1994 Turkish Population and Health Studies, Ministry of Health, Hacettepe
University Institute of Population Studies, and Macro International, Ankara, Turkey, 1993.

Platin N: Contributor.

Pozanti MS, Bruder P: The Turkish healthcare system, *Hosp Topics* 73(2):28,
1995.

Ross HM: Societal/cultural views regarding death and dying, *Top Clin Nurs*
1(1):1, 1981.

Saglik Hizmetleri, Saglik Bakanligi Arastirma Planlama ve Koordinasyon
Kurulu Baskanligi, 535:23, 1989.

Sahin ST: Setting up a maternal child health center: organizational and mar-
keting strategies, *Issues Compr Pediatr Nurs* 9:315, 1986.

Turkiye'de Anne ve Cocuklarin Durum Analizi. Ulke Programi 1991-1995,
Seri No. 2, Yenicag Matbaasi, 1991.

Uyer G: Effect of nursing approach in understanding of physicians' direc-
tions, by the mothers of sick children in an out-patient clinic, *Int J Nurs
Stud* 23(1):79, 1986.

Uyer G: Health for all and nursing in Turkey, *Int Nurs Rev* 34(1):15, 1987.

◆ TURKMENISTAN

MAP PAGE (315)

Location: Once part of the Persian Empire, Turkmenistan
became an independent republic with the dissolution of the

USSR. The country is located in part on the eastern shore of the Caspian Sea, and 80% of the country is desert. Turkmenistan has extensive gas and oil reserves.

Major Languages	Ethnic Groups		Major Religions	
Turkmen	Turkmen	73%	Muslim	87%
Russian	Russian	10%	Eastern Orthodox	11%
Uzbek	Uzbek	9%	Other	2%
	Other	8%		

Ethnic/Race Specific or Endemic Diseases: The AIDS rate per 100,000 is reported by the country as zero.

National Childhood Immunizations: BCG at between 3 and 5 days, at 6 years, and at between 16 and 17 years; DPT at 2, 3, 4, and 18 months, 6 years, between 16 and 17 years, and at 26 years; OPV at birth, 2, 3, and 4 months, between 18 and 20 months, and at 6 years; measles at 9 months.

BIBLIOGRAPHY

No data located.

◆ TUVALU

MAP PAGE (311)

Location: Located just south of the equator in the western Pacific, Tuvalu (formerly the Ellice Islands) is a chain of nine small islands. The people are Polynesian and live in rural villages. Most of the islands are low atolls about 6 feet (1.8 m) above sea level. The country has a tropical climate.

Major Languages	Ethnic Groups		Major Religions	
Tuvaluan	Polynesian	96%	Congregationalist	97%
English	Other	4%	Other	3%

Ethnic/Race Specific or Endemic Diseases: The AIDS rate per 100,000 is reported by the country as zero.

National Childhood Immunizations: BCG at birth; DPT at 6, 10, and 14 weeks; OPV at birth and 6, 10, and 14 weeks; measles at 9 months.

BIBLIOGRAPHY
Natural world, March 30, 1992, Discovery Channel.

◆ UGANDA

MAP PAGE (317)

Location: Situated in central Africa straddling the equator, this landlocked country consists of swampy lowlands, a fertile plateau, a high mountain range, and desert. It is primarily an agricultural nation, with a temperature that is influenced by changes in altitude.

Major Languages	Ethnic Groups		Major Religions	
English	African	99%	Catholic	33%
Luganda	Other	1%	Protestant	33%
Swahili			Indigenous	18%
Bantu Languages			Beliefs	
Nilotic Languages			Muslim	16%

Predominant Sick Care Practices: Bone setters are traditional healers.

Ethnic/Race Specific or Endemic Diseases: ENDEMIC: Diarrhea; hookworm; chloroquine-resistant malaria (including urban areas). RISK: Guinea worm; anemia, affecting an estimated 70% of Ugandan women; schistosomiasis. The AIDS rate per 100,000 is 10.29.

Families' Role in Hospital Care: Bathing, bed changing, and meals are provided by the family. Mothers may sleep under the beds of sick children.

Dominance Patterns: The status of the woman depends on her childbearing potential. Polygamy is acceptable, especially if the woman is infertile or if she has passed her childbearing years. Few households have an adult male present in it to help with family income.

Child Rearing Practices: The husband would reject a wife who practiced birth control. Female circumcision and excision is widespread in some groups.

National Childhood Immunizations: BCG at birth; DPT at 6, 10, and 14 weeks; OPV at birth and 6, 10, and 14 weeks; measles at 9 months; hep B at 2, 3, and 4 months.

BIBLIOGRAPHY

Adler MW, editor: Statistics from the World Health Organization and the Centers for Disease Control, *AIDS* 6(10):1229, 1992.

Anderson SR et al.: AIDS education in rural Uganda: a way forward, *Int J STD AIDS* 1(5):335, 1990.

Blair J: Health teaching in the context of culture: nursing in East Africa, *Kansas Nurse* 6(4):4, 1991.

Kater V: Health education in Jinja, Uganda, *IMAGE: J Nurs Sch* 28(2):161, 1996.

Lambert H: Care of sick children in Uganda: a personal experience, *Midwife Health Visit Comm Nurse* 24(7):293, 1988.

MacNeil JM: Use of culture care theory with Baganda women as AIDS care-givers, *J Transcultural Nurs* 7(2):14, 1996.

Sutton J: AIDS in Uganda, *World Vision Childlife,* Summer 1996, p 2.

Utley G, anchor: Report of the Amsterdam Conference on AIDS, July 18, 1992, *NBC News.*

Wright J: Female genital mutilation: an overview, *J Adv Nurs* 24:251, 1996.

◆ UKRAINE

MAP PAGE (315)

Location: Ukraine regained its independence with the dissolution of the USSR. Located in southeastern Europe, the country has large areas with arable black soil plus the Carpathian and Crimean mountain chains. Chernobyl (where the nuclear power plant disaster occurred in 1986) is located here.

Major Languages	Ethnic Groups		Major Religions
Ukrainian	Ukrainian	73%	Orthodox
Russian	Russian	22%	
	Other	5%	

Predominant Sick Care Practices: Primary and preventive health care and home visits are the focus.

Ethnic/Race Specific or Endemic Diseases: The AIDS rate per 100,000 is 0.07.

Health Team Relationships: Patients may be required to provide gifts of money to hospital caregivers.

Families' Role in Hospital Care: Linens, medications, and food may have to be provided by the family. Analgesics and antibiotics in short supply can be obtained on the black market.

Dominance Patterns: Women have lower status than men do, and nurses are equivalent to housekeepers or aides. With the proper connections and money, certification as a health professional—including that of a physician—can be bought.

Birth Rites: Most deliveries occur in maternity hospitals. Doctors and midwives are available. Labor is sometimes forced by lying on the woman's abdomen and pushing the baby out rather than letting it occur naturally. To assist an infant's first breath, cold water may be thrown on the baby. Infants are washed immediately after birth. Contraceptives are generally unavailable, so the rhythm method and abortion are used for birth control.

Food Practices and Intolerances: Bread and cheese are popular but not meat, in part because of the economics.

BIBLIOGRAPHY

Johnson M: From so much to so little, *Can Nurse* 90(9): 59, 1994.
Morris R, Sinobicher A: Perhaps America can learn a healthcare lesson abroad, *Modern Healthcare* 24(7):60, 1994.
Squires A: Neonatal care in the Ukraine, *Neonatal Net* 13(5):65, 1994.

◆ UNITED ARAB EMIRATES

MAP PAGE (318)

Location: Situated on the eastern side of the Arabian Peninsula, the country is primarily desert and rich in oil. It has one of the highest per-capita incomes in the world.

Major Languages	Ethnic Groups		Major Religions	
Arabic	Asian	50%	Muslim	96%
English	Emirian	19%	Other	4%
Persian	Other Arab	23%		
Hindi	Other	8%		
Urdu				

Ethnic/Race Specific or Endemic Diseases: ENDEMIC: Chloroquine-sensitive malaria. The AIDS rate per 100,000 is reported by the country as zero.

Families' Role in Hospital Care: Family members or close friends accompany the patient and expect to participate in care or take on a vigilant, supervisory role.

Pain Reactions: Immediate pain relief is expected and may be persistently requested. The belief in conserving energy for recovery is in conflict with therapies that require exertion. Pain is expressed only privately or with close relatives and friends; however, during labor and delivery, pain is expressed vehemently.

Death Rites: Muslim belief forbids organ donations or transplants. Muslim physicians may recommend transfusions to save lives. Autopsy is uncommon because the deceased must be buried intact. Cremation is not permitted. For Muslim burial the body is wrapped in special pieces of cloth and buried without a coffin in the ground.

Food Practices and Intolerances: Pork, carrion, and blood are forbidden. Food tends to be spicy. Ramadan fasting is practiced, with exemptions for the sick and children.

National Childhood Immunizations: BCG at birth; DPT at 2, 4, 6, and 18 months; DT at 6 years; OPV at 2, 4, 6, and 18 months and 6 years; measles at 9 and 15 months and 6 years; rubella at 12 years; hep B at birth and 2 and 6 months.

Other Characteristics: Hope, optimism, and the positive advantages of treatment should be stressed.

BIBLIOGRAPHY

Green J: Death with dignity: Islam, *Nurs Times* 85(5):56, 1989.

Reizian A, Meleis AI: Arab-Americans' perceptions of and responses to pain, *Crit Care Nurse* 6(6):30, 1986.

Ross HM: Societal/cultural views regarding death and dying, *Top Clin Nurs* 1(1):1, 1981.

◆ UNITED KINGDOM

MAP PAGE (314)

Location: The United Kingdom is European and is primarily located between the Atlantic Ocean and the North Sea. It consists of England, Scotland, Wales, and Northern Ireland. The climate is temperate.

Major Languages	Ethnic Groups		Major Religions	
English	English	82%	Anglican	85%
Welsh	Scottish	10%	Catholic	8%
Gaelic	Irish	2%	Presbyterian	5%
Scottish	Welsh	2%	Other	2%
	Asian and Other	4%		

Predominant Sick Care Practices: Biomedical. Alternative medical care (for example, acupuncture and chiropractic, homeopathic, naturopathic, and osteopathic care) may be sought for some health care problems.

Health Care Beliefs: Acute sick care; health promotion important. Although health promotion is strongly advocated, physicians in some areas may not actively incorporate these beliefs.

Ethnic/Race Specific or Endemic Diseases: RISK: Small increase in tuberculosis. The death rate from coronary heart disease is one of the highest in the world. The AIDS rate per 100,000 is 2.62.

Health Team Relationships: Clients may consider titles more important than names and use the health professionals' titles when addressing them. In Scotland communication may be cautious or guarded.

Dominance Patterns: In England the father is traditionally the head of the family and his authority may not be questioned. The English have a strong sense of tradition and aristocracy.

Eye Contact Practices: Staring is believed to be a part of good listening. Understanding is indicated by blinking the eyes.

Touch Practices: The English have generally low touch practices.

Perceptions of Time: The past is valued, and traditional approaches to healing are preferred over new procedures or medications.

Food Practices and Intolerances: Organ meats are common in England.

Child Rearing Practices: In English families in which the father is the authority, the children are obedient.

National Childhood Immunizations: BCG at birth and 11 years; DPT at 2, 3, and 4 months; DT/Td at 4 years; TT at 15 years; OPV at 2, 3, and 4 months and 4 and 15 years; measles at between 5 and 16 years.

Other Characteristics: The English do not use space as a refuge from others; they set up internalized barriers to withdraw. Most English have type O blood.

BIBLIOGRAPHY

A shadow from the past: tuberculosis today, *Nurs Stand* 11(1):5, 1996.

Beunza I et al.: Diversity and commonality in international nursing, *Int Nurs Rev* 41(2):47, 1994.

Biley A, Whale Z: Feminist approaches to change and nursing development, *J Clin Nurs* 5(3):159, 1996.

Bingham S: Dietary aspects of a health strategy for England, *BMJ* 303:353, 1991.

Booth J, Waters KR: The multifaceted role of the nurse in the day hospital, *J Adv Nurs* 22:700, 1995.

Buchan J, Thomas S: Profiling 'flexible' nursing staff: bank nurses in Scotland, *Int J Nurs Stud* 32(3):288, 1995.

Coulter A, Schofield T: Prevention in general practice: the views of doctors in the Oxford region, *Br J Gen Pract* 41(345):140, 1991.

Galanti GA: *Caring for patients from different cultures,* ed 2, Philadelphia, 1997, University of Pennsylvania Press.

Giger JN, Davidhizar RE: *Transcultural nursing,* ed 2, St. Louis, 1995, Mosby.

Glasson J: The public image of the mentally ill and community care, *Br J Nurs* 5(10):615, 1996.

Gott M, O'Brien M: Health promotion: practice and the prospect for change, *Nurs Standard* 5(3):30, 1990.

Gott M, O'Brien M: Policy for health promotion, *Nurs Standard* 5(1):30, 1990.

Grove CL: Communications across cultures, Washington, DC, 1976, National Education Association.

Hall ET, Hall MR: *Understanding cultural differences,* Yarmouth, Me, 1989, Intercultural Press.

Martinelli AM: Pain and ethnicity: how people of different cultures experience pain, *AORN J* 46(2):273, 1987.

Mead M: A case history in cross-national communications. In *The communication of ideas,* New York, 1948, Harper & Row.

Menon S: The people of the bog, *Discover* 18(8):60, 1997.

O'Gorman F: Business as usual, *Nurs Times* 86(44):62, 1990.

Paling KJ: Tuberculosis, *Prof Nurse* 12(4):260, 1997.

Price P: Health promotion: health visiting in the field, *Nurs Standard* 5(31):53, 1991.

Prosser MH: *The cultural dialogue,* Washington, DC, 1985, SIETAR.

Samovar LA, Porter RE: *Intercultural communication: a reader,* Belmont, Calif, 1985, Wadsworth.

Smith WC et al.: Development of coronary prevention strategies by health authorities in the United Kingdom, *Community Med* 11(2):108, 1989.

Thomas J, Wainwright P: Community nurses and health promotion: ethical and political perspectives, *Nurs Ethics* 3(2):97, 1996.

Thomas KJ et al.: Use of nonorthodox and conventional health care in Great Britain, *BMJ* 302(6770):207, 1991.

Wardle J, Steptoe A: The European Health and Behaviour Survey: rationale, methods and initial results from the United Kingdom, *Soc Sci Med* 33(8):925, 1991.

Young K: Health, health promotion and the elderly, *J Clin Nurs* 5(4):241, 1996.

◆ URUGUAY

MAP PAGE (314)

Location: Located on the Atlantic Ocean in southern South America, Uruguay has low, rolling, and fertile grassy plains in the south and plateaus in the north. The climate is temperate, and the winter and summer seasons are opposite those in the Northern Hemisphere.

Major Language	Ethnic Groups		Major Religions	
Spanish	White	88%	Catholic	66%
	Mestizo	8%	Protestant	2%
	Black	4%	Jewish	2%
			Unaffiliated and Other	30%

Ethnic/Race Specific or Endemic Diseases: The AIDS rate per 100,000 is 3.98.

National Childhood Immunizations: BCG at birth and 5 years; DPT at 2, 4, 6, and 12 months; Td at 12 years; OPV at 2, 4, 6, and 12 months; MMR at 12 months and 5 years.

BIBLIOGRAPHY

No data located.

◆ UZBEKISTAN

MAP PAGE (315)

Location: Formerly a part of the USSR, Uzbekistan is located in central Asia. Two thirds is semidesert or desert. There are oases and some mountain valleys.

Major Languages	Ethnic Groups		Major Religions
Uzbek	Uzbek	71%	Sunni Muslim
Russian	Russian	8%	Eastern Orthodox
	Other	21%	

Ethnic/Race Specific or Endemic Diseases: The AIDS rate per 100,000 is reported by the country as zero.

National Childhood Immunizations: BCG at between 3 and 6 days, at 7 years, and between 16 and 17 years; DPT at 2, 3, 4, and 16 months; DT at 7 years and between 16 and 17 years; OPV at birth, 2, 3, 4, 16, and 18 months, 7 years, and between 16 and 17 years; measles at 9 and 16 months.

BIBLIOGRAPHY

No data located.

◆ VANUATU

MAP PAGE (311)

Location: Vanuatu (formerly the New Hebrides) is a collection of about 80 islands in the southwestern Pacific Ocean. Much of the land is covered with dense forests.

Major Languages	Ethnic Groups		Major Religions	
Bislama	Melanesian	94%	Christian	90%
French	French	4%	Other	10%
English	Other	2%		

Ethnic/Race Specific or Endemic Diseases: The AIDS rate per 100,000 is reported by the country as zero.

Child Rearing Practices: Education is not compulsory; however, most children attend primary school.

National Childhood Immunizations: BCG at birth and 6 and 12 years; DPT at 6, 10, and 14 weeks; OPV at 6, 10, and 14 weeks and 6 and 12 years; measles at 9 months; hep B at birth and 6 and 14 weeks.

BIBLIOGRAPHY

No data located.

◆ VENEZUELA

MAP PAGE (314)

Location: Venezuela is located on the Caribbean coast of South America. The climate is tropical, but it is influenced by changes in altitude from the coastline, over the plains and high plateaus, to the Andes mountains.

Major Languages	Ethnic Groups		Major Religions	
Spanish	Mestizo	67%	Catholic	96%
Indian Languages	White	21%	Protestant	2%
	Black	10%	Other	2%
	Native American	2%		

Ethnic/Race Specific or Endemic Diseases: ENDEMIC: Yellow fever; chloroquine-resistant malaria (with no risk in urban areas). RISK: Dengue fever. The AIDS rate per 100,000 is 2.83.

National Childhood Immunizations: BCG at birth and first grade; DPT at 2, 4, 6, and 18 months; OPV at birth and 2, 4, and 6 months; measles at 9 months.

BIBLIOGRAPHY

Diamond-De-La-Mata R: Latin American food: more than beans and rice, *Top Clin Nutr* 11(4):57, 1996.

Levine P: Developing a community mental health program in the Venezuelan Andes: implications for international psychosocial rehabilitation, *Psychiatr Rehab J* 19(3):23, 1996.

◆ VIETNAM

MAP PAGE (321)

Location: Located on the Indochinese peninsula in southeastern Asia, Vietnam is long and narrow. Most of the country is covered with mountains and plateaus, and the marshy Mekong River delta is located in the south. The population density is high and concentrated along the coast and delta river ways.

Major Languages	Ethnic Groups		Major Religions	
Vietnamese	Vietnamese	87%	Buddhist	60%
French	Chinese	3%	Confucianist	13%
Chinese	Other	10%	Taoist	12%
English			Catholic	3%
Khmer			Other	12%

Predominant Sick Care Practices: Magico-religious; Eastern medicine. Herbal medicine is an important practice; most Eastern medicines are classified as cool, whereas most Western medicines are considered hot. Water is classified as a cold substance and may be restricted along with other fluids when sick. That may include showers or baths. Traditionally illness is dealt with through self-care and self-medication. Folk remedies include variations of acupuncture, massage, herbal remedies, and dermabrasive practices such as cupping, pinching, rubbing, and burning. In the scarcity of expensive imported pharmaceuticals, the government encourages traditional treatments.

Health Care Beliefs: Acute sick care only. Self-medication and polypharmacy are customary. Injections are more effective than oral medications. Practices such as pinching or scratching the area let the bad winds or the unhealthy air currents out of the body, restore health, and produce marks or red lines. Being given medicine that will restore the yin-yang balance and the hot-cold equilibrium is important.

Ethnic/Race Specific or Endemic Diseases: RISK: Choriocarcinoma; dysentery; tuberculosis; hepatitis; typhoid; dengue fever; Japanese encephalitis; cholera; chloroquine-resistant malaria. Birth defects from elevated Agent Orange levels. The AIDS rate per 100,000 is 0.24.

Health Team Relationships: People stand out of respect when speaking. Pointing the finger at someone is a sign of disrespect. Young, recently educated physicians may be considered incompetent and may be asked the year they completed their training. Older health professionals with 20 years or more since training are considered authority figures and experts, and patients are told little about their conditions, medicines, or diagnostic procedures. Therefore patients may be poor historians and teaching patients and families is not part of nursing's technical role. Sparing someone's feelings is more important than truth, so a "yes" may actually mean "no." In traditional families the oldest male makes decisions about health care.

Families' Role in Hospital Care: The patient is considered a person for whom care needs to be provided by all family members, who essentially live at the bedside and sleep on the patient's bed or on nearby mats. Small wood stoves are used to cook. Feeding, hygiene, and personal comfort are expected to be provided 24 hours a day by the family or a person hired to do it in the family's absence. Thin straw mats may be the mattress.

Dominance Patterns: The extended family is the basic unit and consists of three or four generations that live together. Decision making is influenced by the astrologic/lunar calendar. Although women defer to men, frequently women control the men, the home, the family's health care, and the economic power of the community. An intense identification of self as part of the family and village minimizes the incentive to excel as an individual. Until they die elderly parents are cared for by children.

Eye Contact Practices: Blinking means only that a message has been received. Looking directly into another's eyes when talking is considered disrespectful.

Touch Practices: The head is considered the seat of the soul and should not be touched. Only the elderly are allowed to touch the heads of young children. Touching persons of the same sex is acceptable and between women may be very affectionate. The female breast is accepted dispassionately as the means of infant feeding; however, the lower torso is extremely private. The area between waist and knees is kept covered, even in private. Handshaking has gained wide acceptance with men but not with women. A man will not extend his hand in handshake to a woman or a superior. Sisters and brothers do not touch or kiss each other.

Perceptions of Time: Time is viewed as a recurring circle rather than as moving in a linear direction.

Pain Reactions: Stoic. Pain may be severe before relief is requested. People may remain quiet and even smile while experiencing pain or other forms of inner turmoil.

Birth Rites: Limiting a family to two children is encouraged with disincentives for having a third child. Beliefs may include avoiding weddings and funerals and abstaining from sexual intercourse during pregnancy because harm may come to the mother and baby. The squatting position is preferred for delivery. Some type of blooming (such as the opening of closed flowers) may be used symbolically to help open the cervix during labor. The presence of a female friend may be desired during delivery. Regardless of the temperature the laboring woman drinks only warm or hot water and keeps warm by wearing socks and using blankets. In rural areas, delivery at home with a midwife is preferred. Men, unmarried women, young girls, and the husband are usually not present during birth. Hot coals may be placed under the bed after delivery. At birth the child is thought to be 1 year old. Circumcision is generally unknown. The newborn should not be given compliments, such as being called beautiful, healthy, or smart, for fear of capture by evil spirits.

Death Rites: Preference is for quality of life over length of life because of beliefs in reincarnation and the expectation of less suffering in the next life. Therefore the dying should be helped to recall their past good deeds and to achieve a fitting mental state. Autopsies are permitted and cremation is preferred. Death at home is preferred over death in the hospital. Upon death the body is washed and wrapped in clean white sheets. The wife may prefer to do this to ensure that the rituals are properly conducted. In some areas a coin or jewels (a wealthier family) or rice (a poorer family) will be put in the mouth of the deceased in the belief that this will help the soul go through the encounters with gods and devils and the soul will be born rich in the next life. Relatives sew small pillows that are placed under the neck, feet, and wrists of the deceased. The body is placed in a coffin, and burial is in the ground.

Food Practices and Intolerances: Chopsticks are used to eat. The diet consists of rice at every meal; meat, seafood, fruits, and vegetables are also eaten. Meals are eaten while squatting or sitting on low stools. People may be lactose intolerant. Malnutrition affects perhaps half the population.

Infant Feeding Practices: Because colostrum may be perceived as bad milk, bottle-feeding may be used until the breasts fill. Nearly all women breastfeed, and breastfeeding may continue for 2 years.

Child Rearing Practices: Methods for calculating the age of an infant may vary by as much as 2 years. Parents are relaxed about the development of young children and enjoy it. At approximately age 6 strict upbringing begins, independence is discouraged, and parents demand obedience. The oldest child, boy or girl, is responsible for younger siblings if the parents are dead, old, or ill.

National Childhood Immunizations: BCG at birth; DPT at 2, 3, and 4 months; OPV at 2, 3, and 4 months; measles at 9 months.

Other Characteristics: Belief that illness needs to be drawn out of the body is practiced through coin rubbing. A heated coin or one smeared with oil is vigorously rubbed over the body, producing red welts. The red marks are evidence of the illness's being brought to the surface of the body; it is believed that the red marks will occur only in people who are ill to begin with. Because of stigma against mental illness, emotional disturbances may be manifested somatically. Offensive behaviors include a male stranger touching a female, feet on furniture, and photographs of three people in a group. Names are listed in order by family name, middle name, and given name, reflecting the family as the primary source of identity. Legally women retain their own names after marrying. Age, which is associated with wisdom and experience, is valued and respected. The American signal to beckon another with the finger or the palm of the hand up is offensive because this is the motion used to call a dog.

BIBLIOGRAPHY

Anderson LK: Intercultural communication between Vietnamese and Americans, Unpublished paper, 1988.

Andrews MM, Boyle JS: *Transcultural concepts in nursing care,* ed 2, Philadelphia, 1995, Lippincott.

Bates B, Turner AN: Imagery and symbolism in the birth practices of traditional cultures, *Birth* 12(1):29, 1985.

Clark MJ: *Nursing in the community,* Norwalk, Conn, 1992, Appleton & Lange.

D'Avanzo CE: Barriers to health care for Vietnamese refugees, *J Prof Nurs* 8(4):245, 1992.

Eisenbruch M: Cross-cultural aspects of bereavement. II. Ethnic and cultural variations in the development of bereavement practices, *Cult Med Psychiatry* 8(4):315, 1984.

Farrales S: Vietnamese. In Lipson JG, Dibble SL, Minarik PA: *Culture & nursing care: a pocket guide,* San Francisco, 1997, University of San Francisco Nursing Press.

Fry A, Nguyen T: Culture and the self: implications for the perception of depression by Australian and Vietnamese nursing students, *J Adv Nurs* 23:1147, 1996.

Galanti GA: *Caring for patients from different cultures,* ed 2, Philadelphia, 1997, University of Pennsylvania Press.

Horn BM: Cultural concepts and postpartal care, *Nurs Health Care* 2(9):516, 1981.

Kristy SJ: Health issues in nursing in Vietnam, *Holist Nurs Practice* 9(2):83, 1995.

Lally MM: Last rites and funeral customs of minority groups, *Midwife Health Visit Comm Nurse* 14(7):224, 1978.

Lawson LV: Culturally sensitive support for grieving parents, *MCN Am J Matern Child Nurs* 15:76, 1990.

Li GR: Funeral practices, New York, World Relief, n.d.

Marchione J, Stearne SJ: Ethnic power perspectives for nursing, *Nurs Health Care* 11(6):296, 1990.

Morrow M: Breastfeeding in Vietnam: poverty, tradition, and economic transition, *J Hum Lact* 12(2):97, 1996.

Muecke MA: Caring for Southeast Asian refugee patients in the USA, *Am J Public Health* 73(4):431, 1983.

Nguyen A, Bounthinh T, Mum S: *Folk medicine, folk nutrition, superstitions,* Washington, DC, 1980, Team Associates.

Poremba BA: After the storm: an American nurse visits Vietnam, *Nurs Health Care* 16(3):118, 1995.

Rieu LT: *Modern and traditional medical practices of Vietnam: Vietnamese concepts of illness and treatment,* San Francisco, Calif, Indochinese Mental Health Project, n.d.

Rosenberg J, Givens S: Teaching child health care concepts to Khmer mothers, *J Community Health* 3:157, 1986.

Schreiner D: S.E. Asian folk healing practices/child abuse? Paper presented at the Indochinese Health Care Conference, Eugene, Ore, 1981.

Shanahan M, Brayshaw DL: Are nurses aware of the differing health care needs of Vietnamese patients? *J Adv Nurs* 22:456, 1995.

Stewart EC, Bennett MJ: *American cultural patterns: a cross-cultural perspective,* rev ed, Yarmouth, Me, 1991, Intercultural Press.

Uland E, Smith S: Southeast Asian mental health issues, Unpublished paper, 1984.

U.S. Department of Health, Education, and Welfare Social Security Administration Office of Family Assistance SSA 77-21013: A guide to two cultures: Indochinese, Washington, DC, n.d.

Vandeusen J et al.: South East Asian social and cultural customs: similarities and differences, *J Refugee Resettlement* 1:20, 1980.

◆ WESTERN SAMOA

MAP PAGE (311)

Location: Western Samoa, not to be confused with nearby American Samoa, is the larger and western part of the Samoan archipelago and is located approximately halfway between Hawaii and New Zealand.

Major Languages	**Ethnic Groups**		**Major Religions**	
Samoan	Samoan	93%	Protestant	70%
English	Euronesian	7%	Catholic	20%
			Other	10%

Predominant Sick Care Practices: Traditional. Technologically advanced equipment and supplies are not readily available, even in urban areas. Coconut oil is a common treatment for many minor problems.

Ethnic/Race Specific or Endemic Diseases: RISK: Injuries from fishing and plantation work accidents; malnutrition from lack of vegetables; hypertension; obesity; diabetes. The AIDS rate per 100,000 is 0.58.

Health Team Relationships: Nurses may be referred to as "doctor" in villages without a physician. Hospitals are used primarily for emergencies.

Families' Role in Hospital Care: Family members help care for hospitalized patients, and the facility may provide living quarters for the family.

Dominance Patterns: Male dominance is common; however, it is not universal. The extended family is a strong social force.

Food Practices and Intolerances: Prayers are said and hymns are sung before the evening meal. Taro, green bananas, and breadfruit are dietary staples. Coconut cream is often used for preparing foods. A larger, heavier body build is valued.

National Childhood Immunizations: BCG at 5 years; DPT at 3, 5, and 7 months and 5 years; OPV at 3, 5, and 7 months and 5 years; measles at 9 months and 5 years; hep B at birth, 6 weeks, and between 3 and 4 months.

Other Characteristics: Tattoos symbolize manhood but are worn by both sexes. Homes built on raised platforms and open on all sides are designed for tropical weather. Sitting cross-legged for extended periods of time is common. Religion is an important part of all aspects of life, and Sundays are kept as days of rest and relaxation.

BIBLIOGRAPHY

Collins VR et al.: High prevalence of diabetic retinopathy and nephropathy in Polynesians of Western Samoa, *Diabetes Care* 18(8):1140, 1995.

Ishida DN, Toomata-Mayer TF, Mayer JF: Samoans. In Lipson JC, Dibble SL, Minarik PA: *Culture and nursing care: a pocket guide,* San Francisco, 1996, University of California at San Francisco School of Nursing Press.

Moyle RM: Sexuality in Samoan art forms, *Arch Sex Behav* 4(3):227, 1975.

Shimamoto Y, Ishida D: The elderly Samoan, *Public Health Nurs* 5(4):219, 1988.

Villafuerte A: Samoa: reflections on a cultural adventure, *Courier* (Teachers College, Columbia University Nursing Editors Alumni Association Publication) 60:1, 1992.

◆ YEMEN

MAP PAGE (318)

Location: Yemen (formerly Republic of Yemen and the Yemen Arab Republic) is located on the southwestern end of the Arabian Peninsula along the Red Sea and Arabian Sea. In the drier east the land is arid and supports subsistence farming and nomadic herding. In the fertile highlands of the more heavily populated west, agriculture is the main economy. The highest point is 12,000 feet (3660 m).

Major Language	Ethnic Groups		Major Religions	
Arabic	Arab	95%	Muslim	98%
	East Indian and Other	5%	Other	2%

Ethnic/Race Specific or Endemic Diseases: ENDEMIC: Chloroquine-sensitive malaria. **RISK:** Pneumonia; diarrhea. The AIDS rate per 100,000 is 0.08.

Families' Role in Hospital Care: Family members or close friends accompany the patient and expect to participate in care or take on a vigilant, supervisory role.

Pain Reactions: Immediate pain relief is expected and may be persistently requested. The belief in conserving energy for recovery is in conflict with therapies that require exertion. Pain is expressed only privately or with close relatives and friends. During labor and delivery, pain is expressed vehemently.

Birth Rites: Infant mortality rate is high.

Death Rites: Muslim belief forbids organ donations or transplants. Muslim physicians may recommend transfusions to save lives. Autopsy is uncommon because the deceased must be buried intact. Cremation is not permitted. For Muslim burial the body is wrapped in special pieces of cloth and buried without a coffin in the ground.

Food Practices and Intolerances: Pork, carrion, and blood are forbidden. Food tends to be spicy. Ramadan fasting is practiced, with exemptions for the sick and children. Less economically advantaged women may believe that males should get more and better food.

National Childhood Immunizations: BCG at birth; DPT at 6, 10, and 14 weeks; OPV at birth and 6, 10, and 14 weeks; measles at 9 months.

Other Characteristics: Hope, optimism, and positive advantages of treatment should be stressed.

BIBLIOGRAPHY

Green J: Death with dignity: Islam, *Nurs Times* 85(5):56, 1989.

Lambeth S: Health care in the Yemen Arab Republic, *Int J Nurs Stud* 25(3):1, 1988.

Myntti C: Social determinants of child health in Yemen, *Soc Sci Med* 37(2):233, 1993.

Reizian A, Meleis AI: Arab-Americans' perceptions of and responses to pain, *Crit Care Nurse* 6(6):30, 1986.

Ross HM: Societal/cultural views regarding death and dying, *Top Clin Nurs* 1(1):1, 1981.

◆ ZAIRE (now The Democratic Republic of Congo)

MAP PAGE (317)

Location: Zaire, which was recently renamed The Democratic Republic of Congo, is not to be confused with its neighbor The Republic of Congo, which is located around the equator in central Africa with one small arm extending west and providing a short strip of Atlantic Ocean coastline. The

Zaire (Congo) River traverses the land in The Democratic Republic of Congo. The terrain includes low plateaus covered with a rain forest and grasslands, and high mountains are in the east.

Major Languages	Ethnic Groups		Major Religions	
French	Bantu Groups	80%	Catholic	50%
Kongo	Other	20%	Protestant	20%
Luba			Kimbanguist	10%
Mongo			Muslim	10%
Rwanda and Other			Other	10%

Predominant Sick Care Practices: Use of biomedical health care services has decreased because of cost.

Ethnic/Race Specific or Endemic Diseases: ACTIVE: Cholera; yellow fever. ENDEMIC: Chloroquine-resistant malaria. RISK: Schistosomiasis; posttraumatic stress syndrome. There are five terms to describe symptoms related to different types of diarrhea. The AIDS rate per 100,000 is 4.27.

Health Team Relationships: "Mama" is a title of respect used with female patients.

Food Practices and Intolerances: Diet is heavily vegetarian, which may be inhibitory for iron absorption.

National Childhood Immunizations: BCG at birth; DPT at 6, 10, and 14 weeks; OPV at birth and 6, 10, and 14 weeks; measles at 9 months.

BIBLIOGRAPHY

Boer DD: Just a droplet in the bucket, *Gastroenterol Nurs* 18(5):188, 1995.

Fontaine G: Nurse worked with Rwandan refugees in Zaire, *NURSEweek* 8(17):26, 1995.

Haddad S, Fournier P: Quality, cost and utilization of health services in developing countries: a longitudinal study in Zaire, *Soc Sci Med* 40(6):743, 1995.

Hounsa AM et al.: An application of Ajzen's theory of planned behaviour to predict mothers' intention to use oral rehydration therapy in a rural area of Benin, *Soc Sci Med* 37(2):253, 1993.

Kuvibidila S et al.: Assessment of iron status of Zairean women of childbearing age by serum transferrin receptor, *Am J Clin Nurs* 60(4):603, 1994.

Pittsburgh Post-Gazette: May 23, 1997.

◆ ZAMBIA

MAP PAGE (317)

Location: This landlocked republic (formerly Northern Rhodesia) is located in southern Africa and consists of high, forested plateaus drained by large rivers. The climate is subtropical, and the country is subject to drought and famine.

Major Languages	Ethnic Groups		Major Religions	
English	African	99%	Christian	65%
African Languages	European and Other	1%	Indigenous Beliefs	34%
			Muslim and Hindu	1%

Ethnic/Race Specific or Endemic Diseases: ACTIVE: Cholera; tuberculosis. ENDEMIC: Yellow fever; chloroquine-resistant malaria. RISK: Schistosomiasis. The AIDS rate per 100,000 is 45.33.

Families' Role in Hospital Care: Families may need to provide meals and care.

Birth Rites: Women are valued by their number of children.

Food Practices and Intolerances: A corn meal mush called "nshima" is the main energy food. In a great majority of homes cooking is done over an open fire. Traditional foods are eaten with the hands.

Child Rearing Practices: Breastfeeding is strongly encouraged and continued for about 2 years. As much as 50% of the children experience malnutrition.

National Childhood Immunizations: BCG at birth; DPT at 2, 3, 4, and 12 months; OPV at 2, 3, and 4 months; measles at 9 months.

BIBLIOGRAPHY

Adler MW, editor: Statistics from the World Health Organization and the Centers for Disease Control, *AIDS* 6(10):1229, 1992.

Carlyle MS: I went to Zambia to teach, *Tar Heel Nurse* 55(1):28, 1993.

Pauley J, anchor: *NBC News,* June 22, 1992.

◆ ZIMBABWE

MAP PAGE (317)

Location: This landlocked south central African country (formerly Southern Rhodesia) has high plateaus and mountains in the east. The climate is subtropical. Most people live in small villages and are engaged in subsistence farming.

Major Languages	Ethnic Groups		Major Religions	
English	Shona	71%	Syncretic	50%
Chishona	Ndebele	16%	Christian	25%
Sindebele	White	1%	Indigenous	24%
	Other	12%	Beliefs	
			Muslim	1%

Predominant Sick Care Practices: Many traditional healers.

Health Care Beliefs: In addition to physical causes, diarrhea may also have spiritual causes such as having sex while breastfeeding. A common belief is that breastfeeding when pregnant is pathogenic to the infant. Therefore breastfeeding is immediately terminated and the infant is treated by inducing diarrhea and/or vomiting to clean out the dirty breast milk from the child. The belief that breast milk turns bad if the mother has not fed the child for 1 day also requires termination of breastfeeding or continuation only after performing a ritual. Acceptance of the married mother's breast by an infant is a sign of its legitimacy by the father.

Ethnic/Race Specific or Endemic Diseases: ENDEMIC: Chloroquine-resistant malaria. RISK: Schistosomiasis. Diarrhea is usually treated using medicinal herbs. The AIDS rate per 100,000 is 118.60.

Dominance Patterns: Polygamy is practiced by some. The traditional male role is as decision maker and guardian.

Birth Rites: Breastfeeding, which is very common, is started on the day of birth, and termination usually occurs at 18 to 20 months.

Food Practices and Intolerances: Maize is a staple food. A porridge or gruel (bota) made from maize is often the first food supplement for infants. Groundnuts pounded into peanut butter is an important protein source.

Child Rearing Practices: Some children in a family may be sent to live with grandparents.

National Childhood Immunizations: BCG at birth; DPT at 3, 4, and 5 months; OPV at 3, 4, and 5 months; measles at 9 months; hep B at 3, 4, and 9 months.

BIBLIOGRAPHY

Adler MW, editor: Statistics from the World Health Organization and the Centers for Disease Control, *AIDS* 6(10):1229, 1992.

Cominsky S, Mhlovi M, Ewbank D: Child feeding practices in a rural area of Zimbabwe, *Soc Sci Med* 36(7):937, 1993.

Hounsa AM et al.: An application of Ajzen's theory of planned behaviour to predict mothers' intention to use oral rehydration therapy in a rural area of Benin, *Soc Sci Med* 37(2):253, 1993.

Mafethe I: Perspectives on gender, culture, and power in community health, *Nurs Health Care* 16(4):217, 1995.

Thrasher V: RN learns about school health in Zimbabwe, *NURSEweek* 8(25):11, 1995.

Utley G, anchor: Report of the Amsterdam Conference on AIDS, *NBC News,* July 18, 1992.

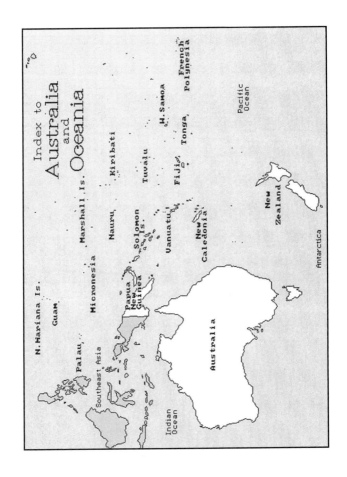

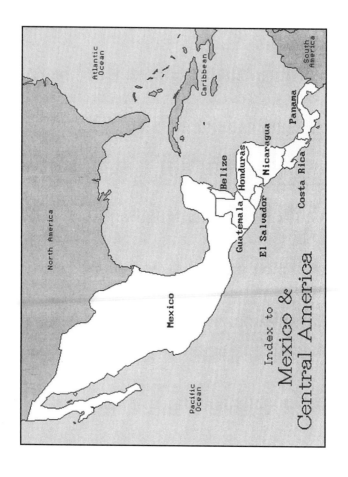

Index to
Mexico &
Central America

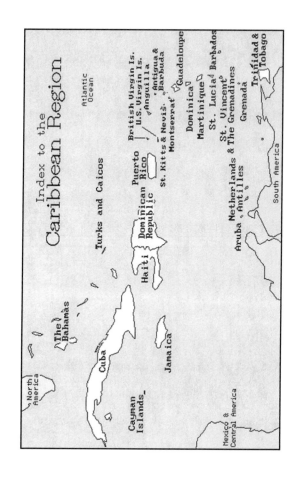

Index to the
Caribbean Region

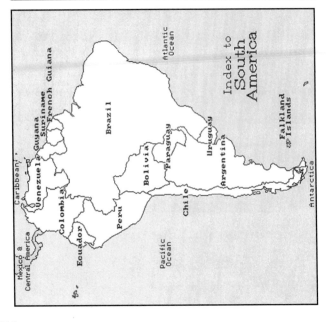

A

B

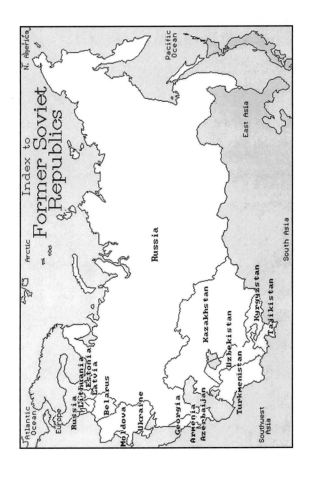

Index to
Former Soviet
Republics

Arctic

N. America

Pacific Ocean

East Asia

South Asia

Russia

Atlantic Ocean

Europe

Russia
Lithuania
Estonia
Latvia

Belarus

Moldova

Ukraine

Georgia

Armenia
Azerbaijan

Southwest Asia

Kazakhstan

Uzbekistan

Turkmenistan

Kyrgyzstan

Tajikistan

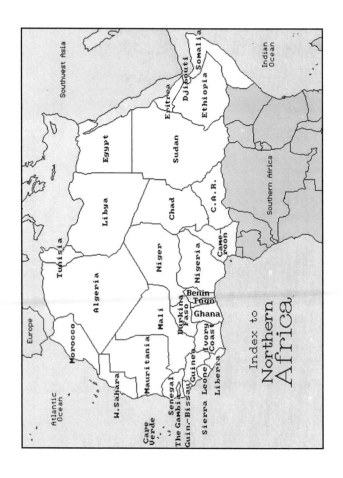

Index to
Northern Africa

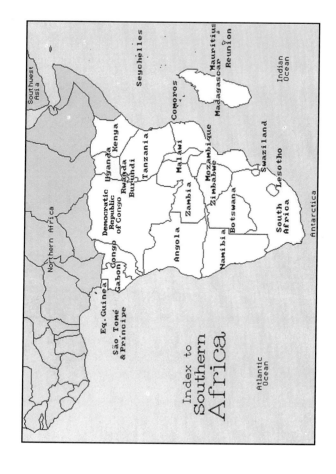

Index to
Southern
Africa

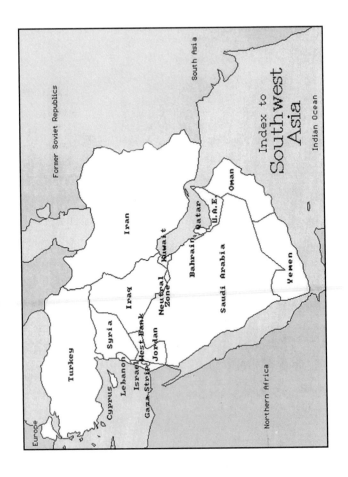

Index to
Southwest
Asia

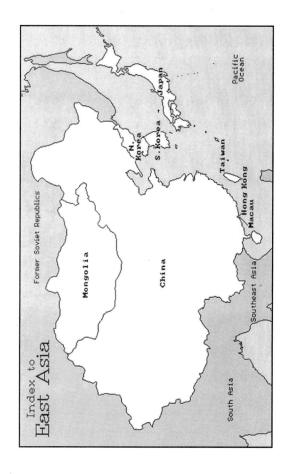

Index to
East Asia

Former Soviet Republics

Mongolia

China

N. Korea

S. Korea

Japan

Pacific Ocean

Taiwan

Hong Kong

Macau

Southeast Asia

South Asia

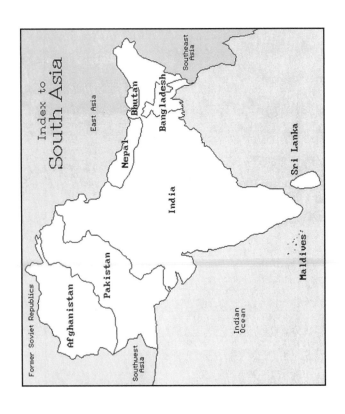

Index to
South Asia

East Asia

Southeast Asia

Former Soviet Republics

Nepal

Bhutan

Bangladesh

Pakistan

Afghanistan

India

Sri Lanka

Maldives

Indian Ocean

Southwest Asia

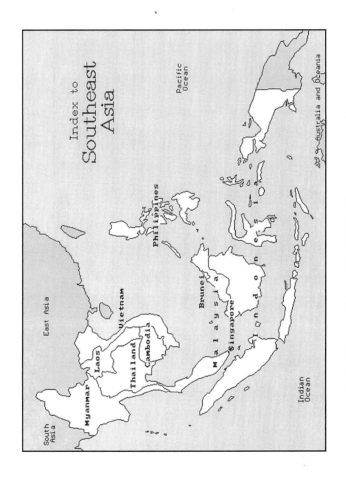

Index to
Southeast
Asia

East Asia

South
Asia

Myanmar

Laos

Vietnam

Thailand

Cambodia

Philippines

Brunei

Malaysia

Singapore

Indonesia

Indian
Ocean

Pacific
Ocean

Australia and Oceania

Ethnic Group Index